Essential Epidemiology and Biostatistics

A Practical Guide for Clinicians

Daniel Hartman MD, MAS

Email for orders, inquiries: Daniel.hartman@yale.edu

For Dawn and Marley, who patiently tolerate my eccentricities

Contents

INTRODUCTION

I remember glancing around at my medical school classmates during our course on Biostatistics some years ago, wondering if they were as bewildered as I was. They were. Much of the course was theoretical and seemed non-relevant to the practice of medicine. It was poorly constructed and poorly organized and did not hold the attention of my colleagues and me; it was as if epidemiology and biostatistics were taught as an afterthought, or from a "let's just get this insignificant requirement out of the way as quickly as possible" perspective. The disconnect between this attitude and the unquestionably vital importance of being able to truly understand the language of the medical literature is disconcerting, and the consequences are vast: it has created a knowledge gap between those who are writing the papers and those to whom they are intended (the medical practitioners), so that the latter is forced to blindly accept what is fed to them by the former. And in so doing, the medical practitioners promulgate potentially erroneous, costly and dangerous experimental conclusions to those whom we are dedicated to serve: our patients who rely on us to tell them what is scientifically proven, and what is not.

After thirty years of frustration watching poorly constructed "scientific" experiments and bad literature work their way into mainstream medical practice I finally decided that I quite literally "couldn't take it anymore" and must do whatever I can to help. This book, then, the happy product of my frustration, is written for my colleagues— the front-line medical practitioners, be they physicians, physician assistants or nurse practitioners. It is *not* written for, and certainly not worthy of biostatisticians and epidemiologists who are experts in these challenging topics. Indeed, full formal courses in biostatistics and epidemiology are not appropriate for most medical clinicians as they are far too in depth and thick on theory and will do nothing but confuse those of us who practice clinical medicine. On the other hand, a course that is too cursory without explaining the theory to a modest degree will leave the clinician too much "in the dark" and at the mercy of the statisticians (who often work for the profit-seeking investigators) who are writing the analyses of the experiments. We need to understand the theory to the level that we are able to question the study authors' methodologies, and to be able, more importantly, to recognize their mistakes: Did they use a Chi-square test when a Fisher's Exact test may have been more appropriate? Did they prove statistical significance using a one-tailed z-score instead of a two-tailed? Are they quoting Relative Risk Reduction instead of Absolute Risk Reduction? And so forth. Therefore, this book is an attempt at that "sweet spot" that provides just enough of the statistical and epidemiologic theory without being overwhelming, while emphasizing real kinds of examples that are found in the medical literature.

My goal was to make the book extremely "readable," using a "just the facts," "how does this relate to literature that you will see?" style, and a tone that is relaxed and conversational. Although there are times when the theory seems to get a bit involved, my goal is to always keep it "grounded" by emphasizing how, when and why it is relevant. I also felt it necessary to weed out for you some topics that you will find in many medical statistics books that are just not relevant to our purposes, and perhaps more importantly, I have included in this books some topics that are very relevant and yet surprisingly difficult to find in the textbooks.

The book is constructed as a synthesis of two fields of study: epidemiology and biostatistics. More often than not they are taught separately, if at all, in medical education, and I think that is an injustice. They are intricately linked, and one simply cannot be learned without the other. And so in this book the various topics of the two disciplines are intertwined, and I have done my best to place them in a logical order so that the biostats topics will reinforce the epidemiology topics, and vice versa. I firmly believe that this unique approach is ideal for the education of medical clinicians seeking to understand the language of the medical literature, whether to guide them in conducting their own research, or to aid them in the noble quest of being better able to serve the people who have entrusted them with their healthcare decisions—decisions that demand nothing less than a strong and confident grasp of the science.

A final and important point: You will notice that the book has somewhat of a "primer" tone to it. I encourage you to *not* skip over the blue interjected "fill-in-the-blanks" sections. Epidemiology and biostatistics are, unlike many other subjects, not overly foundation-based or pyramidal—a good amount of the information presented does not expand upon information already learned. Therefore, a deep understanding of these topics is a challenge for many people. A very useful tool to help grasp this stuff is to mimic the learning we did as children by regurgitating the relevant material right back to the teacher. And that is the purpose of the seemingly easy questions in blue: we make our brains way, "What did I just learn?" and really helps prevents it all from going "in one ear and out the other." In exchange for you completing the blue sections, I promise to avoid *really* treating you like a child and making you do "exercises," which, in my experience reading textbooks, are only included when the author has not done an adequate job teaching the material in the first place.

Biostats 1: Populations and Samples

Section B1.1: Populations

I will begin the discussion about populations by introducing you to a fundamental concept of statistics: the "Normal Distribution." This ubiquitous and versatile phenomenon is the foundation of pretty much everything we know and do in biostatistics, and so a solid grasp is mandatory!

So here is a "normal distribution curve"

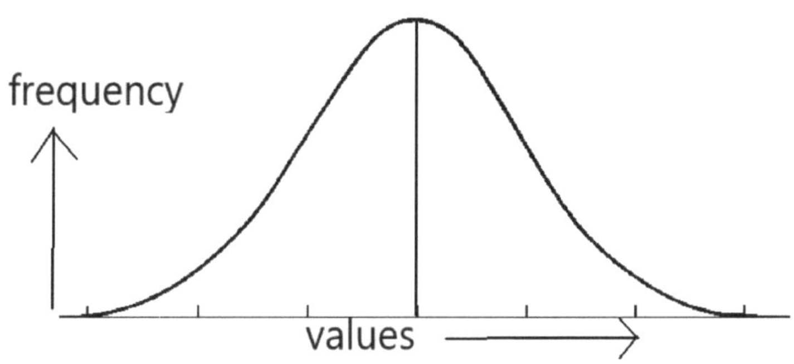

The values that are plotted along the x-axis, and the frequencies that those values occur are plotted along the y-axis. You can think of the area under the normal distribution curve as a histogram (bar-graph) of results—one in which we are able to shrink the x-value "bins" to infinitely small values:

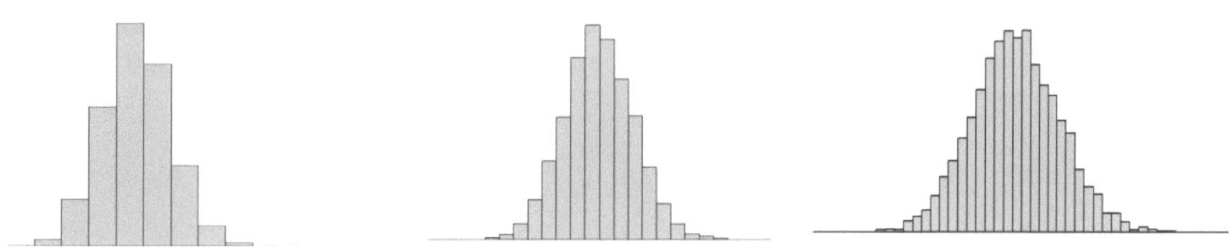

Pretty much everything in human biology that is measurable: height, weight, cholesterol levels, blood pressure, age of menopause, IQ, respiratory tidal volume, hemoglobin, length of time we are sick with the flu, etc. follows a "normal distribution" pattern. The point on the x-axis corresponding to the apex of the curve is the most frequently occurring value (the "mode"). In an ideal normal distribution, this mode is equivalent to both the mean and the median values. (In the real world, they are all similar but may not be identical). All other values occur less and less frequently as we move in either direction away from the apex. This is just how biology is, and so pretty much everything we discuss in statistics revolves around this curve in one way or another.

Let's look at an example. Let's say we are able to measure the systolic blood pressures of all American adults. If we graph the results, it may look like this:

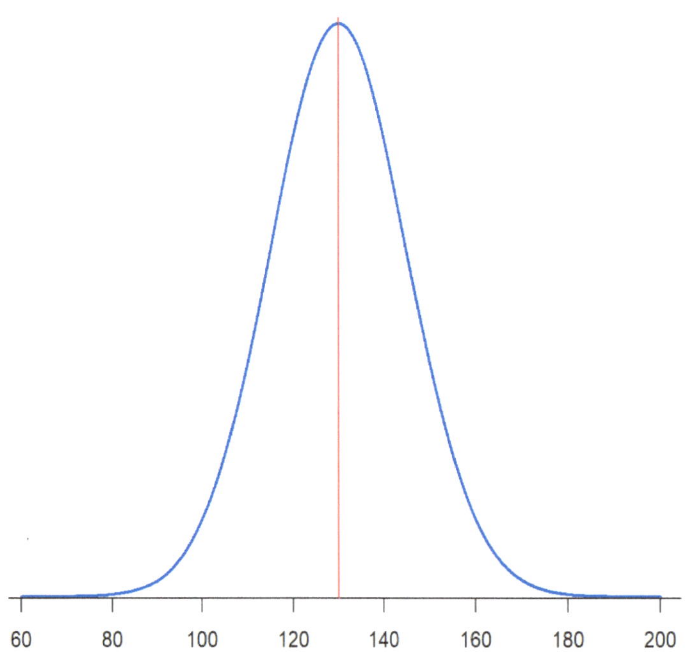

The most common reading ("mode") is 130 mmHg, and that is also the mean and the median readings.

Refresher: the "mean" is what we think of when we say "average." We get that value by summing all the values and dividing by the number of values. The "median" is the middle value in the group. Example: here are 5 values: 1, 2, 2, 4, 5, 9, 10. The "mode" (most common) is 2. The "median" (middle value) is 4, and the "mean" (average) is 1+2+2+4+5+9+10 = 33, divided by 7 = 4.7. (In this very small sample, the mean, median and mode are not the same because the sample is too small to be normally distributed).

Standard deviation

The normal distribution is defined by the mean, median and mode value (in our case 130), and by another thing called the standard deviation. In the graph above, the standard deviation happens to be 15. The important thing to know about the standard deviation is that it is a measure of how *spread out* the data are. A higher standard deviation means that the data are more spread out, and a lower standard deviation means that the data are more closely "clustered" around the mean. The equation for standard deviation is as follows:

$$SD = \sqrt{\frac{\sum_{i=1}^{n}(x_i - \bar{\mu})^2}{n-1}}$$

You certainly don't need to memorize this but is probably a good idea to dissect it just a little bit. The denominator is pretty simple: *n* is the number of people. (So, the more people there are in the population, the smaller is the standard deviation). The $x_i - \bar{\mu}$ thing in the numerator is just the difference between each value (systolic blood pressure) and the mean systolic blood pressure (μ), and the Σ thing means that you just "sum them all up." Oh, and if you take away the square root, the stuff in the middle, $\frac{\sum_{i=1}^{n}(x_i-\bar{\mu})^2}{n-1}$ is the "variance." (So the standard deviation is the square root of the variance).

1. The bigger the standard deviation, the more _______________ the data are.

Because the standard deviation is a measure of how spread out the data are, it is what determines exactly how the curve looks. So, for example, if the standard deviation happened to be 25 instead of 15, here is how the curve would look:

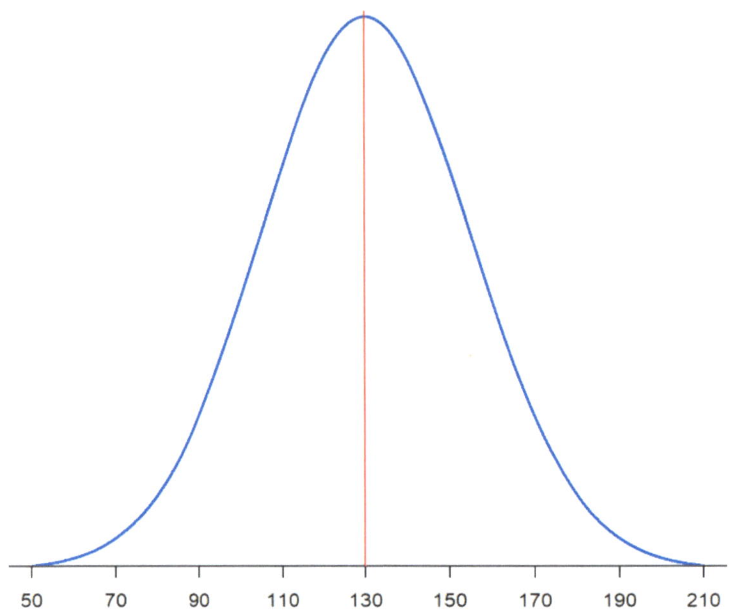

You can see that this curve is a bit “heftier” than the first one, as the values are more spread out.

And finally, what if the standard deviation happened to 8?

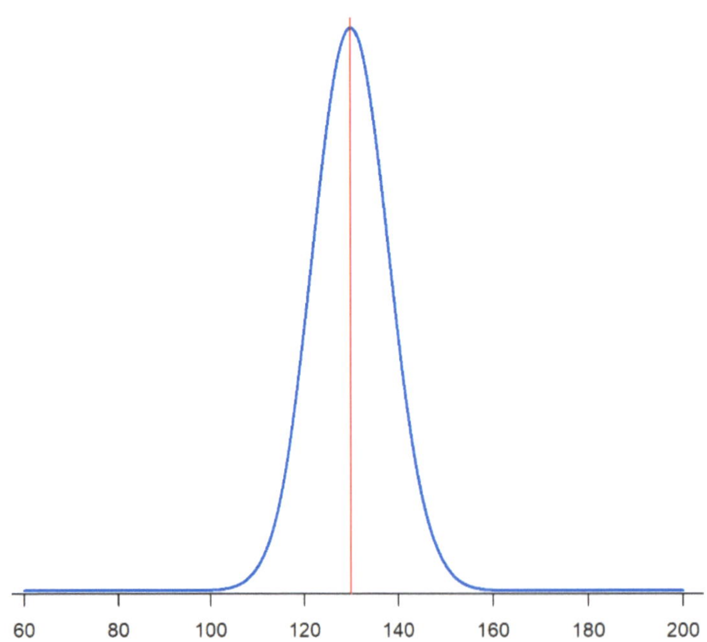

Now the curve is thinner, as the results are more clustered around the mean.

2. As the standard deviation decreases, the normal distribution curve becomes ______________

So what does the normal distribution curve do for us? That is a very good question. And here is one answer: Let's say we want to know the probability that someone in our population has a systolic blood pressure of less than or equal to100 mmHg? It turns out, the answer to this is the *area under the curve* of the value in question. Back to our original example in which the standard deviation is 15.

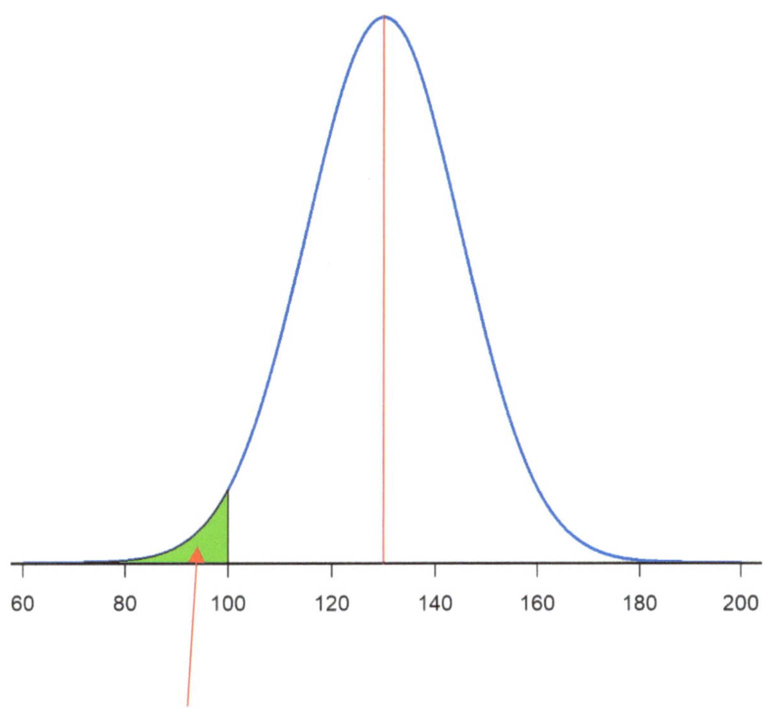

The area of this section in green is the probability that a person in the population has a systolic blood pressure of 100 mmHg or less. (2.3% if you're interested!)

OK, so one last thing about standard deviations and normal distributions. It turns out that the probability of a value occurring between one standard deviation less than the mean and one standard deviation more than the mean is approximately 68.2%. This is true no matter what the standard deviation is, and that is pretty cool.

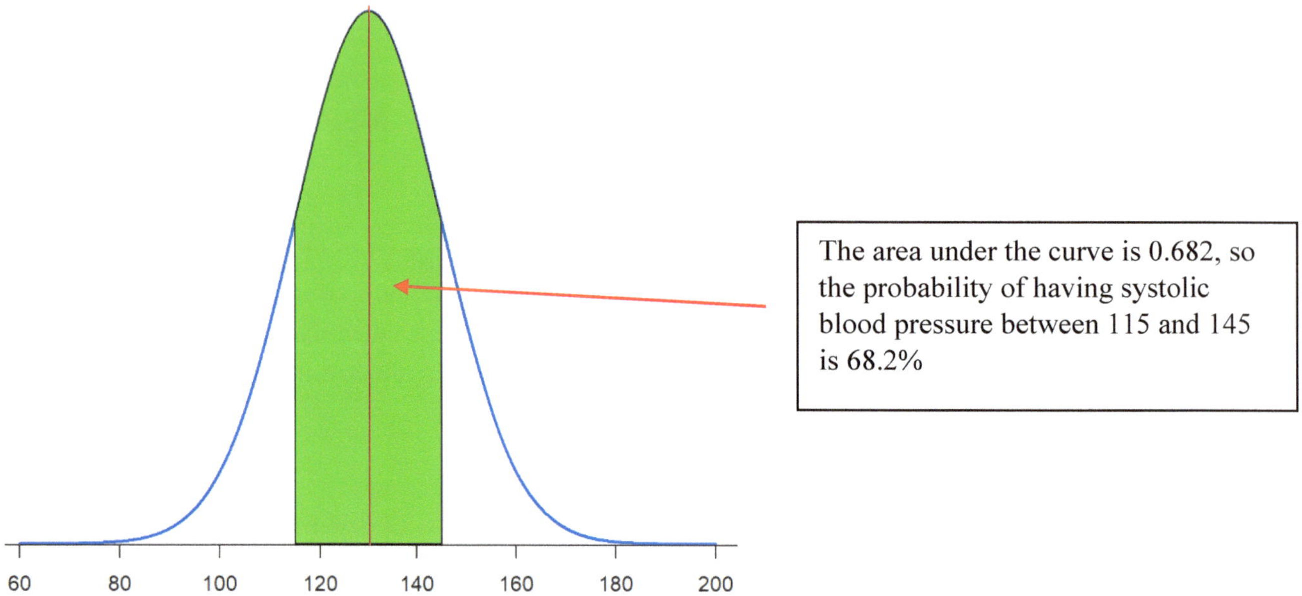

So that is something. But you don't need to memorize 68.2%. Instead memorize the following: the probability of a particular value being between *two* standard deviations below the mean and *two* standard deviations above the mean is 95%. By that I mean this:

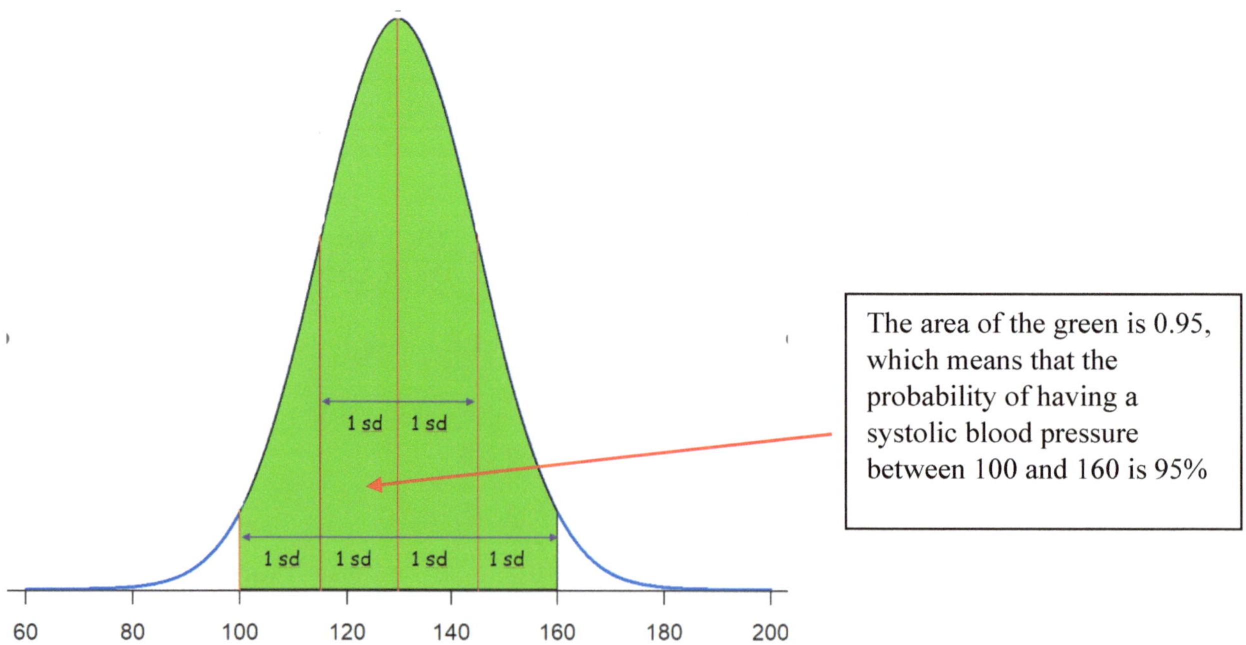

So, remember this one: the probability of a value lying between two standard deviations below and two standard deviations above the mean is 95%. (I lied a little: 2 standard deviations is an approximation; it is actually **1.96** standard deviations below and above the mean that precisely yields the 95%, but who's counting?) And this holds true no matter what the "thinness" of the normal distribution is—no matter what the standard deviation is. And that is a cool thing!

3. The really important thing to remember about normal distributions is that between (approximately) two standard deviations below the mean and two standard deviations above the mean lies ________ % of the data.

Section B1.2: Samples

The problem that we deal with all the time in medical research is that unfortunately we cannot include every person of interest in our study. There are usually way too many people in the population. So instead of enrolling all 150 million or so adult Americans into our study, we pick a *sample* that we *hope* well represents the *entire* population. Remember that what we really want is the mean of the entire population, but the best we can do is take a sample of the population, and hope that the mean of the sample is close to the mean of the population. Obviously no sample that we pick will be *exactly* identical to the entire population, but we hope that it comes close! I would like to illustrate this with a couple of examples. The first sample we randomly choose has only four people in it, and here are their systolic blood pressures:

Person 1: 157 mmHg

Person 2: 141 mmHg

Person 3: 136 mmHg

Person 4: 118 mmHg

What is the mean of the sample? Recall that the mean is calculated by summing up all the numbers and dividing by how many numbers there are.

When discussing the mean of a sample, we use the symbol $\bar{x}$.

$$\bar{x} = \frac{162+141+136+118}{4} = 139.3$$

So the mean of our sample is 139.3. In our pretend situation we know the mean of the entire population, and it is 130, but remember that usually we do *not* know the mean of the entire population and so we estimate it with our sample mean. So we would say that we *think* the mean of the entire population is somewhere around 139.3 mm Hg, based on our very small sample of four people. And the next thing we would do is calculate the standard deviation of our sample.

Recall the equation:

$$s = \sqrt{\frac{\sum_{i=1}^{n}(x_i - \bar{x})^2}{n-1}}$$

("s" means standard deviation of a sample). *n* is the number of people, and the $x_i - \bar{x}$ thing is just the difference (subtraction) between each reading and the mean.

And the big Σ thing means just sum them all up. So,

$(162 - 139.3)^2 = 515.3$

$(141 - 139.3)^2 = 2.9$

$(136 - 138)^2 = 10.9$

$(118 - 139.3)^2 = 453.7$

Add them all up, and get 982.8. Divide this by n – 1 = 3 and you get 327.6. Take square root of this and get: 18.1

So our very small sample did, well…OK. The mean is kind of off, but not horrible (139.3 vs the "true" mean of 130), and the standard deviation of our sample is 18.1 (as opposed to the "true" standard deviation of the entire population, which we know to be 15). And that is typical of very small samples. The values tend to be all over the place, and we need to be quite lucky for a very small sample to be truly representative of the entire population.

Now let's see if we can improve things a bit by taking a larger sample of n = 20.

Systolic Blood pressure readings:

162, 168, 136, 152,108, 111, 141,137,128,147,119,133,138,130,106,135,129,120,128,134

The mean is **133.1.** Well, that seems more reasonable than the 139.3 we got from the first sample.

If you're a glutton for punishment, and decide to calculate the standard deviation by hand, you would do this:

Value	x_i	$x_i - x$	$(x_i - x)^2$
x_1	162	28.9	835.21
x_2	168	34.9	1218.01
x_3	136	2.9	8.41
x_4	152	18.9	357.21
x_5	108	-25.1	630.01
x_6	111	-22.1	488.41
x_7	141	7.9	62.41
x_8	137	3.9	15.21
x_9	128	-5.1	26.01
x_{10}	147	13.9	193.21
x_{11}	119	-14.1	198.81
x_{12}	133	-0.1	0.01
x_{13}	138	4.9	24.01
x_{14}	130	-3.1	9.61
x_{15}	106	-27.1	734.41
x_{16}	135	1.9	3.61
x_{17}	129	-4.1	16.81
x_{18}	120	-13.1	171.61
x_{19}	128	-5.1	26.01
x_{20}	134	-0.9	0.81
Total			**5019.8**

We then plug in the 5019.8 into the formula for standard deviation:

$$SD = \sqrt{\frac{\sum_{i=1}^{n}(x_i - \bar{x})^2}{n-1}}$$

$$SD = \sqrt{\frac{5019.8}{19}} = \mathbf{16.25}$$

(Of course, there is absolutely no reason for you to do this by hand; there are calculators all over the place on the internet that will do it for you).

You can see that the results for this sample are much better! An average (mean) of about 133 with a standard deviation of about 16. So, not surprisingly, we have better results now as compared to our first sample of 4. And that makes intuitive sense: as we increase the sample size, we expect that the sample is more "true." We would feel a bit more comfortable now reporting that the mean of the *entire population* is somewhere around 133mmHg.

Let's look at a bar-graph (histogram) of the data:

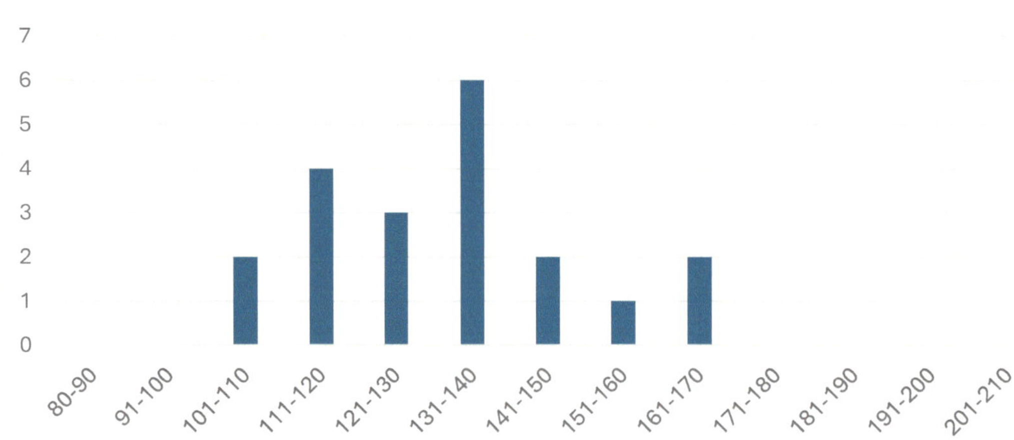

Well....we see...*sort of* like a normal distribution. As you can see, a sample size of 20, although much better than 4, is still a bit of a "stretch" to say it's "normal", but you can at least imagine it!

Take home point: As we increase the sample size, we expect that the mean of our sample would more closely represents the "true" mean of the entire population. Just *how* close will be the subject of the next section!

4. In general, the greater the n, the closer are the mean and standard deviation of our particular______________ compared to the mean of the entire __________________.

Section B1.3: Comparing samples to the entire population

As mentioned above, our study sample we hope is a good representation of the *entire population.* But exactly *how* good a representation is it? This is a general concept that will hold all through this book, as we must remember that in the world of medical research, experiments and papers, we always deal with a *sample* of the entire population of interest. It is the authors' and experimenters' job to choose good samples that are representative of the entire population, or else their data are meaningless to us. For example, in our example of a sample size of 20 people, we calculated the mean systolic blood pressure to be 133.1 mmHg. But remember that we don't really care about the mean of our sample, we want to know the mean of the *entire population.* We know that the mean of the entire population is very unlikely to be exactly 133.1, but we hope that it is somewhere close to that. So when we report out the mean of our sample, we have to add some kind of uncertainty...we need to calculate how certain we are that our population mean is somewhere around this. We need a *confidence interval* of the mean. That is, we report the mean of our sample with some interval around it – an interval that we can be fairly sure would include the actual mean of the entire population. And so the next section will explain how we calculate this interval.

To define how good a sample is, we define something known as the *Standard Error (SE).*

The Standard Error of a mean is defined as:

$$SE_{mean} = \frac{s}{\sqrt{n}}$$

Lower case s is the sample's standard deviation. Strictly speaking, we should actually be using σ (sigma), which is the precise standard deviation of the *entire* population. But usually we do not know the precise standard deviation of the entire population, so we are allowed to use s, the standard deviation of our sample. (We are allowed to use this because the standard deviation of our sample is in general close to that of the entire population). As you can see, the higher the n, the smaller the standard error. So there are only two things that determine how good a sample is: the standard deviation and the number of subjects in the sample. The higher the n, the better is the sample, and the lower the s, the better is the sample. This makes intuitive sense: if our sample has more people it is more likely to be "like" the entire population. Similarly, if our sample has a low s, and thus the values are not spread out wildly on either side of the mean, then our sample is also more "like" that of the true population. If a sample has a relatively high standard error, then the sample is not so good, and we are less confident that the mean of our sample truly represents the mean of the entire population. A sample with a lower standard error is "better" and we are more comfortable that the mean of our sample represents the true mean.

5. The Standard Error of the mean is our sample's ________________ ____________________ divided by the ________________________________ . The Standard Error of the mean is a way to measure how well our particular sample resembles the entire _______________________ .

The concept of standard error (SE) is an extremely important concept to grasp fully as it is fundamental to how we evaluate samples (or comparisons of samples, as will be covered later). The standard error in our previous example is specifically the standard error of the mean (SE_{mean}), but there are many other standard errors that I will discuss as we move forward. So we need to dive into the concept of the standard error a bit more. I have already explained what it does for us: it "evaluates" the quality of a sample…it tells us how confident we are that our sample represents the entire population. And I have described that the standard error of the mean is described by the standard deviation of the sample, and the n of the sample. So you know how it is defined, and what it does for us, but now I would like to begin a discussion of exactly *what it is*: where it comes from and how it is derived. Again, I cannot over-emphasize the importance of fully understanding this fundamental and vital concept.

An illustrative example

To begin our discussion, I am going to present an example. This is a full "population" of approximately 13,000 hospitalized patients and their lengths of stay in the hospital. And here is the histogram:

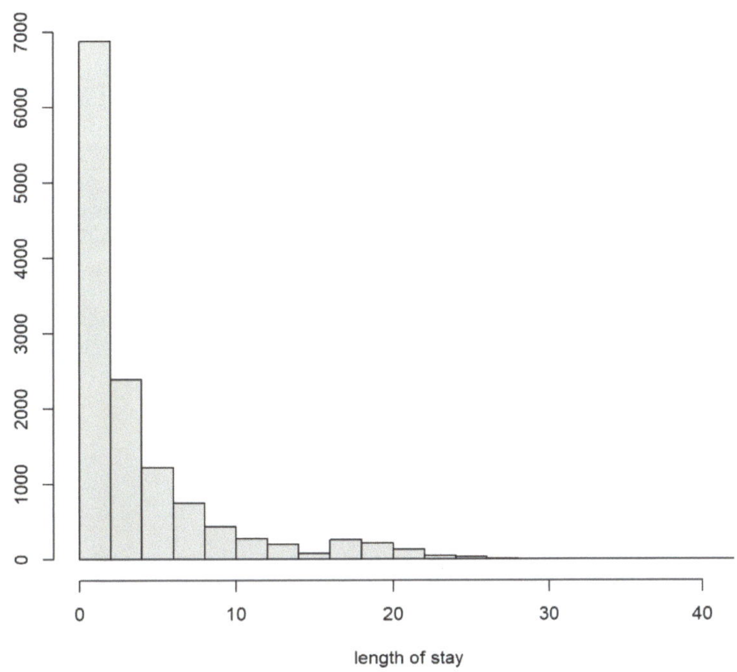

Figure B1.1 The entire population

The first thing to notice about this histogram is that it does not follow the normal distribution pattern that we have already talked about. A distribution pattern, like this one, in which there are far more lower results (ones and twos here) vs higher results (ten to twenty here) is called "right skewed). Recall that in a normal distribution, the mean, median and mode and all approximately equal. In a right-skewed distribution, the median is *less* than the mean, and the mode is even less than the median. In this population of hospital lengths of stay, the mean value is **4.29.** The median (middle) value is 2, and the mode (most frequently occurring value) is 1.

Here is a general graph of right-skewed distributions:

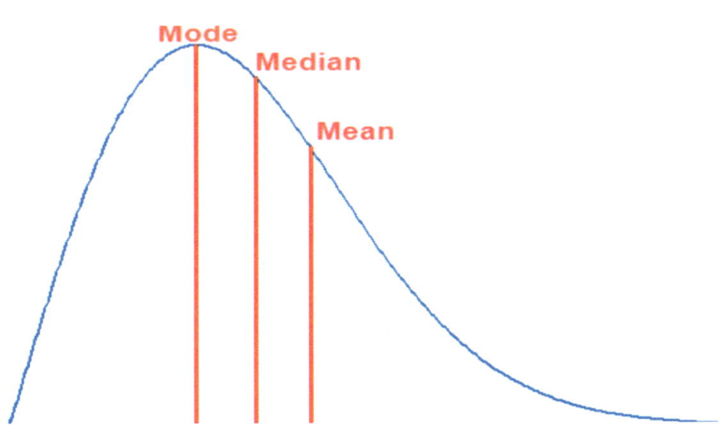

And so you can see that our example of hospital admission days of stay is *way* right-skewed. And (by the way) here is a left-skewed distribution:

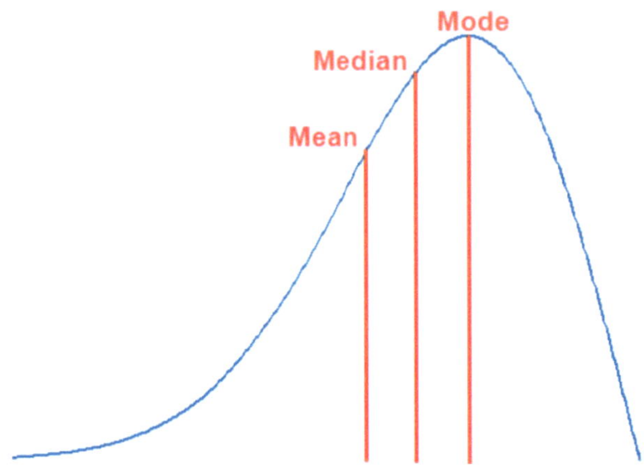

Here you see that the mean is now less than the median, which in turn is less than the mode.

6. In a right-skewed distribution, there are more values at the __________ end of the distribution, so the median value is _______________ than the mean.

So, back to our example. We see the entire distribution of the full population of 13,000 people. But let us now pretend we are doing a study and we cannot enroll all 13,000 people, and let us also pretend that we do not know the mean of our complete population (which is usually the case in the real world!). And so we would take a *sample* of those 13,000 people and use that sample to *estimate* the values of the entire population. We start by asking the computer to take one random sample of 50 people, and the resulting histogram looks like this:

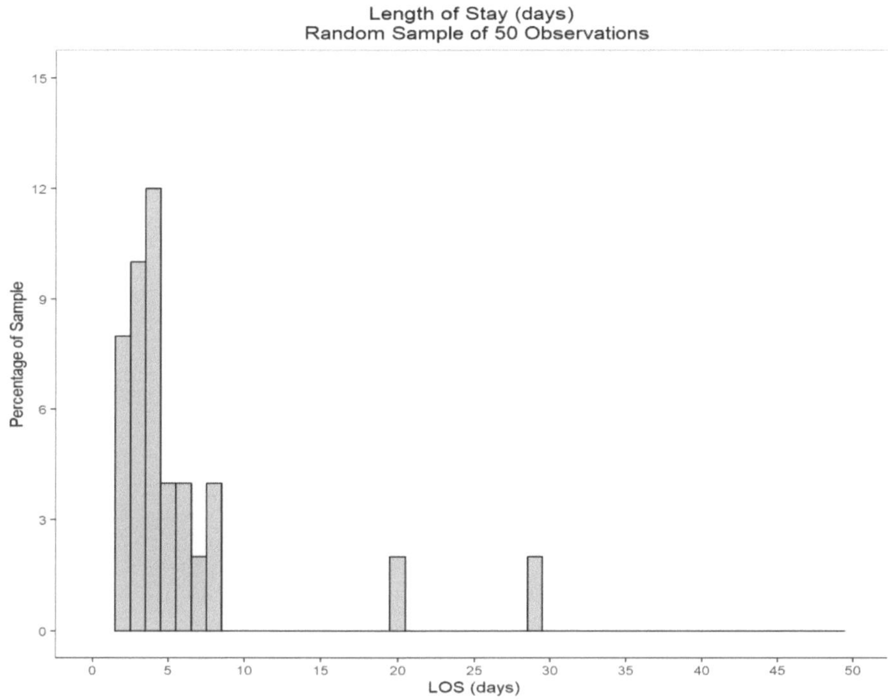

Figure B1.2 First sample

Notice that the histogram *sort of* looks like the histogram of our entire population. The mean of this sample is **3.34.** And so, in the real world in which we do not know the mean of the entire population, the best we can do is hope that our sample mean, 3.34, is close to the actual mean of the entire population. Recall that in our little unreal world we actually know that the true mean is 4.29. And so as luck would have it, our random sample was sort of an unlucky one, because our mean is considerably less than the true mean.

Let's ask the computer to take another random sample of 50 people

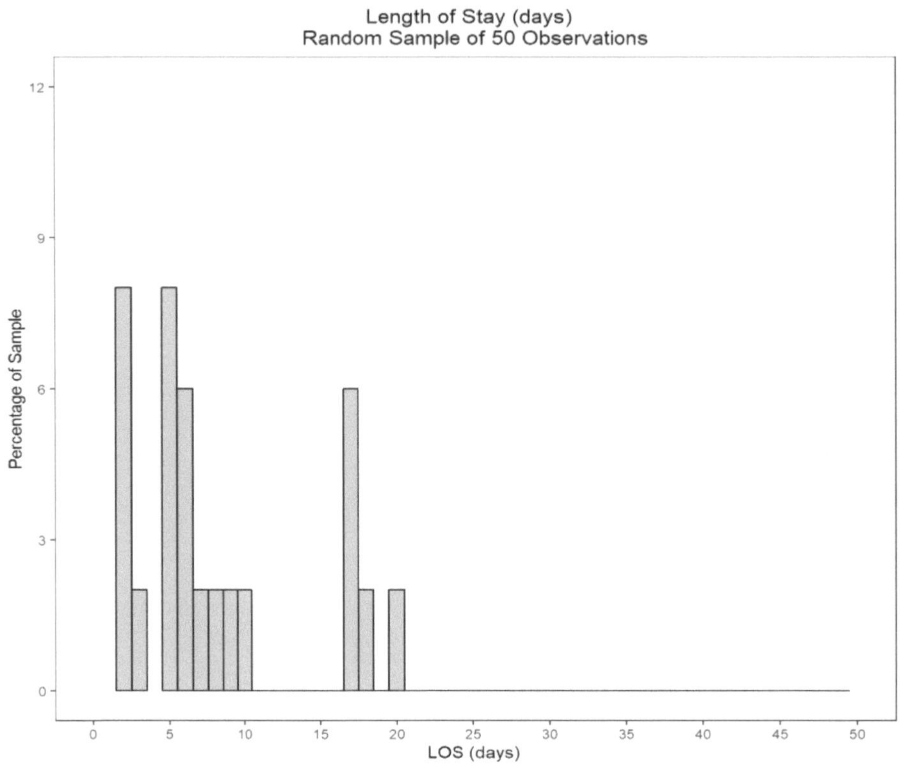

Figure B1.3 (2nd sample)

In this random sample, the mean is **4.62.** So all we could say based on this sample is that the true mean of the population is somewhere around 4.62. (We got luckier with this sample…it is closer to the true mean!).

Let's do one more and see what happens! Here is a third random sample:

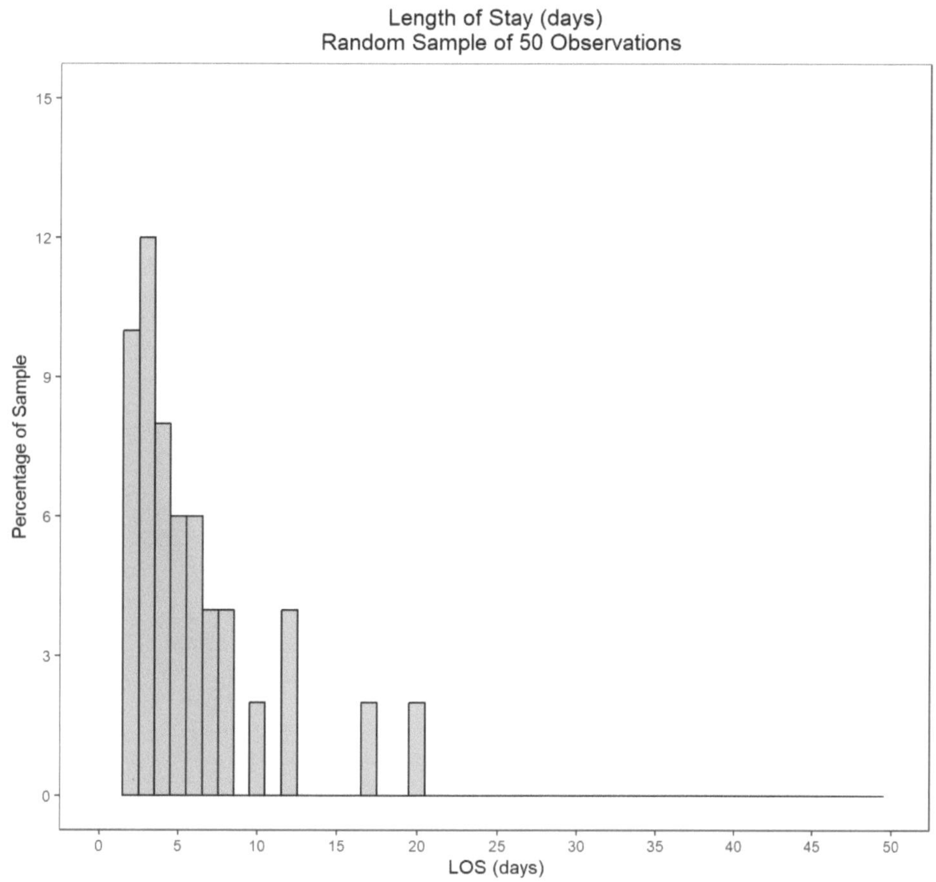

Figure B1.4 (3rd sample)

The mean of this random is sample is **3.96**.

So the means of the random samples tend to jump around the true mean, some close and some not so close.

OK, so now comes the big step, so pay close attention! What do you think would happen if we took 10 of these random samples, and graphed a histogram of the *means* of all the samples? Remember, now we are not graphing the actual data points of the samples, we are graphing the *means* of the samples.

Here is what we get:

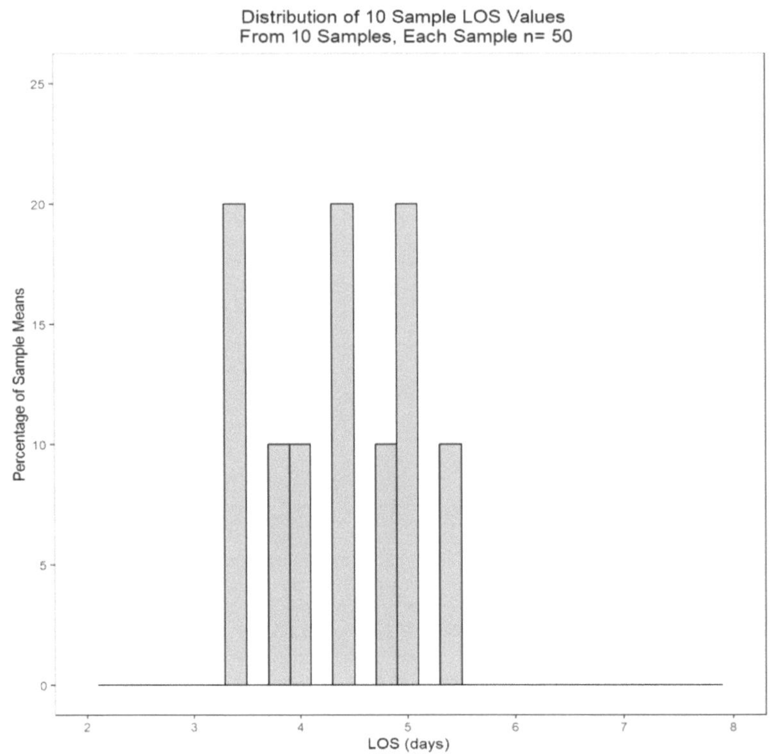

So, again what you are looking at is a graph of the *means* of ten random samples. The mean of this graph, by the way, is 4.17, which is the mean *of the means* or our sample. Notice that the graph no longer has a right-skewed appearance. And that is because we are not graphing the actual results of the samples, i.e. the individual lengths of stay. Rather, we are graphing the *means* of the samples.

So get ready for some magic. Let's now take a look at 100 random samples (of 50 each), and graph the results of the means of all 100 samples. We get this:

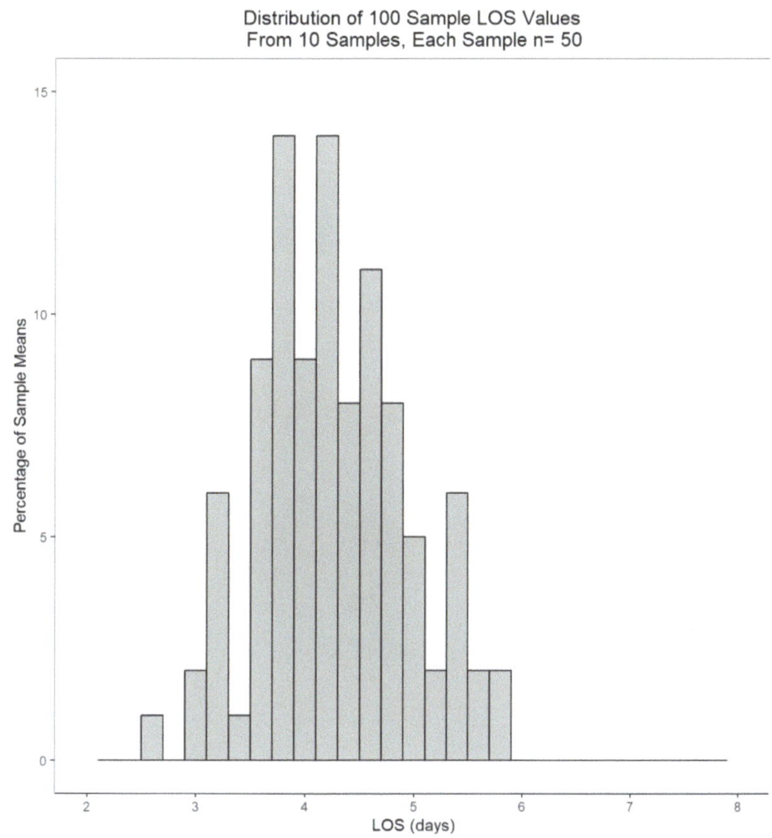

What do we see happening? If you think the graph is looking like a normal distribution, you are absolutely correct, and you are demonstrating the theorem that statisticians call "magic," and love to talk about: the **Central Limit Theorem.** The Central Limit Theorem states what you just witnessed: If we take any population distribution—and it can *any* distribution: a normal distribution, a distribution skewed to the left or right (no matter how heavily skewed), or even a distribution that follows no discernible pattern, just complete "willy-nilly, " i.e something like this:

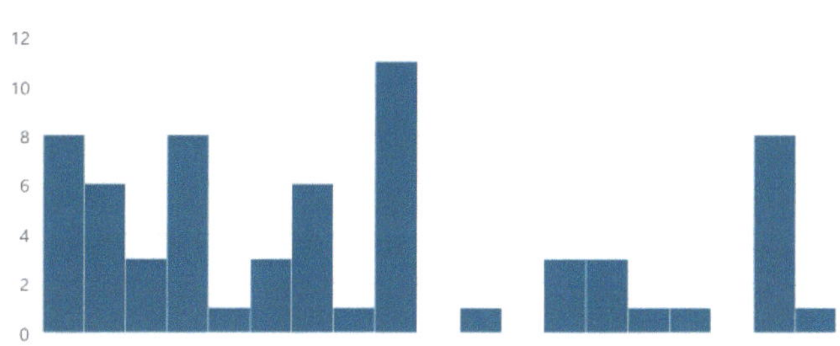

– *whatever* the distribution of the population, if we take a bunch of random samples from that population and graph the *means* of those samples, then the graph of the means will *always* be normally distributed. That is pretty amazing, isn't it?

7. The Central Limit Theorem states that no matter what the distribution of values in the population, if we take random samples of the population and graph the means of the samples, the graph of the means will always be ___________________________ distributed!

In our graph of 100 random samples above, the mean is 4.20. This is pretty close to the mean of the entire population, which you recall is 4.29.

Now let's ask the computer to take 5000 random samples from the population (each with n=50)

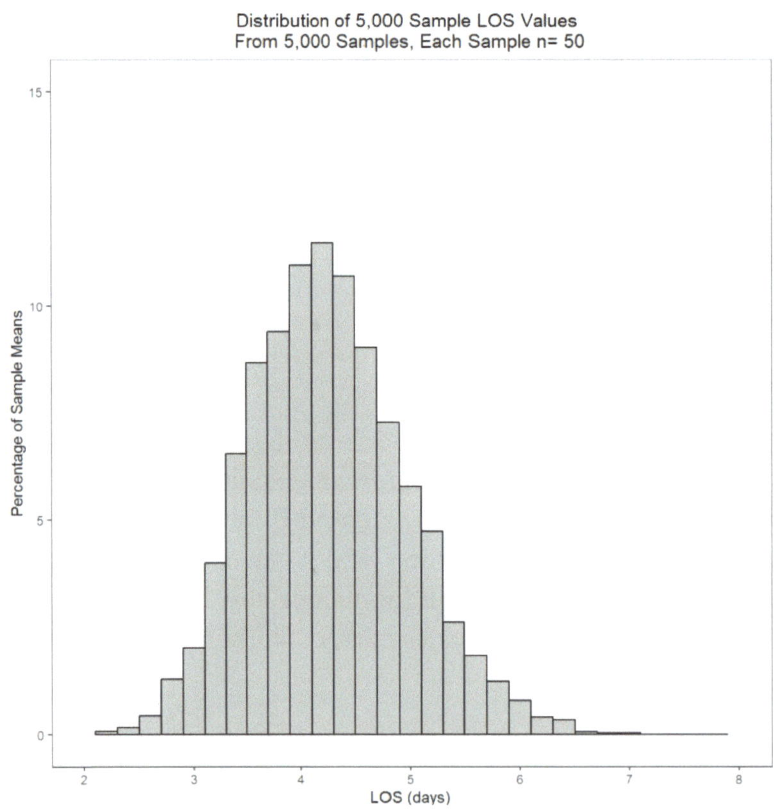

Figure B1.5

An almost perfect normal distribution! The mean of this distribution is 4.26…now *very* close to the actual population mean of 4.29. And so, yes, if we took an *infinite* amount of random samples, we would get a mean of 4.29.

Let's take a step back. What does all this have to do with what we are talking about? Recall that we are discussing the *standard error,* and specifically the standard error of the mean of a particular sample. And the random particular sample we were talking about has an n = 50.

So here is how the Central Limit Theorem is relevant to our one random sample

The distribution of the means of 5000 random samples shown above, each sample with an n = 50, has a mean of 4.26, and a standard deviation of 0.710. Recall what the standard deviation of the distribution means. It is how "spread out" the values are. But more importantly for our purposes, recall that 95% of the values lie between (approximately) 2 standard deviations below and 2 standard deviations above the mean. So I will now show the distribution with the mean value shown by a red line, and the 95% of values bordered by blue lines:

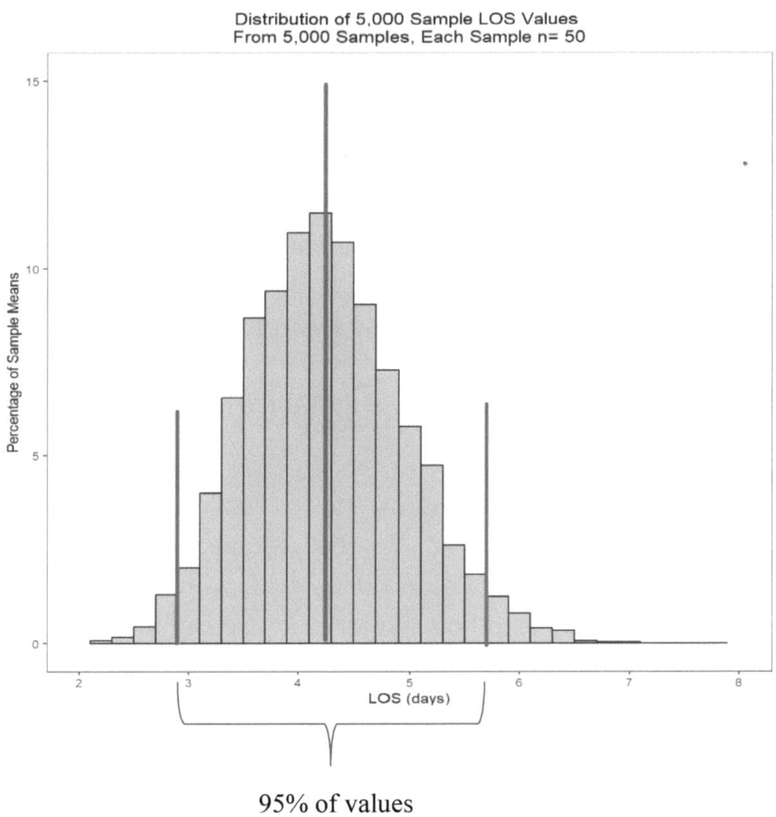

So what does this mean? If we take random samples of n = 50 from our population, then 95% of the samples will have a mean somewhere between 2.89 and 5.68. Indeed, remember the three random samples we pulled out of the population? (figures 1.2, 1.3 and 1.4) the means were **3.34**, **4.62** and **3.96,** all in the range. But if we pulled enough samples, we would eventually get "unlucky," and the mean would fall out of the range.

But here is the important point: the standard error of the mean for a sample is the standard deviation of the distribution of sample means. Ugh. That is a lot to digest. So look again at figure B1.5. This is the distribution of sample means of 5000 samples, all of 50 observations.

The standard deviation is 0.71. So, 0.71 is the *standard error of the mean* for *any random sample* of n = 50.

8. The standard error of a sample of say, n = 50 is the standard deviation of the __________ of a whole bunch of samples of n=50.

So let's go back to our first random sample of n = 50 (figure B1.2). The mean of this sample was 3.34. Since our n is equal to 50, we know that the standard error is 0.71. So just like we did for standard deviations, we take 2 standard errors below our mean, and 2 standard errors above our mean, and we report that interval as our 95% confidence interval. (Strictly speaking, it's 1.96 standard errors below to 1.96 standard errors above, but who's counting?)

So, our sample's mean is 3.34. But, again, we don't really care what our sample mean is, we want to know what the mean of the entire population is! (I know I already told you that our population's mean is 4.29, but that is just for learning purposes—in the real world we *don't know* the mean of the true population). So, anyway, we can't just say that we think the mean of the entire population is 3.34 based on our sample. We have to give a confidence range. So we say: the mean is 3.34, with a 95% confidence interval from $3.34 - 2(0.71)$ to $3.34 + 2(0.71)$; or (**1.92 to 4.76**). This translates to "we are reasonably confident that the *true* mean of *the entire population* falls somewhere between 1.92 and 4.76." How confident are we? Oh, about 95% confident! And, since we are not in the real world and actually know that the true mean of the entire population is 4.29, well…we were right!

Now let's look at our second random sample of n = 50 (figure B1.3). In this random sample, the mean happened to be 4.62. But again, that mean is meaningless! We just care about the mean of the entire population, so once again, we calculate our 95% confidence interval, which is $4.62 - 2(0.71)$ to $4.62 - 2(0.71)$; or (**3.20 to 6.04**). So now, based on *this* sample, we say that we are reasonably confident that the *true* mean of the entire population falls somewhere between 3.20 and 6.04. And, in our make-believe world in which we know that the true mean of the entire population is 4.29, again we are right!

And our third random sample (figure B1.4)? The mean of this sample was 3.96. Here is an exercise for you:

9. In our third random sample of n =50, the mean was 3.96. Since we know that the standard error of a sample of n=50 is 0.71, then we calculate our 95% confidence interval to be ______ to _______.

Did you get a confidence interval of (2.54 to 5.38)? If you did, you are correct! And, once again our 95% certainly held true, since the mean of the entire population is indeed in this interval.

So, we are three-for-three, batting 1000!

BUT, if I continue to take random samples of n = 50, eventually, our 95% confidence interval will not hold true. For example, let's say we took a random sample, and the mean happened to be 5.75. Well, same drill: we would calculate the 95% confidence interval to be between 4.33 and 7.17. And all we can say is that we are reasonably confident that the true mean of the entire population falls between 4.33 and 7.17. But, alas, this time our reasonable confidence does not hold true, as the true mean is not included in this interval. Aww!!

Well, come on, now, there is a reason we say 95% and not 100%!!

So, bottom line: Whenever we report the mean of a sample, it is meaningless without its 95% confidence interval, and here is exactly what a 95% confidence interval is:

If we take 100 random samples, all of the same size (in our example, we used n=50), then in 95 of those samples, the true mean of the population lies within the 95% confident interval, but in the other 5, the true mean of the population does *not* lie within the 95% confidence interval.

Extending the discussion: What do you suppose would happen if we took a distribution of 5000 samples as we did before, but instead of each sample having an n = 50, we now let each sample have an n = 250? We ask the computer to do this, and here is the histogram:

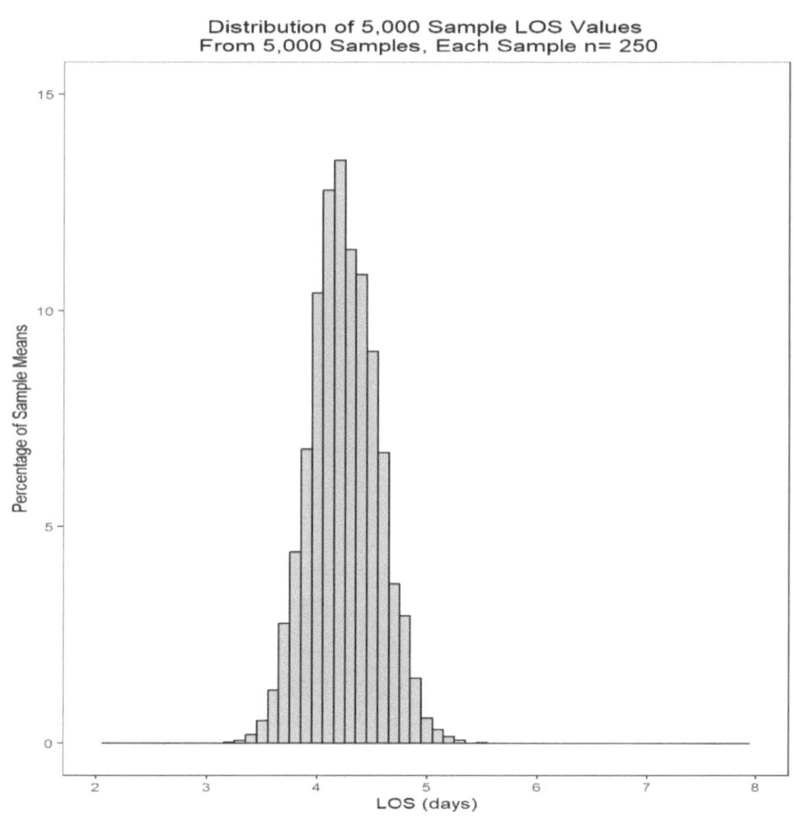

Figure B1.6

Notice that compared to figure B1.5, the histogram is a lot thinner, and clustered around the mean. The mean of this histogram, which, remember, is the mean *of the mean* of all 5000 samples is 4.25, and the standard deviation of this histogram is 0.30. Notice the difference between this and figure B1.5, which had 5000 samples, but n = 50. The standard deviation went from 0.71 to 0.30. Our standard deviation is much smaller, which is a good thing…it means our results are more clustered around the mean, and more "reliable." And remember, the standard deviation of the means of a whole bunch of samples of n = 250 is what we define as the **standard error** of a sample of n = 250. So, for a sample size of n = 250, the standard error would be **0.30**. Let's play around now with one random sample of n = 250. We ask the computer to generate one random sample, and we get:

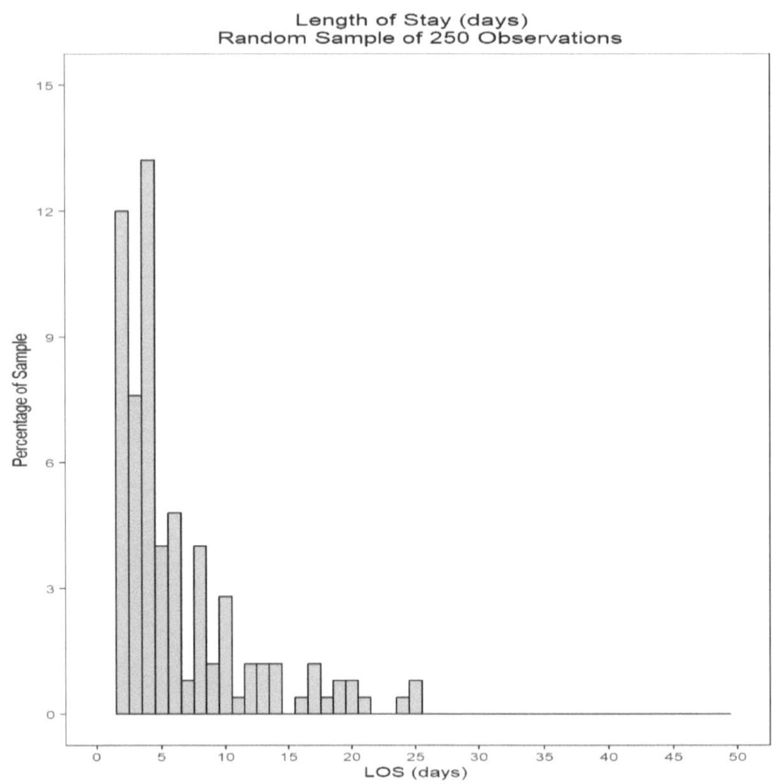

Figure B1.7

So, you see it is right-skewed, which makes sense, because the histogram of the entire population is right-skewed. The mean of this one sample is **4.20**, and the standard deviation of the sample is **4.81**. Remember that the mean of one sample is not want we want: we want the mean of the entire population, so we would report that the mean of the entire population is likely 4.20 with a 95% confidence interval. And how do we estimate the 95% confidence interval? It is twice the standard error above the mean and twice the standard error below the mean. We say that the 95% confidence interval is 4.20 – 2(0.30) to 4.20 + 2(0.30), or (**3.60 to 4.80**). So we are reasonably certain that the true mean of the population is between 3.60 and 4.80. And were lucky this time, because we know that the true mean of the entire population is 4.29, so we were right! Remember what the 95% confidence interval means: if we had the computer take 100 random samples, each of n = 250, in 95 of them, the confidence interval generated would in fact contain the true mean of the population, but in 5 of them, we would be "unlucky" because the 95% confidence interval would not contain the true mean. (Of course, we would have no way of knowing whether our one sample is lucky or not, because we usually do not know the mean of the entire population.

Important take home point: When we compare a random sample of n = 50 with a random sample of n = 250, we see that the *standard error decreases.* The bigger our sample the better, because with bigger samples comes smaller standard errors, and thus *narrower* 95% confidence intervals. And narrower 95% confidence intervals are more precise: the true mean of the entire population (likely) lies within a smaller interval.

10. The bigger the sample, the better, because as we increase the sample size, the standard error ________________________, and the 95% confidence interval becomes more ____________________, thus increasing the precision of our estimate.

One last bit of magic.

Recall at the beginning of the section, I defined the standard error like this:

$$SE_{mean} = \frac{s}{\sqrt{n}}$$

But then I kind of ignored this and explained to you the precise definition of the standard error of a particular sample size: it is the standard deviation of a distribution of the means of a whole bunch of samples all of that particular sample size. Figure B1.6 showed that distribution for a whole bunch of samples of n = 250. The standard deviation of that distribution was 0.30. Now watch: Recall that *s* is the standard deviation of our one sample (because in general we do not know the standard deviation of the entire population). In figure 1.7, we had one sample of n = 250, and its standard deviation (s) is 4.81. So watch:

$$SE_{mean} = \frac{s}{\sqrt{n}} = \frac{4.81}{\sqrt{250}} = \mathbf{0.30}!!!$$

Got it? So the actual precise definition of the standard error (sorry to be redundant!) is that it is the standard deviation of the means of whole lot of random samples. That is the precise and conceptual thing to understand. But the shortcut mathematical formula for the standard error is simply the equation above. They are the same thing!

Summary of Biostats 1

There was a lot in this chapter, and I hope you made it through unscathed! Indeed, samples, and how they relate to populations on the whole is one of the basic fundamentals of biostats and epidemiology. Here is a summary:

- Many things in medicine (but not all) follow a normal distribution pattern.
- The standard deviation of the sample is a measure of how spread out the data are around the mean. A smaller standard deviation means a better quality sample.
- A sample is a portion of the whole population, and we use our sample to make inferences about the whole population.
- We hope our sample is as representative as possible of the entire population.
- We hope that the mean of our sample is close to the mean of the entire population..
- We report the mean of our sample with its 95% confidence interval, which tells us with some certainty that the true population mean lies within that interval.
- We obtain our confidence interval by using the standard error of the sample, which is the standard deviation of the means of many samples of that size.
- Large samples are more representative of the entire population than are small samples because they have a smaller standard error, and therefore a narrower 95% confidence interval.

Epidemiology 1: Types of Epidemiologic Studies
Part 1: Observational Studies

Now that we have gone through the basics of biostats, it is logical to introduce the fundamental concepts of epidemiologic research studies, so that you will begin to see what the biostatistical methods are used for.

The goal of any epidemiologic study is to explore the relationship between factors. We might ask, for example, is cigarette smoking associated with lung cancer? Well of course we now know the answer to this, but fifty years ago we did not, and the association needed to be studied. After many years of research, we can say with certainty that cigarette smoking is indeed associated with lung cancer, and we even go so far as saying that cigarette smoking *causes* lung cancer. Note that the difference between *association* and *causation* is important in epidemiology, and I would like to clarify this with another example: Let's say that we want to explore the association between cigarette smoking and depression. If more smokers are depressed than non-smokers, we might report a positive association or relationship between the two, but we cannot say for certain that cigarette smoking *causes* depression. It is equally possible that being depressed makes people want to smoke cigarettes, and if that were the case, then depression causes cigarette smoking. And that is an important point to keep in mind when considering epidemiologic studies: while the ultimate goal may be to try to prove *causality*, the studies themselves often fall short of this, and only show that the two factors are related to each other. One may be a "risk factor" for the other, but there are many other requirements that must be satisfied before one can prove causality. As we go through the different kinds of epidemiologic studies in the next section, you will notice a sort of "hierarchy" of studies, with those in the upper echelons coming closest to being able to establish causality.

1. Although the ultimate goal of epidemiologic research is to explore causality, in general, epidemiologic studies can only show that two factors are _______________ to each other.

Epidemiologic studies are generally divided into two major types: experimental and **observational**. And the difference is as it sounds: in experimental studies, the researchers are "experimenting" on some of the people in the study, and following them forward in time for an outcome. The experiment can be anything you can think of: perhaps some people are given a certain medicine and watched for an effect, while others are given a placebo and the two groups are compared; perhaps some people are given advice on preventing a disease, while another group is not, and the rates of the disease occurrence in each group are compared; perhaps some people are started on an exercise program and a diet while others are started on a diet alone, and the two groups are compared for weight loss after a trial period; or really anything else researchers can think of. The key is that the researchers are deciding who is experimented on (who is "exposed" in the language of epidemiology), and who is not. In observational research, on the other hand, nothing is "being done" to anyone. Certain groups are simply analyzed as they are. For example, cigarette smokers may be compared to non-smokers, or males compared to females, etc. As you can see below, there is only one kind of experimental trial (which is considered the "gold-standard" of epidemiologic research): the randomized controlled trial. But there are several different kinds of observational studies.

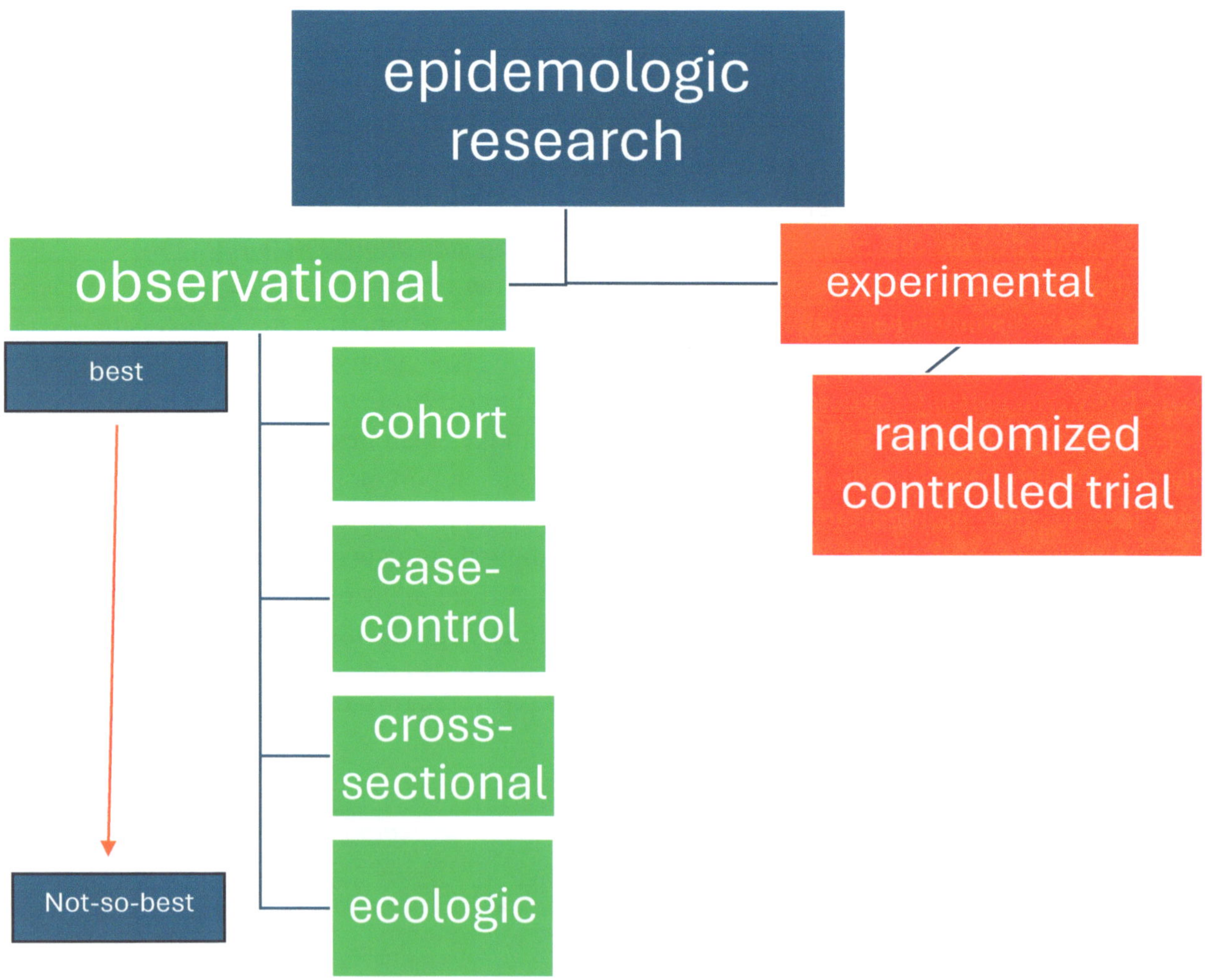

I would like to begin by discussing observational studies, and I will proceed down the line, from cohort to ecological. And as you will see that is a logical order; in general, cohort studies are considered a "higher" order study than case-control, which are "higher" order than cross-sectional, which are "higher" order than ecologic. The reason for the hierarchy is that the studies of the higher order do the most to establish *causality,* while those at the bottom do little, if anything to establish *causality.*

Section E1.1: The cohort study

OK, remember that the word "cohort" means "group." In a cohort study, the goal is to see if some kind of factor (called the "exposure") leads to some kind of "outcome." The outcome can be pretty much anything: a disease occurring, a hospitalization required, a cure, etc. Often, cohort studies are designed to compare two groups: one group is the "exposed" group, and the other is the "control" group (people who do not have the exposure). The cohort, or cohorts, are followed forward in time and observed (it's an *observational* study, remember?) for an event occurring. And then the two groups are compared. Did more events occur in the exposed group or the control group? Or are they the same?

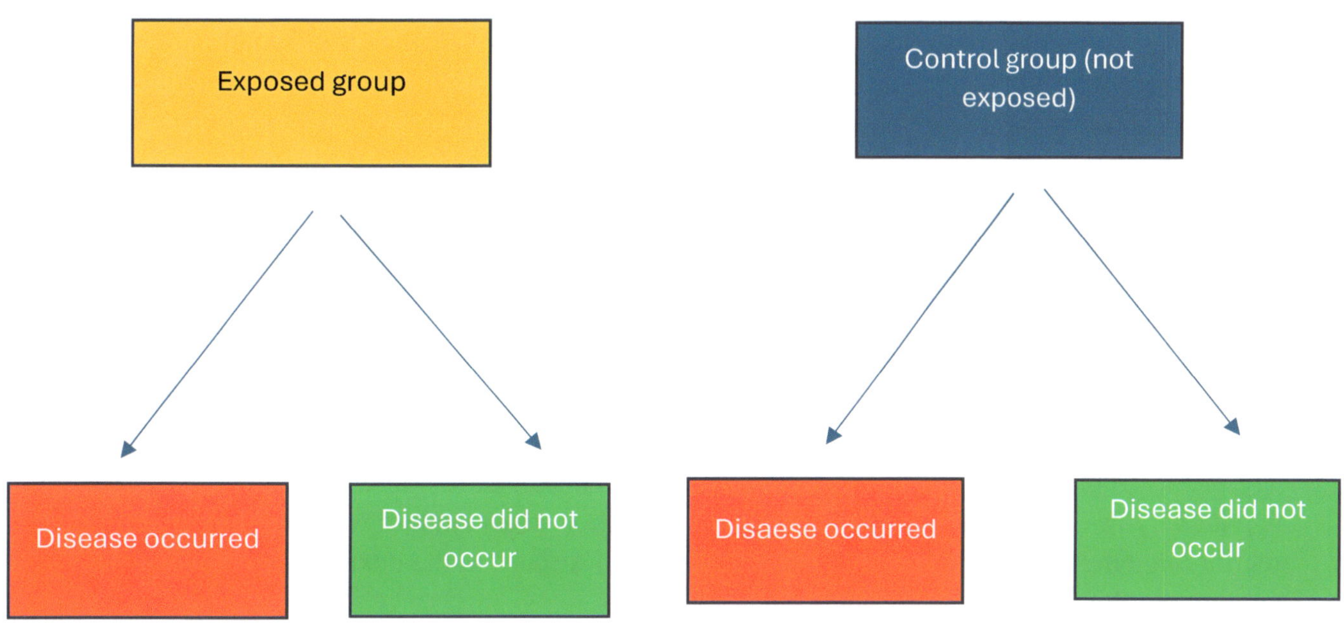

Here is an example of a cohort study.

> Henquet et al. Prospective cohort study of cannabis use, predisposition for psychosis, and psychotic symptoms in young people. *BMJ* 2004; 330:11

In this study, the researchers sought to explore the relationship, if there is one, between cannabis use and psychosis. To do this, they identified a group of people who were cannabis users and a group of people who were not cannabis users and followed them for four years, and then tabulated the number of psychotic episodes that occurred in each group. So it is a cohort study because the researchers defined the cohorts (cannabis use or not), and observed them for disease occurrence (psychosis). And specifically, this is a *prospective* cohort study, as the groups were followed forward in time.

2. In a cohort study, groups are first defined in terms of whether or not they have an ____________________ to a factor, and then followed along in time to see if they develop an ________________________, which can be some event occurring like a disease or a death or a hospitalization, etc.

Cohort studies are in general considered high quality for achieving the goal of determining whether an association between an exposure and an outcome exists. But you can imagine the inherent problems in trying to conduct a cohort study. The first problem is that the outcome in question cannot be a rare outcome. Why is that? If the outcome is rare, you would need to recruit a very large number of people into your study, so that a reasonable number of them will have the outcome. For example, let's say we conducted a study with 1000 people in the exposure group, and 1000 people in the non-exposed group, and we followed them for say five years for the occurrence of an event. We found that at the end of our study period, the outcome was so rare so that there were 3 events in the exposed group and 2 events in the unexposed group. Well, how can we compare 3 cases out of 1000 vs 2 cases out of 1000? We cannot say anything at all about that difference: the numbers are so small that it is meaningless. On the other hand, if the outcome is not rare, and say there were 452 events in the exposed group vs say 312 events in the unexposed group, well, now we can make some inferences! So, if the outcome is relatively rare, we have a problem conducting a cohort study, unless we have the capability to recruit *huge* numbers of people into our study. (I will discuss in the next section how we circumvent this).

3. It is difficult to conduct a cohort study if the outcome is relatively ____________.

The other problem associated with cohort studies is a logistic one. You can imagine that following a relatively large group of people over a relatively long period of time requires a relatively large amount of resources (and patience). One way around this is instead of conducting a *prospective* cohort study, the researchers conduct a *retrospective* cohort study. In a retrospective cohort study, the researchers start with two or more groups, depending on exposure status, but instead of identifying the groups on day one and follow them forward in time to day x, (and spending much money), the researchers get very lucky and are able to identify cohorts that *already existed at some time in the past*, and follow them up to the *present day*. Here is an example of a *retrospective* cohort study:

> Schuurman AG, et al. Increased risk of Parkinson's disease after depression. *Neurology* 2002; 58(10), 1501-1504.

In this study, the authors sought to examine the association between the existence of depression and the subsequent development of Parkinson's disease. They knew that the outcome, Parkinson's disease, is relatively rare, so they would have to recruit a lot of people and follow them for a good amount of time for there to be a significant number of cases. But the researchers were very lucky as they were able to identify a large cohort that *already existed in the past.*

Here is the description of what they did; it is from the "Methods" section of the paper:

> A retrospective cohort study was carried out based on the Registration Network Family Practices (RegistratieNet Huisartspraktijken [RNH]). The RNH is a continuous and computerized database in which 53 general practitioners working in 21 practices in the south of the Netherlands are participating.12 In the RNH, all relevant health problems are registered, including all relevant past health problems of a patient.

Well, this was amazing for the researchers! They had a ready-made database of about 200,000 patients, all with various diagnoses, from thirty years ago till the present! (The "present" is the year this paper was written, 2002). Indeed, among this very large database they were able to identify 1375 people who were diagnosed with depression between 1975 and 1990. They then identified a "control" group from this database, which consisted of 67,608 people who were born in the same years as the 1375 people, but were not depressed. They then followed both these cohorts…not into the future, as in a prospective study, but *up to the present day* (in this case, 2002), to see how many in each group were subsequently diagnosed with Parkinson's disease. And so that is the difference: in a *prospective* cohort study, the researchers start in the present day, recruit their cohorts, and follow them into the future. In a *retrospective* cohort study, the researchers identify a cohort that existed in the past and follow them to the present via some kind of electronic records-keeping. It should not come as surprise that the past twenty years or so we have seen a huge increase in the amount of retrospective cohort studies in the medical literature. Medical practices are now heavily computer-based; vast amounts of patient data are available now via insurance claims information, national and regional databases, etc. As in the quoted study, is now quite easy for researchers to gain access to diagnoses and demographic information on thousands, if not millions of patients at some point in the past. The time and monetary savings to researchers is vast. By conducting a retrospective study, the researchers are able to accomplish in say, one month or so of data analysis, what would take ten or more years and countless dollars if they had conducted a prospective study.

4. Because the cohorts already exist in the past, retrospective studies save researchers both ___________ and ____________.

Of course, as with all things in life, there is "no such thing as a free lunch," and the huge benefit gained in efficiency with a retrospective study comes with a cost. Let's think for a minute about the Parkinson's study. They identified people with depression based on electronic records from some time in the past. And then they simply calculated how many of those people were subsequently (from the time when they were diagnosed with depression to the present) diagnosed with Parkinson's. (And they did the same for the control group: those without depression). Although they know the demographics of the trial participants, they know nothing else. What if, for example, many of the those in the exposed group were exposed to some poisonous chemical at some point during the study period that could predispose them to Parkinson's? Had they conducted a prospective study, they would follow each participant carefully into the future and would make sure the participant informed them if something like that occurred, and adjusted the results accordingly. Or what if they suffered a serious head injury, or were started on some medication during the time period? Etc. The point is that when we do a retrospective study, we lose details about each participant that may be affecting the hypothesis in question. Our gains in time and money may come with the cost of lack of *precision* of our data. In addition, a retrospective trial uses data already collected in the past by others, and often for other reasons that our interests. So, again, there may be a lack of precision in the selection process.

Section E1.2: Case-control Studies

The case-control study is entirely different than the cohort study. In a case-control study, participants are first identified based on whether or not they are a "case." That is, do they have the *outcome* in question? (usually some disease state). They are then followed *back in time* to see if they ever had a particular *exposure* that the researchers wanted to study.

Here is an example of a case-control trial:

> D'Souza et al. Case–Control Study of Human Papillomavirus and Oropharyngeal Cancer. *NEJM 2007; 356:1944-1956.*

Here is quote from their methods section:

> Our case–control study was nested within a longitudinal cohort study of patients with newly diagnosed squamous-cell carcinomas of the head and neck in the outpatient otolaryngology clinic of the Johns Hopkins Hospital in Baltimore from 2000 through 2005. Eligible case patients included those with a confirmed diagnosis of oropharyngeal squamous-cell carcinoma.
>
> The control group consisted of patients without a history of cancer who were seen for benign conditions between 2000 and 2005 in the same clinic from which the case patients were enrolled

So the cases (those with oropharyngeal cancer), and the controls (those without oropharyngeal cancer) were identified, and then the researchers looked *back in time* to see if certain exposures occurred. Here again is the method:

> All patients completed an audio, computer-assisted self-administered interview that obtained information about demographic characteristics, oral hygiene, medical history, family history of cancer, lifetime sexual behaviors, and lifetime history of marijuana, tobacco, and alcohol use…

So those are the exposures the researchers were interested in: demographics, oral hygiene, etc. There are two important points about case-control trials that are illustrated by this study:

1. Case-control studies are used when the outcome (the "cases") is something that is very rare. Oropharyngeal cancer is a rare condition, and so it would take lots of trial participants and lots of time for enough cases to occur that would make data analysis meaningful.

2. Case-control studies allow researchers to evaluate many different exposures. (in our example, researchers were examining eight different exposures!).

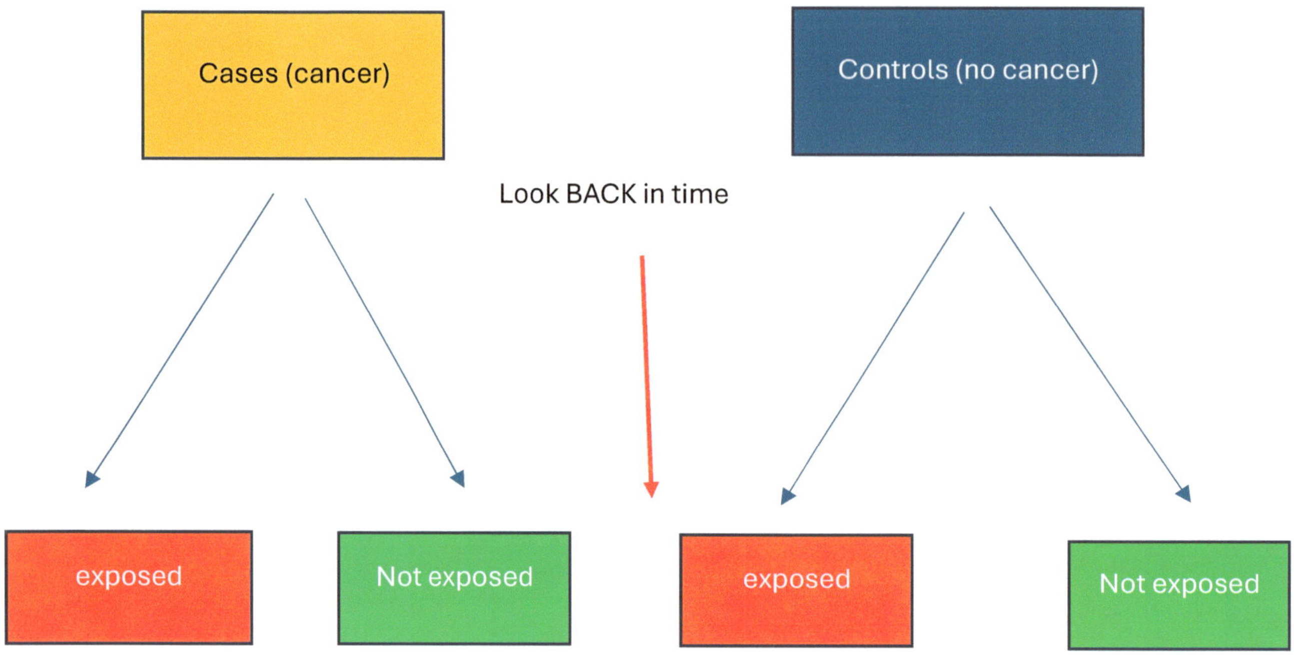

I would like to once again review the difference between case-control studies and cohort studies.

Cohort studies identify a specific cohort, or group, based on the presence of a particular factor known as the "exposure." The group or groups are followed forward in time to see if an outcome occurs. The exposure can be a relatively rare occurrence, but if the outcome is very rare, logistics will make conducting a cohort study very difficult. (Unless you happen to have access to very large previously created databases, and can run a *retrospective* cohort study, as explained above).

Case-control studies are the opposite: people are identified who have a particular outcome ("case") and followed backward in time to see if they had an exposure. Studies of this design are not quite as good as cohort studies, for reasons that I will discuss Epidemiology 4, but are necessary when studying an outcome that is relatively rare.

5. While case-control studies are generally not preferred, they are often necessary when the ____________________ in question is very rare.

Section E1.3: Cross-sectional studies

As we move down the hierarchy of observational studies, we next come to cross-sectional studies. These studies completely remove the element of *time.* Recall that the cohort study follows people forward in time, and the case-control study follows people backward in time. The cross-sectional study is present time only. Think of it as a "snapshot" in time in which we measure the *prevalence* of a disease (or whatever we are studying) at a particular moment in time. For example, there are approximately 1,000,000 Americans currently living with Parkinson's disease. Since there are approximately 250,000,000 adult Americans, we can say that the prevalence of Parkinson's disease is approximately 1 case per 250 people. (They would likely convert this to 4 cases per 1000 people, since convention usually uses multiples of 10 in the denominator).

Cross-sectional studies can also compare two groups. Recall our retrospective cohort study of Parkinson's disease and depression. The same type of study could have been done as a cross-sectional analysis as follows: A sample of 1250 people with depression and a sample of 1250 people without depression were surveyed and asked if they currently also carry a diagnosis of Parkinson's disease. They might find that the prevalence of Parkinson's among people with depression is 7 cases per 1250 people, and the prevalence of Parkinson's among people without depression is 3 cases per 1250 people. But again the key take-home message is that we have no element of time. We are assessing the concurrent existence of two factors. Since the prevalence of Parkinson's is higher among depressed people than among not depressed people, we may be able to conclude that there is indeed some kind of connection between the two. We may be able to say that depression is a *risk factor* for Parkinson's. But because we are talking about two simultaneous factors existing, we can say nothing about possible *causality*. It is just as likely that the Parkinson's caused the depression, rather than vice-versa. And that is the great limitation of cross-sectional studies.

6. Cross-sectional studies are a snap_____ in time, and therefore cannot say anything about ___________________________.

Section E1.4: Ecological studies

Lowest on our hierarchy is the ecological study, which shows data on a population level, rather than an individual level. And that is precisely why we gain the least useful information from these studies. Here is an example:

> Zhang, J: Egg Consumption and Mortality From Colon and Rectal Cancers: An Ecological Study. *Nutrition and Cancer: 2003;46(2), 158-65.*

And here is the main result figure:

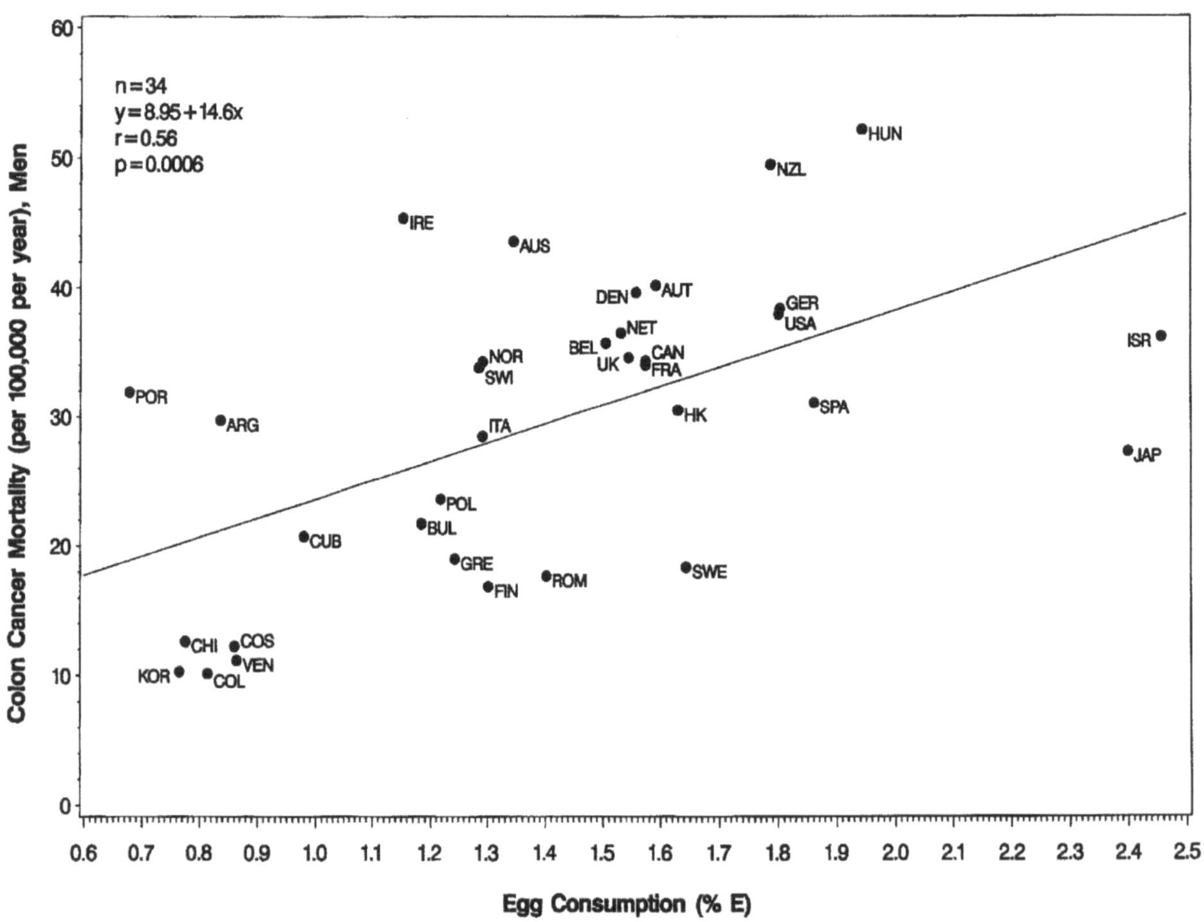

On the y-axis is colon cancer mortality rates, and on the x-axis is egg consumption in each country surveyed (measured as percentage of diet that is eggs). What do we learn here? Well, there really does appear to be a relationship between the two: although there is some variability, in general countries that have a higher percentage of consumption have a higher rate of colon cancer mortality. Korea, in the lower left corner, has a relatively low percentage of egg consumption, and a relatively low rate of colon cancer mortality, while Hungary, in the upper right, has relatively high results of both.

OK. So…what do we learn? Do we think, given this data, that eggs increase colon cancer mortality? That is, can we say from this data, that if I eat significantly more eggs than my neighbor, that I am more likely to die from colon cancer than she? Is egg consumption a "risk factor" for dying from colon cancer? No, of course not. And that is the great limitation of ecological studies. We only can make conclusions at the *population* level, and not at the *individual* level. This is known as the "ecological fallacy." What specifically do we learn from these data? We learn that *living in a country with a high egg consumption is associated with dying from colon cancer.* That is all. Although Hungary has a high egg consumption, it is quite possible that a lot of processed meats are consumed there, (and it would make sense that processed meat consumption and egg consumption go together) or it is possible that oncologic health care is not as good there as it is in some other countries. And it is possible that the countries with higher egg consumption also have higher levels of obesity: Korea, on the far left of the figure, may have healthier people in general or lower levels of obesity, etc.

So, yes, we can say that there is an *association* between living in a country with high egg consumption and higher levels of colon cancer deaths, but that is all we can say. We can say nothing about any association on an *individual* level.

7. Ecological studies only give us data on a population level, not on an individual level; this limitation is known as the ________________ ________________________.

Summary of Epidemiology 1

This chapter presented an overview of observational studies, which are studies that observe things in nature, and how they behave without us (the researcher) intervening in any way. Remember that *prospective* studies are the best (prospective cohort studies), followed by retrospective studies (retrospective cohort studies and case-control studies), followed by cross-sectional studies, followed by ecological studies. In the next epidemiology chapter, I will introduce the "gold standard" of ecological studies, the randomized controlled trial.

Epidemiology 2: Types of Epidemiologic Studies
Part 2: Experimental trials

We now turn our attention to what is commonly referred to as the "gold standard" of epidemiologic trials. In the previous chapter, I discussed observational studies. I will now discuss "experimental" studies. The main difference is that in experimental studies, the researchers are *doing something* to a group or groups of people and observing them into the future for any pre-specified outcomes. Oftentimes, the researchers are comparing participants who receive the "intervention" (the "exposed" group) with participants who do not (the "control group"). Recall that this is the main difference: in all the types of observational trials mentioned in the previous chapter, the researchers did nothing to the participants: they were observed in the natural state, whatever that may be.

Experimental trials are also called "randomized controlled trials." "Randomization" is the key to why these trials are considered the gold standard.

Section E2.1: Randomization

Randomization is an extremely important component of these trials, and I would like to use a fictitious example to show why. Suppose researchers are studying a new blood thinner medicine for people with atrial fibrillation. The primary endpoint (the reason atrial fibrillation is often treated with a blood thinner) is whether or not stroke occurred during a ten-year period. Here is what they found:

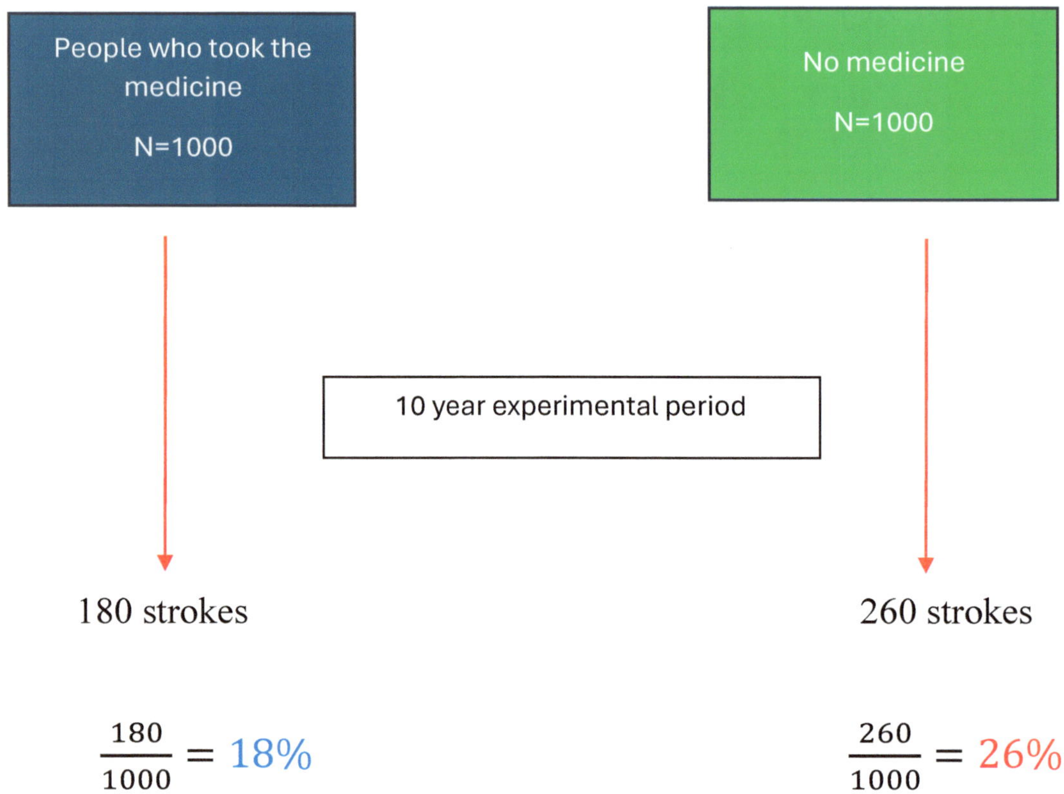

Figure 3.1

So we see a rather significant difference in the two groups. 18% of the group treated with the medication suffered a stroke, while 26% of the group that was not treated suffered a stroke. You can imagine that the pharmaceutical company that makes the drug would be quite happy with these results.

Now, let's say it just so happened that in the treated group, 200 of the 1000 people were smokers, while in the untreated group, 400 of the 1000 were smokers. We know that smoking is strongly associated with risk of stroke. So here is what we might find (we might estimate that 50% of smokers develop a stroke, while 10% of non-smokers develop a stroke).

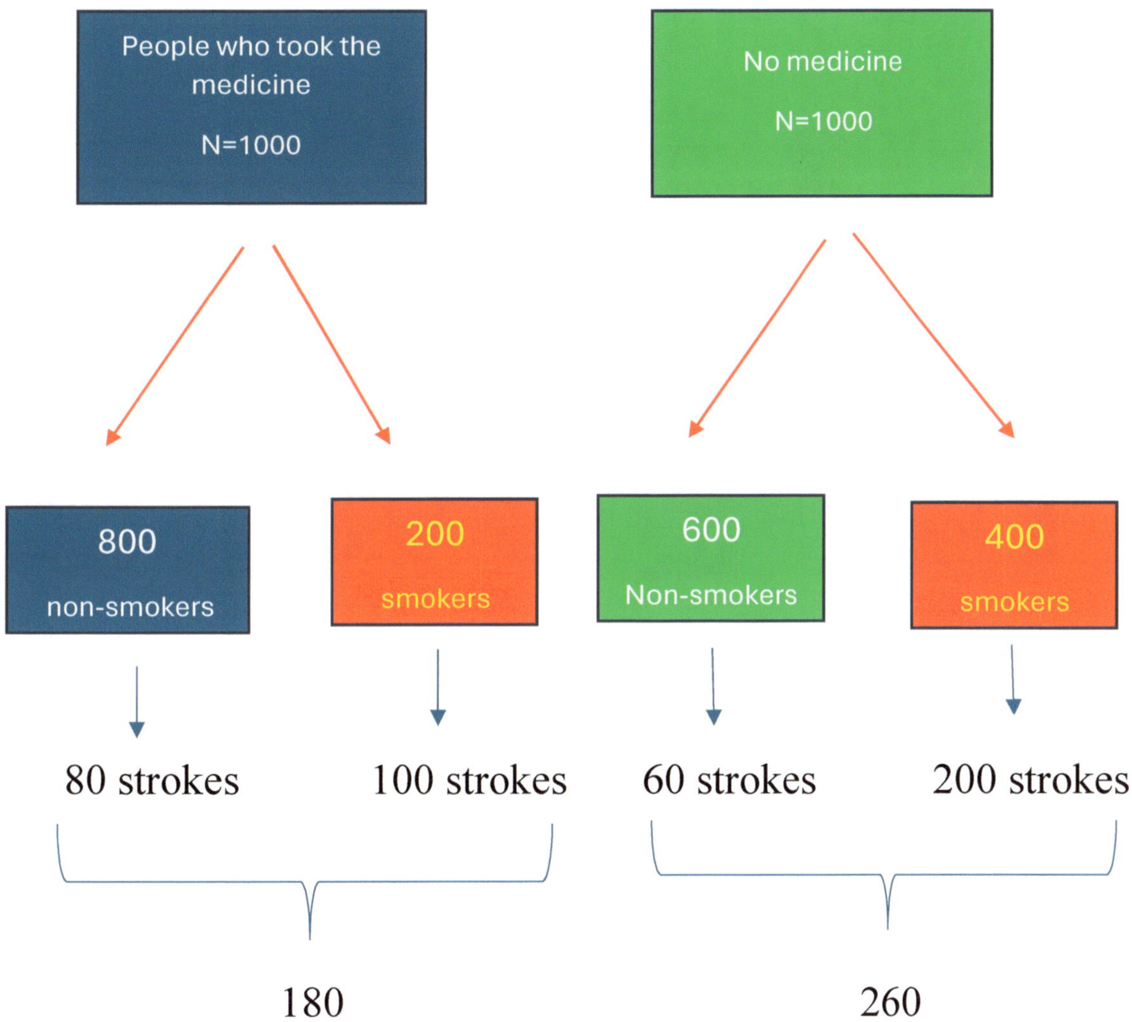

Figure 3.2

So, you see the problem. It *appears* as if a significantly smaller percentage of those who took the drug developed a stroke. But as you can see, the difference was a mirage: it was due entirely to the fact that there were more smokers in the untreated group compared to the treated group, and it was this difference (the smoking) that caused the difference in stroke outcome.

Here is what would have happened if the participants were randomized, and an equal amount of smokers were in each group:

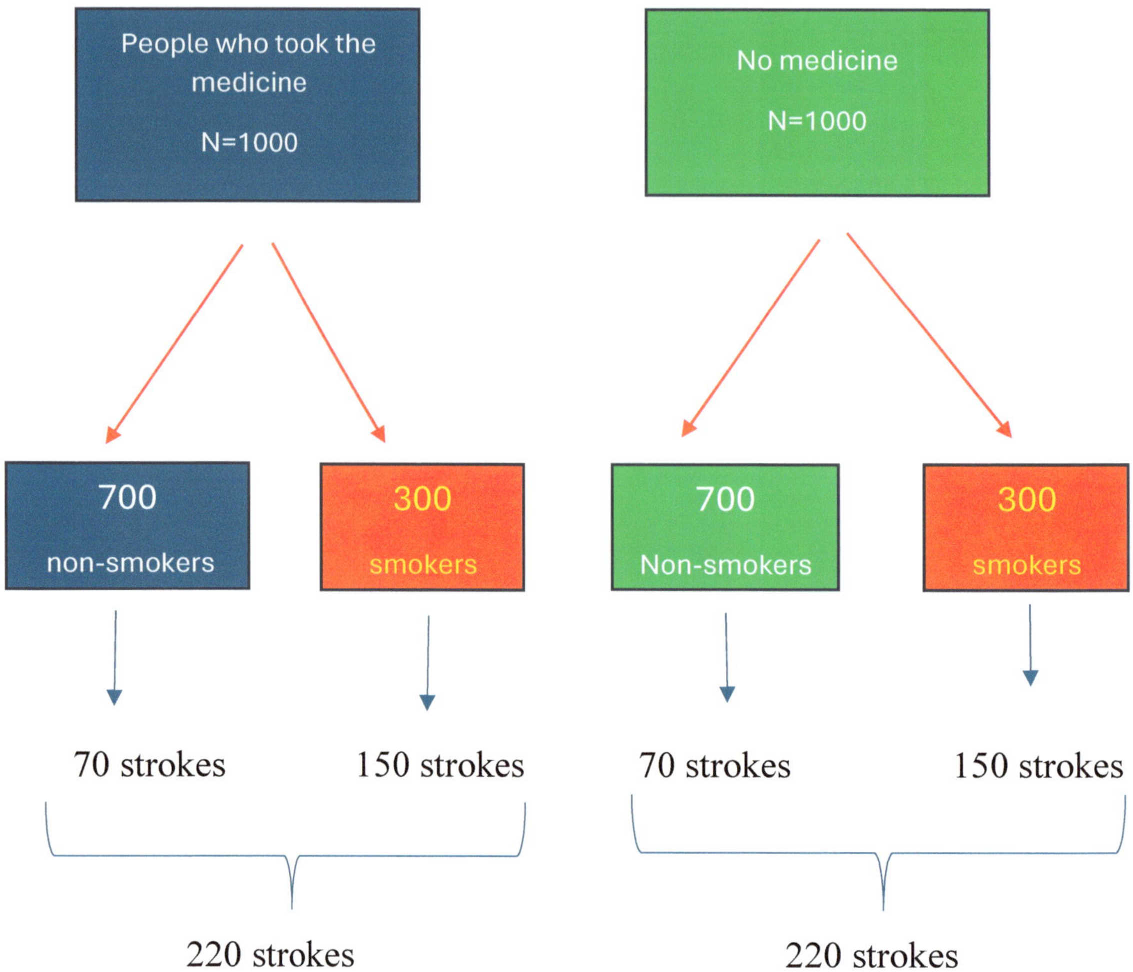

And this is where randomization comes in, and why it's so important. At the start of the trial, the researchers would be very careful to make sure that the participants were assigned to each group in a random manner. This would ensure that a (roughly) equal number of smokers were assigned to each group. Smoking here is referred to as a "confounder," and although I will talk more about confounding in a later chapter, for our current purposes just understand that a confounder is something that "screws up" the results of an experiment if the confounder is not evenly distributed among the groups. And so by randomly assigning groups, the researchers will know that the confounder is most likely evenly distributed and therefore won't screw up their results. And of course there are likely other confounders that need to be evenly distributed: things that are associated with stroke such as diabetes, family history, etc. If the groups are truly assigned randomly then *all* possible confounders should end up more or less evenly distributed. (There is of course always the chance that luck alone would cause more of a particular confounder in one of the groups, even if totally random. The more people that are recruited the less of a chance that this will happen, thus laying further credence to the recurrent theme of epidemiology and biostats: the more the better! But even if the researchers get unlucky, and despite randomly assigning the groups, there ends up more of a particular confounder in one of the groups, there are biostatistical techniques for accounting for that…I will discuss these techniques later!)

1. Randomization is vitally important when conducting an experimental trial. It assures that all confounders are more or less ________________________ distributed among the groups. This ensures that the confounders are not "screwing up" the results.

Section E2.2: Blinding

Good clinical trials strive to eliminate all forms of *bias* in their studies. Bias can take many forms, and will be discussed more in a later chapter, but it basically refers to any systematic error in the design, conduct, or analysis of a study that leads to an incorrect estimate of the true association between an exposure and an outcome. That is, our study may show a significant association, but because of one or more *biases*, this association is actually not true.

In experimental trials, blinding is one important way of preventing bias. Let's think again about our example with atrial fibrillation and the new drug to prevent stroke. Let's say the researchers are able to recruit 100 different primary care practices to participate in the research. When a patient presents to their clinician with atrial fibrillation, they are asked if they would like to participate in the trial. If they agree, the patient's clinician refers them to the researchers who will, on a random basis, assign the patient to either the treatment group or the control group. The point is that the practicing clinician has no say whatsoever in deciding which group the patient is assigned to. This prevents the bias that may occur if the clinician "wants" those who are perhaps the highest risk to get the actual drug. You can see how this would lead to a spurious association if more of the high-risk participants were given the drug, and the lower risk were not (or vice-versa, if the treating clinicians were worried about the higher risk patients suffering bleeding complications from the drug).

In addition to the treating clinicians being blinded to which patient is assigned to which group, the researchers themselves must also be blinded. And the researchers must be blinded *twice:* first, they must not know anything about the participant's medical history when they assign him or her to a group, and second, they must not know the group assignments when analyzing the results. Why? Well, unfortunately humans are humans. Researchers are, unfortunately, often paid by the industry that made the drug and hope to profit from it, and therefore hope for a positive result. Thus the poor researchers are often under pressure to do research that yields a positive result. And so you can appreciate that a researcher may consciously or subconsciously "fudge" results a bit: perhaps that "mini-stroke" reported in a patient's chart who received the medication was actually not a stroke…So, to really prevent bias in the analysis, the researchers themselves must be blinded as to which patients are in which group.

Lastly, the participants themselves must be blinded as to which group they are in. This is because of the very fascinating topic known as the placebo effect, of which I will not discuss in detail here, but there have been many interesting books written on this if you are interested! The participants in the non-treated group must, whenever possible, be given some kind of placebo. If they are not – if they are just given *nothing* – then invariably the treated group will do better, even if the intervention is doing *nothing at all biologically.* And that is the placebo effect, and it extends to all kinds of interventions: patients who are given a "sham" surgery, (they are actually taken to the OR, and given anesthesia, and incisions made but nothing is actually done), will consistently do better than those not given the sham surgery. Patients given sham acupuncture, in which the clinician places the needles at completely random places, will experience relief. So the placebo effect is real, and quite powerful, and a good experimental trial compares the intervention in question not with *nothing* but with a placebo – a pill or a treatment that looks or appears just like the actual treatment, so that the patient truly does not know which she is getting. (You can imagine then that the patient who knows for sure that she is receiving the placebo would not do as well as the patient who knows for sure that she is receiving the actual intervention).

2. Blinding is necessary to help prevent bias in experimental trials. All three major components of the research study must be blinded: the clinicians, the ____________________, and the ____________________________ .

Section E2.3: Intention-to-Treat vs Per-protocol

One of the inherent problems in conducting interventional studies is that many of the participants do not follow the treatment arm that they are assigned to. Perhaps they stop the intervention (and thus become part of the placebo group). Perhaps they started out in the placebo group and then start the intervention later on in the study. (You can envision this happening in an experimental trial comparing the efficacy of NSAIDs vs placebo in the treatment of back pain). And this of course affects our data analysis. We must decide, when we analyze the data, what to do with the results of the participants who do not follow the protocol that was assigned to them.

Option 1: Intention-to-treat analysis

In this analysis, we basically ignore the fact that some participants do not follow the protocol, and include these non-compliers in with the others who maintained their protocol. So for example, if we knew that 5% of our placebo group actually started taking NSAIDs during the study, we disregard this and still count their results as if they maintained their placebo status.

Option 2: Per-protocol analysis

> In this analysis, we count the non-compliers by the treatment that they got or did not get. Thus, if 5% of the placebo group start taking NSAIDs on their own, they are counted in the *treated* group.

Which should we choose? The short answer is Option 1. And this may seem counterintuitive because it seems that the per-protocol approach is more "precise," because, after all, what we're really after is whether the treatment is effective or not. And of course our results are more "precise" if we analyze the data based on exactly which treatment the participant received. But we pay a considerable penalty for this perceived precision. If people leave their treatment group on their own, then basically the study morphs from an experimental trial to an observational trial. Remember the key difference: the one thing that sets apart experimental trials from all the others is *randomization.* When we, the researcher, assigns the treatment arms, we are able to do it randomly, so that all the possible confounders will randomly balance themselves out between the two groups. And that is a huge thing. Once we in effect allow the participants to determine their own group, we have lost our randomization, and bias sets in. You can imagine, for example, that the people in the placebo group who switch to the treatment group may be the sickest, and so now we have sicker people (who might benefit the most) in the treatment group, and we will have biased results. And vice versa: those in the treatment group who switch to placebo may be the healthiest, and thus healthier people are now in the placebo group. And that is why, despite the apparent improvement in precision, the FDA considers the industry "standard" to be the intention-to-treat protocol.

But of course intention-to-treat has its drawbacks as well. If we keep everyone in their original groups for data analysis, how do you think it will affect the results? Imagine if 10% of the treatment group actually stops the treatment. Well, the benefit resulted in the treatment arm will be falsely low. And if 10% of those in the placebo group started the treatment, then the placebo group on the whole would appear to do better than they actually did. And so the measure of association between the groups, say for example the relative risk, would be dulled, or would be closer to the null. But the FDA has correctly determined that this sacrifice, resulting in a dulling of a possible significant response, is an appropriate sacrifice to maintain the sanctity of the bias-free results that our randomization allowed.

The main reason I bring all this up is for you to be aware that when you read the results of an experimental trial that you are reading the intention-to-treat results, and not the per-protocol results, as the per-protocol results will be biased, and will often show a significantly stronger measure of effect. (Many authors will present the results from both protocols in their analysis…but just beware of the pharmaceutical company-funded studies claiming statistical significance based on per-protocol analysis!).

Section E2.4: Summary and synthesis with EI

In this chapter I discussed the "gold standard" of epidemiologic trials, the randomized controlled trial. In the previous chapter (E1) I discussed observational trials. Here is the overall hierarchy:

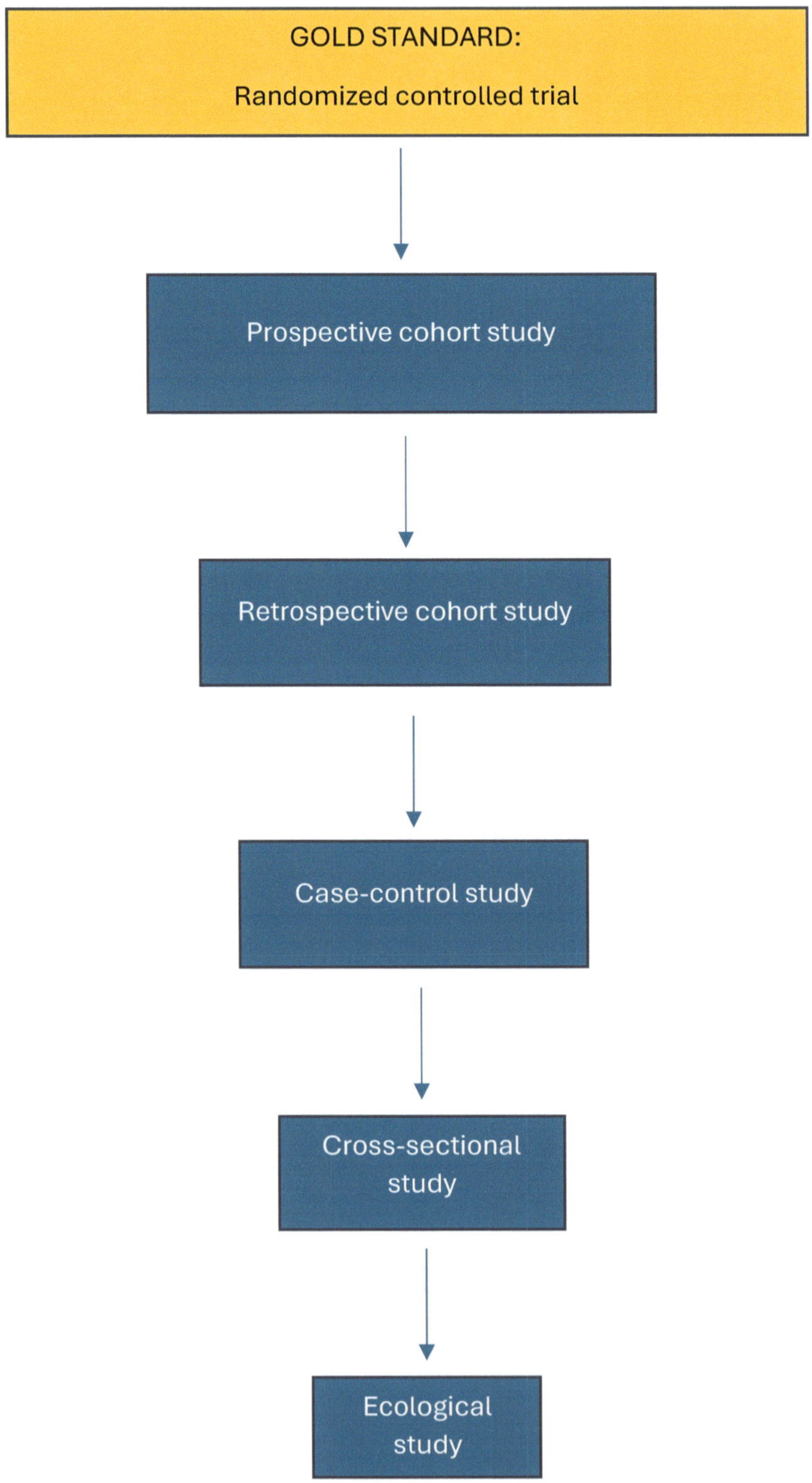

Again, the big difference between the randomized controlled trial—what separates it from all of the observational trials—is randomization. In the observational studies, we, the researchers are not "doing anything" to any of the groups being studied and therefore cannot determine who is in which group. The participants determine this themselves. If we want to compare for example the exposure of cigarette smoking to no smoking, the people themselves determine which of those two groups they are in. There is no randomization, and therefore the groups compared may show an imbalance of one or many confounders. Although researchers will try their best to account for as many of these confounders as they can when they do the data analyses of the observational trials, there are always additional "unmeasured" confounders that may be messing up the results.

But this is not at all to disparage the study types that are at the bottom of the hierarchy. There is much to be learned from all types of studies. For example, let's say I conducted an ecological study based on country populations, and found that there appears to be an association between prevalence of multiple sclerosis and levels of organophosphates in the soil—that is, countries with the most organophosphates had more people suffering from multiple sclerosis. I might then develop the hypothesis that organophosphates in the soil is a *risk* factor for multiple sclerosis for each induvial person, and to help prove this hypothesis, I would conduct a case-control study by recruiting 1000 people with multiple sclerosis, and 1000 people without, and examine the soil in their geographic areas for organophosphates. Or, even better, if I had the funding I would conduct a long-term prospective cohort study of 1000 people who live in an area of high organophosphates, and compare them with 1000 people who live in an area of low organophosphate, and watch them for twenty years to see who develops multiple sclerosis.

Or, perhaps I conduct a cross-sectional study and find that there appears to be an association between hearing loss and Alzheimer's disease. Since this is a cross-sectional analysis (a "snapshot in time") it says nothing about causality. I could then develop the hypothesis that hearing loss causes—or is part of a "causal mechanism" for the development of—Alzheimer's disease. To attempt to prove my hypothesis, I would conduct prospective cohort study by recruiting, say 1000 people with hearing loss and 1000 people without hearing loss, and watch them for a period of time (as long as I can!) for the development of Alzheimer's disease. Or, if I don't have the funding for doing a research project that may last many years, I could run a case-control study by recruiting 1000 people with Alzheimer's and 1000 people without Alzheimer's and go back in time to determine who had hearing loss and who did not. Or, better yet, if I had access to some very large data bank of patients with their past diagnoses, I could identify say 1000 patients who were diagnosed with hearing loss twenty years ago and follow them up to the present day to see how many eventually were diagnosed with Alzheimer's.

3. The above study that I just mentioned is an example of a ______________________ ________________ study.

And I think that pretty much completes the introduction to types of epidemiologic studies; they will of course be referred to many times again in future chapters!

Biostats 2: Comparing Continuous Outcomes

Now that we have the basics of the biostats, and how samples relate to an entire population, and now that we explored the basics of epidemiologic studies, we will begin to combine the two by demonstrating how we analyze data from epidemiologic studies that present results from *two or more samples.* And specifically, in this chapter, I will show how we compare two or more samples with *continuous outcomes.* A continuous outcome is any measure that is numerical, and continuous. Like for example, weight, or height, or blood pressure, head circumference, etc. Really any measurement where if you take a whole group of them, you would measure the mean of the values. This is opposed to *categorical* outcomes, which will be discussed later. For now just know that categorical outcomes are most commonly "yes" or "no" outcomes, i.e. did an outcome occur, or did it not?

Let's start our discussion on comparing continuous outcomes – and now I will refer to this as "comparing means" – with a study from the literature. Here is the study:

> Lam et al (2016). Efficacy of bright light treatment, fluoxetine, and the combination in patients with nonseasonal major depressive disorder: A randomized clinical trial. *JAMA Psychiatry,* 73(1), 56-63

So, first let's use what you learned from the previous chapter. This is the "gold-standard" of trials, the randomized trial. The researchers randomly assigned participants to one of four groups: one group received bright light treatment, one group received fluoxetine, one group received a combination of the two, and one group received a placebo therapy. And here are the results that they reported:

Table 2. Outcome Measures[a]

Measure	Treatment Group: Placebo (n = 30)	Fluoxetine Monotherapy (n = 31)	Light Monotherapy (n = 32)	Combination Therapy (n = 29)
Change in MADRS score from wk 0 to end point, mean (SD)	6.5 (9.6)	8.8 (9.9)	13.4 (7.5)	16.9 (9.2)

The MADR score is the Montgomery-Asberg Depression Rating Scale. The higher the score, the worse the depression. They followed the participants for 8 weeks and measured their scores at the beginning of the trial, and then again at the end of the 8-week period, and the numbers are the *change* in score. Notice that all the numbers are reported as positive numbers. To clarify, all four groups showed an improvement in their scores, so that the numbers at the end were lower than the numbers at the beginning, so strictly speaking the numbers reported should be negative numbers, but the authors for whatever reason chose to report the numbers as positive numbers. So, for example, the placebo group showed a 6.5 point improvement (lessening of their score by an average of 6.5 points), while the combination therapy group showed a 16.9 point improvement (lessening their scores by an average of 16.9 points). So the numbers, 6.5, 8.8, 13.4, and 16.9 are all means of the groups' changes. And so of course it is a "continuous" numerical result. (The numbers in parentheses after the numbers are the standard deviations of the groups).

Section B2.1: Confidence intervals of difference of means

Let's look at comparing the placebo group with the group that received combination therapy. The mean improvement score for the placebo group was 6.5, and the mean improvement score of the combination therapy group was 16.9. We now say that the *difference in the means* between the two groups is 16.9 – 6.5 = 10.4. You will often see the difference in two means represented as : $\bar{x}_1 - \bar{x}_2$. But remember, we are talking about samples. And whenever we talk about samples we must remember that we don't really care about the samples themselves, we care about the population as a whole. That is, we hope our results can be generalized to the *entire population* of depressed people. So the difference of 10.4 in our two groups is really meaningless and must come with some mention of a confidence interval. That is, how precise is our result of 10.4, with respect to the entire population? We hope that the result for the entire population is somewhere around 10.4, but how confident are we? And of course, just like when we calculated the confidence interval for a single mean in section BI.3, we need a *standard error.* For one mean of one sample, recall that we defined the standard error of the mean as the standard deviation of the means of a whole bunch of samples (all of the same size). And we defined it mathematically as

$$SE_{mean} = \frac{s}{\sqrt{n}}$$

Similarly, the standard error of the *difference of two means* is the standard deviation of the differences if we ran the same experiment (with the same numbers in each group) many many times. And mathematically, this is

$$SE_{(\bar{x}_1 - \bar{x}_2)} = \sqrt{\frac{s_1^2}{n_1} + \frac{s_2^2}{n_2}}$$

Equation 4.1

So, let's run this in our example and see what we get. Notice that the authors gave us the n's and the SD's which is very helpful!

$$SE_{(\bar{x}_1 - \bar{x}_2)} = \sqrt{\frac{s_1^2}{n_1} + \frac{s_2^2}{n_2}} = \sqrt{\frac{9.6^2}{30} + \frac{9.2^2}{29}} = 2.45$$

Remember, we would like to know what 95% of the results would lie, and that is between 2 standard errors above and two standard errors below our result. So, our result of 10.4 has a 95% confidence interval of 10.4 – 2(2.45) to 10.4 + 2(2.45) = **(5.5 to 15.3).** We can be reasonably certain that the true difference between the two groups if we measured the *entire population* is somewhere between 5.5 and 15.3. Notice that our 95% confidence interval does not include zero. This means that we are reasonably certain that the true difference does not include zero…that in fact there *is* a difference between the groups, and we say our results are "statistically significant."

1. When analyzing the difference of two means, if the 95% confidence interval does not include zero, we say the results are "____________________ ____________________."

Now let's compare the group that received fluoxetine monotherapy with the placebo group. In this case. $\bar{x}_1 - \bar{x}_2 = 8.8 - 6.5 = 2.3$, but again this is meaningless because we are talking about one small sample. So, same drill.

$$SE_{(\bar{x}_1-\bar{x}_2)} = \sqrt{\frac{s_1^2}{n_1} + \frac{s_2^2}{n_2}} = \sqrt{\frac{9.6^2}{30} + \frac{9.9^2}{31}} = 2.50$$

So, our result of 2.3 has a 95% confidence interval of 2.3 – 2(2.50) to 2.3 + 2(2.50) = **(-2.7 to 7.3).** We can now be reasonably certain that the true difference of the entire population lies somewhere between -2.7 and 7.3. Notice now that the 95% confidence interval *does* include zero. So there is a good chance that there is no difference at all between the groups. When the 95% confidence does include zero, we cannot say that we have a statistically significant result. Our difference of 2.3 in our sample is considered "non-significant."

2. When analyzing the difference of two means, if the 95% confidence interval includes _______________, there is too much of chance that there is no difference at all between the two groups, and our result is ____ - __________________________.

Section B2.2: Hypothesis testing

It is necessary first for you to digest some basic terminology of biostats. When we do an epidemiologic trial, we set out to prove our hypothesis. Say, for example, that smoking causes lung cancer, or an exercise program results in weight loss, or our new blood pressure medication causes a lowering of blood pressure. But strictly speaking in the world of biostats, we are trying to "reject the null hypothesis." The null hypothesis is that there is *no* difference between the two groups being compared. In our drug study, we would give one group the drug and the other group a placebo, and monitor their blood pressures before treatment is started, and after a period of say, six weeks after treatment is started. The null hypothesis states that there is no difference between the two groups, and is referred to as:

The Null Hypothesis: H_0: $\bar{x}_a - \bar{x}_b = 0$

The null hypothesis is referred to as H_0, and it means that there is no difference between the means of the two groups being compared.

The "alternative hypothesis" is referred to as H_A, and is that there *is* a difference between the means of the two groups, or: $\bar{x}_a - \bar{x}_b \neq 0$

I know this all may seem silly right now, but trust me it will be beneficial to solidify this in your mind: In epidemiology and biostats we *assume that the null hypothesis is true* (that is, we assume that there is no difference between the two groups), and in our experiment we hope (or usually hope) that we can *reject the null hypothesis.* That is, we can show that it is quite unlikely that there is no difference between the groups.

To demonstrate hypothesis testing, I would like to present a fictitious study. Let's say I'm interested in whether or not the practice of Tai Chi can lower blood pressure. I enrolled 100 people into the study and randomized them to one of two groups: the first group is enrolled in a Tai Chi program, and the second group is not. Consistent with all good experimental trials, the participants are randomly assigned to the two groups. At the end of six weeks, their systolic blood pressures are measured. Nice and simple. Now, astute readers will pick up on the obvious weaknesses in this study, namely that the sample sizes are small (50 in each group), so that even with randomization, there is a possibility that possible confounders will not be evenly distributed (just by chance), and also you will notice that the control group is not treated with a placebo. Because of the powerful placebo effect, it would really be necessary to give the control group some kind of placebo (which you can imagine would be quite a challenge…some kind of "sham" Tai Chi, in which participants, I guess, were shown some totally random exercises/poses that are not Tai Chi, or any other marshal art). Well, at any rate, despite these weaknesses, we go ahead and run our study, and find the following results:

No Tai Chi: 50 adults	**Tai Chi: 50 adults**
$\bar{x}_A = 132.4$	$\bar{x}_B = 127.2$
$s = 10.7$	$s = 10.1$

$$\boldsymbol{\bar{x}_A - \bar{x}_B = 5.2}$$

The first step of hypothesis testing is to assume that the null hypothesis is true. That is, we assume that $\boldsymbol{\bar{x}_A - \bar{x}_B = 0}$. In our small sample, the result was 5.2. Did that just occur randomly? What is the chance of a result of 5.2 occurring just by random chance? Another quick analogy: Let's say I drop 100 pennies onto a table. If I do this many many times, I would expect, on average, that 50 pennies land on heads and 50 land on tails. But if I do it just once, I might expect, say, 53 heads and 47 tails, or 44 heads and 56 tails, etc. I would not be the least bit surprised to see this, and I would know that the difference just occurred by random chance. But…if I dropped 100 pennies on the table, and it came up 90 heads and 10 tails, I would think that something "fishy" is going on…perhaps the coins are "weighted" or something so that they are more likely to come up heads. 90 heads just seems very unlikely to have occurred by random chance. At some point we draw the line and say…nah, that much of a difference is just too unlikely.

In our experiment, we have a result of 5.2, and we must ask ourselves if that is just too far away from 0 to have just occurred randomly or not.

Here is what I mean. If we ran our little experiment many many times—and remember that the "truth" we are assuming is the null hypothesis, that there is no difference—we would get a histogram of results that looks like this:

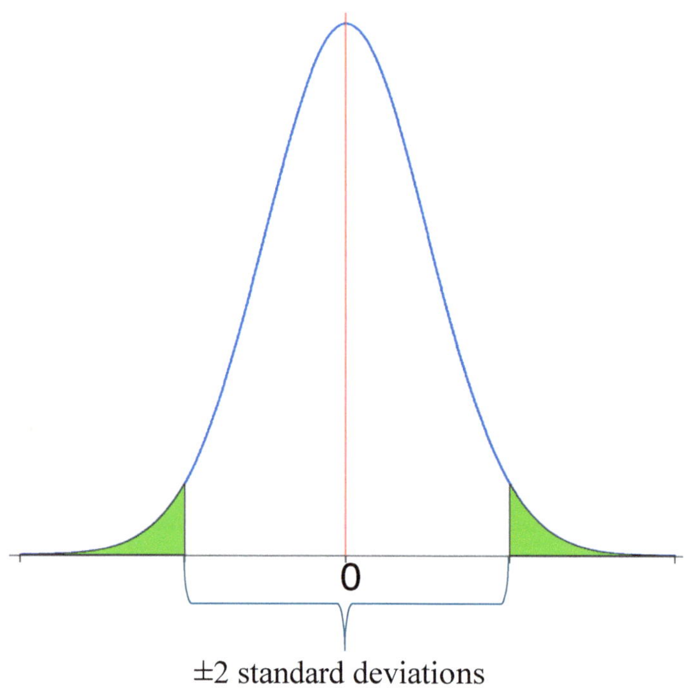

The mean of all the many, many experiments is 0. Why? Um…did you forget? We're assuming the null hypothesis! There is no difference! What are the little green areas? That is the area under the curve beyond two standard deviations from the mean (in either direction). Recall that the area under the curve *within* 2 SDs from the mean is where 95% of the results will fall. In our experiment, we need to determine where on the curve 5.2 falls. Is it in the white area above, where 95% of the values are? Or is it the green area, where 5% of the values are? Remember what the standard deviation of the means of many many samples is called? It is the standard error!

3. We need to determine if our result is within, or not within two ____________ ________________ from the mean of 0.

So it's simple: is our result of 5.2 more than two standard errors away from the mean or not? Because remember, that 5% is sort of the "magic" number in biostats… Well, then, I guess we need first to calculate the standard error. What standard error is it? It is the standard error of the difference of two means, which is equation 4.1. So here we go:

$$SE_{(\bar{x}_1-\bar{x}_2)} = \sqrt{\frac{s_1^2}{n_1}+\frac{s_2^2}{n_2}} = \sqrt{\frac{10.7^2}{50}+\frac{10.1^2}{50}}$$

$$SE_{(\bar{x}_1-\bar{x}_2)} = \mathbf{2.08}$$

So there you go…to see how many standard errors away from the mean our result of 5.2 is, we just divide:

$$\frac{5.2}{2.08} = 2.50$$

So our result of 5.2 is 2.50 standard errors away from the mean. On the graph, it would be here:

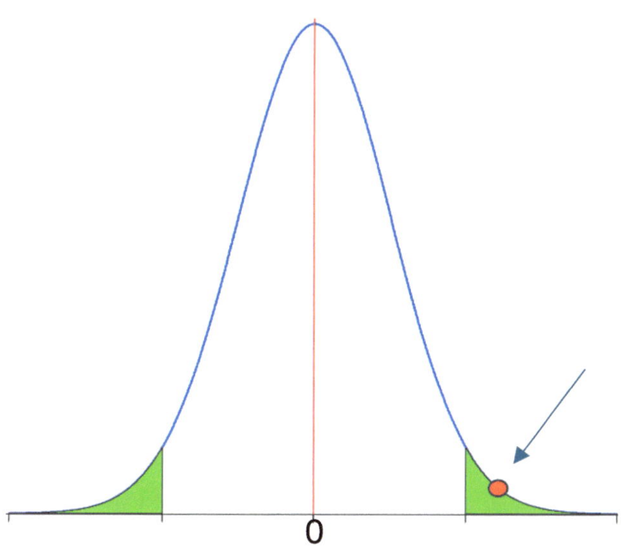

So it's in the green! That means 5.2 is indeed "far away" from 0, and very unlikely to have just occurred by chance. By the way, this whole thing we just did is actually a very famous test in statistics, called the "student's t-test," (now shortened to just a "t-test"). It was invented by a guy named William Sealy Gosset around the turn of the century. (That is, the turn of *last* century!).

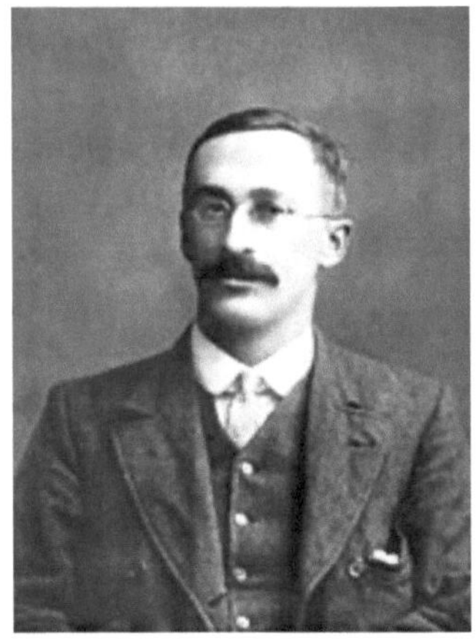

Now listen carefully, because it is not too often we can experience something amusing in the world of biostats! Mr. Gosset worked for Guiness Brewery in Dublin, and was a really smart mathematician and chemist who actually invented the student's t-test as a method of making predictions about large samples of brews based on experiments done on small samples. (I kid you not!). Guiness was nervous about making public the origins of this statistical technique, so when the method was published, Mr. Gosset used the pseudonym "student's t-test." Thanks to Mr. Gosset, biostats and beer are intimately related!

Section B2.3: The p-value

You have probably heard of this. "P" basically stands for probability, and is the probability that the value occurs where it is on the curve. Our result of 5.2 is in the green section, so we know that the probability will be less than 5% (remember the green areas represent 5%). The exact probability is calculated via the t-distribution, which is very similar to the normal distribution. It is a really really complex mathematical formula that is not even worth showing here, but fortunately our computers now can calculate it very easily.

Here is medcalc.org doing the calculation:

Comparison of means calculator

Sample 1

Mean:	132.4
Standard deviation:	10.7
Sample size:	50

Sample 2

Mean:	127.2
Standard deviation:	10.1
Sample size:	50

Test

Results

Difference	-5.200
Standard error	2.081
95% CI	-9.3294 to -1.0706
t-statistic	-2.499
DF	98
Significance level	P = 0.0141

So our p-value is 0.014, which means that our probability of our result of 5.2 is only 1.4%. That is a very small chance, and so, we say that we are allowed to "reject the null hypothesis." 5.2 is just not the same as 0, statistically speaking. As long as our p-value is less than 5%, we can reject the null hypothesis. We can also say that our result of 5.2 is "statistically significant."

4. If the probability of our result occurring is less than ________ %, we can __________________ the null hypothesis and declare our results to be __________________ significant.

In the olden days, we did not have powerful computers that could calculate this instantaneously for us. Instead, we relied on a distribution table, which looked like this:

t-test table

cum. prob	$t_{.50}$	$t_{.75}$	$t_{.80}$	$t_{.85}$	$t_{.90}$	$t_{.95}$	$t_{.975}$	$t_{.99}$	$t_{.995}$	$t_{.999}$	$t_{.9995}$
one-tail	0.50	0.25	0.20	0.15	0.10	0.05	0.025	0.01	0.005	0.001	0.0005
two-tails	1.00	0.50	0.40	0.30	0.20	0.10	0.05	0.02	0.01	0.002	0.001
df											
1	0.000	1.000	1.376	1.963	3.078	6.314	12.71	31.82	63.66	318.31	636.62
2	0.000	0.816	1.061	1.386	1.886	2.920	4.303	6.965	9.925	22.327	31.599
3	0.000	0.765	0.978	1.250	1.638	2.353	3.182	4.541	5.841	10.215	12.924
4	0.000	0.741	0.941	1.190	1.533	2.132	2.776	3.747	4.604	7.173	8.610
5	0.000	0.727	0.920	1.156	1.476	2.015	2.571	3.365	4.032	5.893	6.869
6	0.000	0.718	0.906	1.134	1.440	1.943	2.447	3.143	3.707	5.208	5.959
7	0.000	0.711	0.896	1.119	1.415	1.895	2.365	2.998	3.499	4.785	5.408
8	0.000	0.706	0.889	1.108	1.397	1.860	2.306	2.896	3.355	4.501	5.041
9	0.000	0.703	0.883	1.100	1.383	1.833	2.262	2.821	3.250	4.297	4.781
10	0.000	0.700	0.879	1.093	1.372	1.812	2.228	2.764	3.169	4.144	4.587
11	0.000	0.697	0.876	1.088	1.363	1.796	2.201	2.718	3.106	4.025	4.437
12	0.000	0.695	0.873	1.083	1.356	1.782	2.179	2.681	3.055	3.930	4.318
13	0.000	0.694	0.870	1.079	1.350	1.771	2.160	2.650	3.012	3.852	4.221
14	0.000	0.692	0.868	1.076	1.345	1.761	2.145	2.624	2.977	3.787	4.140
15	0.000	0.691	0.866	1.074	1.341	1.753	2.131	2.602	2.947	3.733	4.073
16	0.000	0.690	0.865	1.071	1.337	1.746	2.120	2.583	2.921	3.686	4.015
17	0.000	0.689	0.863	1.069	1.333	1.740	2.110	2.567	2.898	3.646	3.965
18	0.000	0.688	0.862	1.067	1.330	1.734	2.101	2.552	2.878	3.610	3.922
19	0.000	0.688	0.861	1.066	1.328	1.729	2.093	2.539	2.861	3.579	3.883
20	0.000	0.687	0.860	1.064	1.325	1.725	2.086	2.528	2.845	3.552	3.850
21	0.000	0.686	0.859	1.063	1.323	1.721	2.080	2.518	2.831	3.527	3.819
22	0.000	0.686	0.858	1.061	1.321	1.717	2.074	2.508	2.819	3.505	3.792
23	0.000	0.685	0.858	1.060	1.319	1.714	2.069	2.500	2.807	3.485	3.768
24	0.000	0.685	0.857	1.059	1.318	1.711	2.064	2.492	2.797	3.467	3.745
25	0.000	0.684	0.856	1.058	1.316	1.708	2.060	2.485	2.787	3.450	3.725
26	0.000	0.684	0.856	1.058	1.315	1.706	2.056	2.479	2.779	3.435	3.707
27	0.000	0.684	0.855	1.057	1.314	1.703	2.052	2.473	2.771	3.421	3.690
28	0.000	0.683	0.855	1.056	1.313	1.701	2.048	2.467	2.763	3.408	3.674
29	0.000	0.683	0.854	1.055	1.311	1.699	2.045	2.462	2.756	3.396	3.659
30	0.000	0.683	0.854	1.055	1.310	1.697	2.042	2.457	2.750	3.385	3.646
40	0.000	0.681	0.851	1.050	1.303	1.684	2.021	2.423	2.704	3.307	3.551
60	0.000	0.679	0.848	1.045	1.296	1.671	2.000	2.390	2.660	3.232	3.460
80	0.000	0.678	0.846	1.043	1.292	1.664	1.990	2.374	2.639	3.195	3.416
100	0.000	0.677	0.845	1.042	1.290	1.660	1.984	2.364	2.626	3.174	3.390
1000	0.000	0.675	0.842	1.037	1.282	1.646	1.962	2.330	2.581	3.098	3.300
z	0.000	0.674	0.842	1.036	1.282	1.645	1.960	2.326	2.576	3.090	3.291
	0%	50%	60%	70%	80%	90%	95%	98%	99%	99.8%	99.9%
	Confidence Level										

Even though this table is old-fashioned, it is worth examining for learning purposes. On the very left column, please notice the little letters "df." Those are "degrees of freedom." The degrees of freedom is one less than the sample size. So, in our case, we have two samples of 50 each, so the degrees of freedom would be 98. At the very bottom of the left column, you notice "z." The z is the theoretical t-score when we have an infinite amount of subjects in our sample, and therefore is exactly like a normal distribution. Notice that as sample size gets bigger and bigger, the t-score gets closer and closer to the z-score. Now, notice the little red rectangle that encompasses 2.364 and 2.626. This is highlighted because it's our result: our t-score was **2.50,** which is somewhere between 2.364 and 2.626, and our degrees of freedom is 98 (so we use 100…close enough!), and then the red rectangle as the top gives us our p-value probability, which is somewhere between 0.01 and 0.02. So although in the olden days we didn't know the exact p-value, we knew it was less than 0.05, so we could reject the null hypothesis.

One last thing before we leave the old-fashioned table. Notice that as we move up in a particular column (toward smaller degree of freedom and thus smaller sample size), we see the t-scores gradually increasing. This makes sense: as the sample size gets smaller, our values are less precise, and so we need a larger t-score (we need to be further away from 0) to say that we have statistically significant results. Here are the distributions graphically: (courtesy of Graphpad.com)

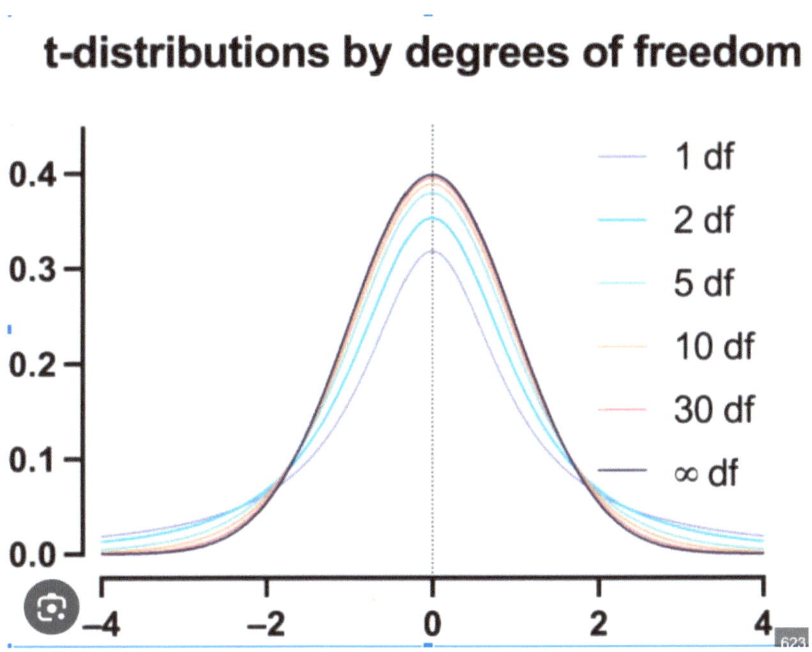

The black curve at the top is the normal standard normal distribution, and the colored curves below it are the t-test distributions depending on degrees of freedom. You see how there is a slight difference; the curve "flattens out" as we get smaller sample sizes.

Degrees of freedom explained (optional)

If you are wondering what the heck this "degrees of freedom" thing is, I will explain in here. If you are OK with just accepting the fact that the degrees of freedom is the sample size less one, then feel free to skip this little section!

> I'll use the mean blood pressure in the Tai-Chi group, which was 127.2. There are 50 people in this group. The first 49 people in our sample could have any reading (within reason). But after the first 49 people are measured, there is only ONE value that the 50th person has to have in order to give us our mean of 127.2. So 49 of them are "free" and one is not. So a sample size of 50 has 49 "degrees of freedom."
> That's it.

Section B2.4: Two-tailed vs one-tailed testing

This is kind of a big deal and worth talking about, because it has traditionally been abused by researchers trying to do whatever they can to show statistical significance. A pharmaceutical company is testing their new antihypertension drug. They give the drug to one group of 50 participants, and they give a placebo to another group of 50 participants. They measured systolic blood pressures at the end of six weeks of treatment.

Results:

Group A: Treated	**Group B: Placebo**
$\bar{x}_A = 124.4\ mmHg$	$\bar{x}_B = 128.2\ mmHg$
s = 10.1	s = 10.7

The difference of the means is -3.8. They tested for statistical significance using a student's t-test. They would likely use a calculator, but I will take you through the steps one more time. First we calculate the standard error of the difference of the means:

$$SE_{(\bar{x}_A - \bar{x}_B)} = \sqrt{\frac{s_A^2}{n_1} + \frac{s_B^2}{n_2}} = \sqrt{\frac{10.7^2}{50} + \frac{10.1^2}{50}} = \mathbf{2.08}$$

The t-score (how many standard errors away from the mean is our result of -3.8) is

$$\frac{-3.8}{2.08} = -1.83$$

So, we are here on the curve:

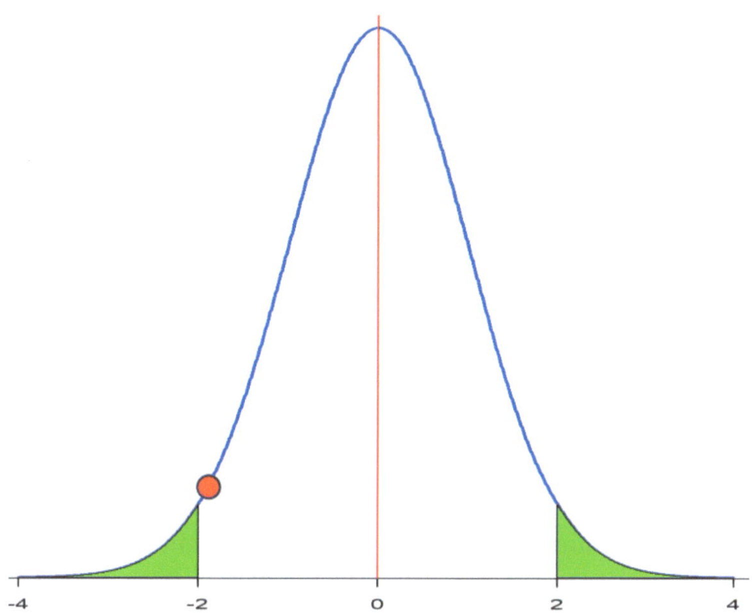

As you can see, a t-score of -1.83 is not quite in the green, so they cannot reject the null hypothesis, and have to report that their results on not statistically significant. Using a calculator, we find that the p-value = **0.07.** But the researchers are under a lot of pressure by the pharmaceutical company that makes the drug to produce statistically significant results, so they decide to do a "one-tailed t-test" instead of a "two-tailed t-test." I will start by saying that pretty much all studies in medicine should be two-tailed. Two-tailed basically means that the results can go in either direction. The green areas, outside of the 95% probability results, are both the left and right tails of the curve. And this makes sense: the drug could certainly also *raise* people's blood pressures. But if the researchers ran a one-tailed t-test, they are basically asserting that they only consider the possibility that their drug *lowers* blood pressure, so only the left tail exists, the right tail does not. All that uncertainty on the right (the right tail) now gets shifted over to the left, so that all the 5% is in the left tail:

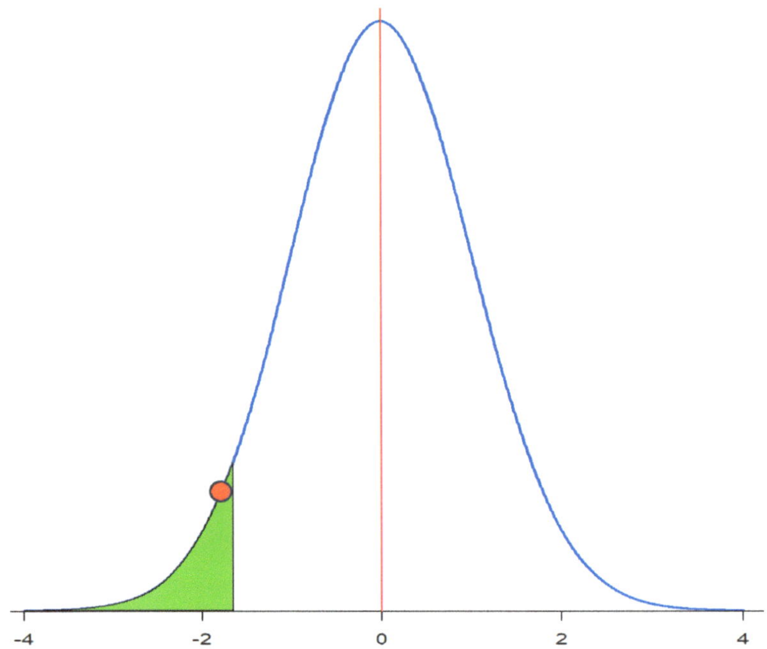

Well, guess what? Now the t-score of -1.83 lies within the green! Indeed, if we ask our calculator to run a one-tailed-test, the p-value comes out to $\boldsymbol{p} = \mathbf{0.035}$**!!** The ecstatic researchers now report statistically significant results to the pharmaceutical industry that is funding the study, and everyone is happy.

Fortunately, shenanigans of this sort are less common nowadays as the FDA and many of the major journals have strongly discouraged the use of one-tailed testing. But, you will still find it on occasion!

5. __________-tailed t-tests are basically boloney, and should not really exist in the literature, but they still do!

Section B2.5: Paired t-tests

So far in this chapter, I have discussed experiments in which the two samples are *independent* of each other. That is, they are different people. One group of people get the experimental drug (or whatever), and the other group of people do not. Thus the two groups are considered "independent." But there are other studies in which there is *only one group*. In the world of statistics, this is referred to as "matched samples." What kind of a study just has one sample?

Well let's say we are trying to test a new cholesterol drug, and rather than a placebo-controlled trial, we just have one group of participants. Each participant's cholesterol level is measured before starting the new medicine, and then measured again say six weeks later. (One major advantage of doing a study of this type is that each participant serves as her own control…so that any possible confounding is eliminated!)

The formulas for the paired t-test are a bit different:

$\boldsymbol{t} = \frac{\bar{\boldsymbol{d}}}{\boldsymbol{SE}}$ where $\bar{d}$ is the mean of all the differences (take each patient's differences in their two cholesterol levels and divide by n), and SE is our old friend the "standard error," which in this case is $SE = \frac{s_d}{\sqrt{n}}$ where s_d is the standard deviation of the differences. And, just as before, if the sample size is small, use t-score with degrees of freedom (n–1).

Section B2.6: Analysis of Variance (ANOVA)

I have thus far discussed hypothesis testing when comparing two means. But very often, investigators would like to compare means from three or more groups. That is what ANOVA is for, and it is an important topic to understand.

Let's say I am curious how blood pressures might vary among socioeconomic groups. So I create 4 groups based on the participants' socioeconomic levels, and the results are as follows:

GroupA: 50 adults	Group B: 50 adults	Group C: 50 adults	Group D: 50 adults
$\bar{x}_A = 133.4$	$\bar{x}_B = 129.8$	$\bar{x}_c = 128.8$	$\bar{x}_D = 127.2$
$s = 10.7$	$s = 10.4$	$s = 10.1$	$s = 9.9$

So now we have *four* different means to compare. How do we go about hypothesis testing? When comparing more than 2 means, we want to know if any of the means are different from any of the others. So the null hypothesis is that all of them are basically the same:

Null: H_0: $\bar{x}_A = \bar{x}_B = \bar{x}_c = \bar{x}_D$

The alternative hypothesis is:Type equation here.

H_a: $\bar{x}_A \neq \bar{x}_B$, or $\bar{x}_A \neq \bar{x}_C$, or $\bar{x}_A \neq \bar{x}_D$, or $\bar{x}_B \neq \bar{x}_C$, or $\bar{x}_B \neq \bar{x}_D$, or $\bar{x}_c \neq \bar{x}_D$

The key is those "ors." If only one of these is true, then we reject the null hypothesis

6. In ANOVA testing, we can only determine if at least one of the means is ____________ than any of the others. If so, then we ____________ the null hypothesis.

In ANOVA, we basically take the total variation in the blood pressures and divide it into 2 parts:

1. The variation among the four groups (the "between groups variation")
2. The variation *within* each group that is due to sampling error (the "within groups variation").

(Is #2 clear to you? Remember there are 50 people in each group and we are only reporting one mean for each group. Within each group, there is variation around that mean…they are not all exactly the mean. That is what is meant by "within groups variation.")

The variations are found via a "sum of squares" method, thus we say

$SS_{total} = SS_{groups} + SS_{error}$

The formulae for these are as follows:

$$SS_{groups} = \sum_{groups} n_i(\bar{x}_i - \bar{x})^2$$

where n_i is the number of observations in the group, $\bar{x}_i$ is the mean of the group, and $\bar{x}$ is the mean of the entire thing (all groups combined).

$$SS_{error} = \sum_{groups} (n_i - 1)s_i^2$$

Where s_i^2 is the variance of the group.

Ultimately, ANOVA testing sets out to see if SS_{groups} is large relative to the SS_{error}. If it is, then an actual difference in the blood pressures between the groups explains a significant portion of the observed variability. We use a term called "mean squares" which is defined as follows:

$MS_{groups} = \frac{SS_{groups}}{k-1}$ where k is the number of groups (4 in our example)

$MS_{error} = \frac{SS_{error}}{N-k}$ where N is total amount of observations (200 in our example)

We then define an "F statistic," which is the ratio: $\frac{MS_{groups}}{MS_{error}}$

The higher the F statistic, the more likely we can reject the null hypothesis.

Once we get our F statistic, we ask the computer to calculate the probability (p-value) and there you have it!

7. In ANOVA testing, if the difference between groups is relatively large compared to the error within groups, then it is likely we can ____________________ the null hypothesis.

You might wonder why we need this. If the alternative hypothesis is that at least one of the groups is different from the others, why can't we just run several t-tests? That is, compare group A to group B, then compare group A to group C, then compare groups A to group D, then compare group B to group C, then compare group B to group D, then compare group C to group D? Well, the problem is something called "type-I error," which I will discuss in more detail in Biostats 4. Recall that our "statistical significance" level is set at 0.05. That means if the probability of our result occurring is less than 5%, we reject the null hypothesis. But of course, there is a chance we are wrong, which is up to 5%. (Our result had a 5% chance of occurring by random chance alone). If we have several tests, then our chance of being wrong is actually multiplied by the following relationship:

$1-(1-\alpha)^n$

Where α is our significance level, and n is the number of trials. Thus in our case we would have to run 6 trials, and our chance of being wrong is a whopping 26.5%!

Summary of Biostats 2

This chapter showed how to analyze and compare data of continuous measure. That is, anything with a mean. You should understand how to calculate a 95% confidence interval of the *difference* of two means. You should understand how we use the student's t-test to see if we can reject the null hypothesis (which assumes no difference between the two groups). And you should have a basic understanding of ANOVA (analysis of variance) testing when there are more than two groups that are being compared.

Epidemiology 3: Measures of Association

In Epidemiology 1 and 2, I discussed the various kinds of studies in epidemiology, and so now it is time to explore the measures of association—that is, how the outcomes of the various kinds of trials are presented. It is how we make comparisons between groups in epidemiologic studies, so that we can decide if there is an association between an exposure and outcome, or perhaps if the exposure causes the outcome.

Section E3.1: Cohort studies and Randomized trials

When discussing measures of association, we can group together cohort studies and randomized trials. Recall that cohort studies first identify a cohort that has an exposure and compares it with a cohort that does not have the exposure. Recall that in a randomized trial, one group has an "intervention" and the other group does not. Both these types of trials compare one group "with" and one group "without," with the purpose of trying to determine if the exposure or the intervention has any effect on the outcome. In these trials, we generally compare the group with the exposure or intervention with a control group, because ultimately what we really want to know is: What would have happened to the exposed group if they did *not* have the exposure? Would they still have had the outcome? If so, how much? And usually the only way we can estimate this is by identifying a control group that is as similar to the exposed group as possible. The only difference between the two groups ideally would be just whether or not they had the exposure. By identifying such a similar control group, we get as close as we can to estimating what would have happened to the exposed group if they were not exposed.

Here is the schematic for cohort studies and randomized controlled trials:

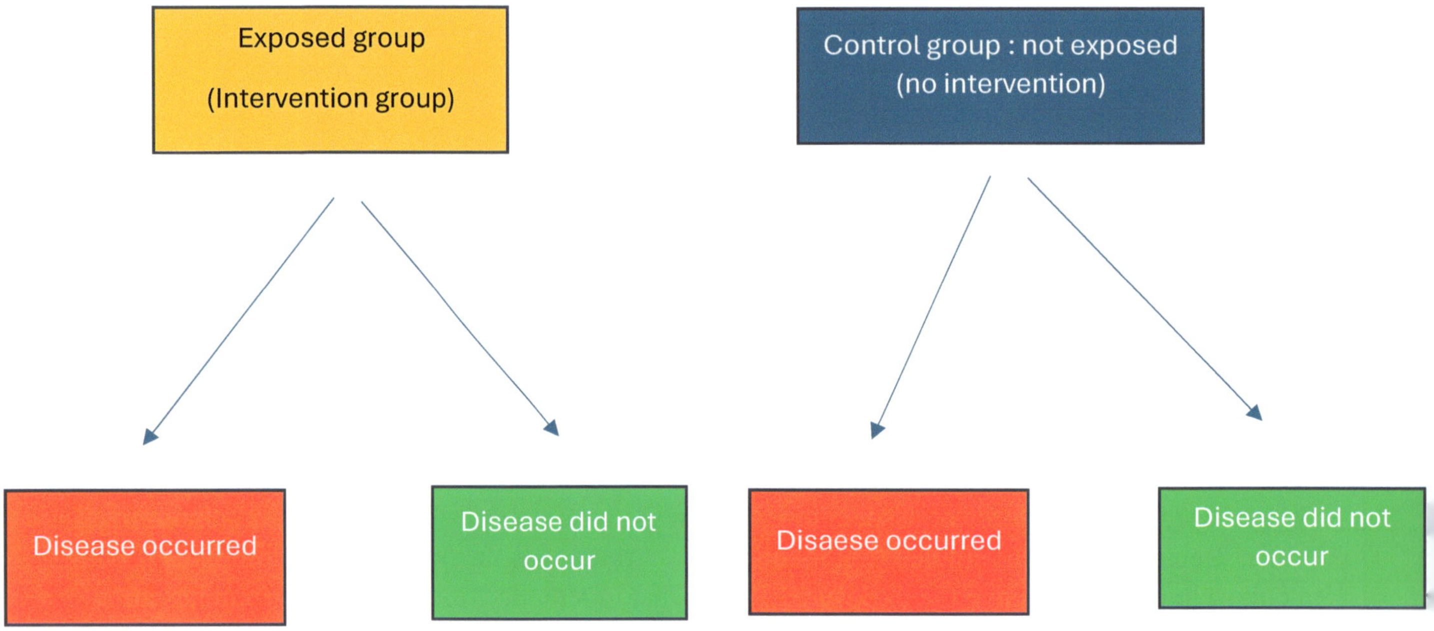

In each group, we need a measure on how much the disease (or other outcome) is occurring.

Section E3.2 Cumulative Incidence (risk)

One measurement of this is the *cumulative incidence*. This is denoted as I_c and is simply the total amount of outcomes that occurred in the trial period, divided by the total amount of people at risk. For example, let's say we are doing a cohort study and the exposed group is smokers, and the outcome is heart attack. If over a ten-year period, 1000 smokers are followed and 200 of them have a heart attack, then we would say

$$I_c = \frac{200}{1000} = 0.2\ (or\ 20\%)$$

The cumulative incidence is also known as the **risk**, and is a ratio. It does not take into account the element of time; it is simply the total amount of outcomes that occurred during the trial period. You can also think of the risk as the "probability" of the outcome. That is, for one smoker followed for 10 years, the probability of a heart attack of 20%.

1. The cumulative incidence is also commonly called "___________", and is the ratio of the total amount of outcomes divided by the total number at ____________ of the outcome.

Comparing the cumulative incidence of two groups: Relative Risk

Since we are comparing two groups, we have two different cumulative incidences. One way to compare them is with the **relative risk.** The relative risk is the ratio of one group's risk relative to the other group's risk. It is, by definition, the "cumulative incidence ratio," but is much more commonly known as the relative risk.

	Outcome occurred	**Outcome did not occur**
Exposed	a	b
Not exposed	c	d

You will see 2x2 tables pop up many times in the world of epidemiology and biostats; please remember to *always* construct them this way – that is, the rows are exposed/not exposed, and the columns are outcomes/no outcomes.

2. When constructing 2x2 tables remember to always construct them so that the rows represent ________________________ status, and the columns represent ______________________ status.

The I_c of the exposed group is the total outcomes divided by the total # at risk, or $\frac{a}{a+b}$

The I_c of the unexposed group is the total outcomes divided by the total # at risk, or $\frac{c}{c+d}$

The relative risk is $\frac{\boldsymbol{I_c(exposed)}}{\boldsymbol{I_c(unexsposed)}} = \frac{a/_{a+b}}{c/_{c+d}}$

Let's say in our study 200 smokers had an outcome (heart attack), while 120 nonsmokers had an outcome.

	Outcome occurred	**Outcome did not occur**
Exposed (n=1000)	200	800
Not exposed (n=1000)	120	880

Example E3.1

$$risk_{exposed} = \frac{200}{200+800} = 0.20$$

$$risk_{unexposed} = \frac{120}{120+880} = 0.12$$

$$\boldsymbol{Relative\ risk} = \frac{200/_{200+800}}{120/_{120+880}} = \mathbf{1.67}$$

How do we interpret the relative risk of 1.67? We can say that a

In general if the relative risk (RR) >1, then the risk in the exposed is greater than the risk in the un-exposed, and so there is a "positive association" between exposure and outcome, and the exposure may be a risk for the outcome to occur. If the RR = 1, we would say that the risk in the exposed group is equal to the risk in the non-exposed group, and so there is no association between the exposure and the outcome. And if the RR < 1, the risk in the exposed is less than the risk in the non-exposed, and there is a protective effect of the exposure. (This commonly occurs in randomized controlled trials, when the exposure is actually an intervention that is designed to reduce an outcome). In this case, the RR < 1 can be called a "negative association," but remember that a negative association does not mean that the RR is a negative number. The RR cannot be a negative number! Oh, also note that RR has no units; it is just a ratio.

3. In cohort studies, the exposure tends to be a bad thing, like for example smoking, and so the RR is ________________ than one, meaning the exposure increases the risk of the outcome. But in experimental randomized trials, the exposure (the intervention) is often a good thing designed to decrease an outcome, so the RR is often ____________ than one.

Comparing the cumulative incidence of two groups: Risk difference

Sometimes it is more useful to calculate the actual difference in the risks rather than calculating the ratio.

$$Risk\ difference = risk_{exposed} - risk_{non-exposed}$$

In our example,

$$Risk\ difference = 0.20 - 0.12 = 0.08$$

But unlike our relative risk, the risk difference has units that we must specify. We can't just say that the risk difference is "0.08." If we did, the correct response would be, "0.08 what?" So we have to do a bit more calculating. The 0.08 is the risk per person, so by convention, we multiply this by 1000 people to get 80 heart attacks per 1000 people, and then we would add the time period:
"The risk difference is 80 heart attacks per 1000 population over a ten-year period."

And so a risk difference that is > 0 means that the exposure increases the risk of the outcome. A risk difference that = 0 means that there is no association between exposure and outcome, and a risk difference that is < 0 means that the exposure has a protective effect against the outcome.

The risk difference is an important measure; it is also known as "attributable risk" because it tell us how much of the outcome in question is attributed to the exposure. We would say in our example that "**80 heart attacks per 1000 population in a 10-year period are attributed to smoking**."

Perhaps even more information might be gained by calculating the risk difference as a percent. This is know as "**attributable risk percent,"** and is defined as

$$attributale\ risk\ percent = \frac{risk_{exposed} - risk_{unexposed}}{risk_{exposed}}$$

Attributable risk percent is often seen in cohort studies, as opposed to experimental studies. How do we interpret the attributable risk percent? Note that the denominator is $risk_{exposed}$. So what this means then, is the percent of the risk of the outcome *in the exposed group* is due to the exposure itself. So in our example,

$$attributale\ risk\ percent = \frac{0.20 - 0.12}{0.20} = 0.4$$

Interpretation: **"Among smokers, 40% of the risk of heart attack is due to smoking."**

4. The "attributable risk percent" tells us what percent of the risk of an ____________________ among people with the ____________________ is attributed to that exposure.

Absolute vs relative risk reduction

As I mentioned, in randomized controlled trials, researchers are often trying to prove that an exposure (actually, an "intervention") is causing a reduction in the outcome. That is, they are hoping that their intervention results in a protective effect, or a negative risk difference. For example, back in the 1990s several pharmaceutical companies manufactured and heavily touted a new class of cholesterol-lowering drugs called statins. There had already been other types of cholesterol-lowering drugs on the market that dramatically reduced blood cholesterol levels, but these drugs consistently showed disappointing results on the endpoints that really mattered: the reduction of heart disease. The statin drugs were marketed as accomplishing just that: they would lower blood cholesterol levels AND lower the rate of heart disease. But the data analyses of these studies were perfect examples of a little mathematical manipulation (bordering on deception) that duped many doctors into jumping on the statin band wagon, and is important to explore that manipulation.

Many of the trials enrolled a group of people (the intervention group) to take the drug, and a group of people (the controls) to take a placebo, and followed both groups for five years and see if they developed heart disease. They often found results like this:

	Outcome occurred	**Outcome did not occur**
Intervention (n=1000)	20	980
Control (n=1000)	30	970

Let's apply these results to the measures of association described above.

First, risk difference:

$$Risk\ difference = risk_{exposed} - risk_{unexposed}$$

$$Risk\ difference = \frac{20}{1000} - \frac{30}{1000} = \frac{-10}{1000} = -1\%$$

So, the drug lowered the outcomes by 1%

Now, let's do relative risk:

$$\frac{\boldsymbol{I_c(exposed)}}{\boldsymbol{I_c(unexsposed)}} = \frac{\boldsymbol{a/_{a+b}}}{\boldsymbol{c/_{c+d}}}$$

$$RR = \frac{20/_{1000}}{30/_{1000}} = 0.67$$

How is this interpreted? Since the RR is < 1, we say that the intervention reduces the risk of heart attack. We can say that the risk of heart attack if you take the drug is 0.67 the risk if you take placebo. We can also say that there is a 33% less risk of heart attack if you take the drug as compared with placebo. So you can well imagine that the pharmaceutical industry who is trying to tout the drug (and make countless profits) is not too happy with the risk difference of 1%, but they love how 33% sounds. So guess what happened? And here is an example:

This is one of the first studies from the 1990s that compared a statin drug with a placebo, and reported the incidence of heart disease in the two groups:

> (Downs, et al. Primary Prevention of Acute Coronary Events with Lovastatin in Men and Women with Average Cholesterol Levels. *JAMA* 1998: 279(20); 1615-1622.)

Here is quote from their results: **"lovastatin therapy significantly reduced the risk for fatal or nonfatal myocardial infarction by 40% and unstable angina by 32%."**

Yes… those numbers, 40% and 32% are relative risks. You have to look hard in the paper to find the risk differences, but there they are on page 1260. For fatal or nonfatal myocardial infarction, the risk for those who took the drug was $\frac{57}{3304} = 0.017 = 1.7\%$, and for controls the risk was $\frac{95}{3301} = 0.029 = 2.9\%$. A risk difference of 1.2% does not *sound* that good, so all throughout the paper, the authors talk about the relative risk, which is

$$RR = \frac{57/3305}{95/3301} = 0.60$$

A relative risk of 0.60 does indeed mean that the risk of MI is 40% less for people taking the drug. But this is certainly deceiving when it is mentioned without also mentioning the small risk difference of 1.2%. It should be up to the reader to decide how important that 40% relative risk reduction is. For example, what if the risk in the treated group was 0.2%, while the risk of the placebo group was 0.4%. Well, that is a relative risk of 50%! But what does that actually mean given a risk difference of only 0.2%? Probably not very much at all. Indeed, it is the risk difference that relates the most important information about the efficacy of a treatment. I think this is best demonstrated by introducing another concept closely related to the risk difference: the number needed to treat.

Number needed to treat

The number needed to treat is defined as $\frac{1}{Risk\ difference}$. It is the number of people that need to be treated in order for one person to show benefit. In the example from the Downs paper, then, for the endpoint of fatal or nonfatal MI, the risk difference was 0.029 – 0.017 = 0.012. So the NNT (number needed to treat) is $\frac{1}{0.012} = 83.3$. So this means that approximately 83 people would have to be treated with the drug in order for one to benefit. I'm sure you'll agree that having to treat 83 people for one to benefit is a far cry from "a 40% decreased risk!"

5. The "number needed to treat" is defined mathematically as one divided by the ____________ ____________________.

Does it make sense to you that the NNT is $\frac{1}{Risk\ difference}$? If it does not, then read the next paragraph. If it does make sense to you, then skip the next paragraph!

Optional paragraph: NNT explained:

Consider a simple example of two groups each of n=100. One group is given the drug, and 10 of the 100 had an event. The other group of 100 is given a placebo, and 20 of this group had an event. There were 10 fewer events in the treated group, so we can say that 10 people benefited – these 10 people would have had an event if they were not treated. We had to treat 100 people to have

10 people benefit, and that is the same as saying we needed to treat 10 people to have one benefit. The NNT is 10. Mathematically, the risk difference would be 0.2 – 0.1 = 0.1. And 1/0.1 = 10.

So really the take home message of this whole absolute vs relative risk reduction thing is to watch out for the manipulations that can occur when you read the papers—especially those funded by the pharmaceutical industry—and understand the differences between absolute (the risk difference), and relative (the relative risk).

Population Attributable risk

Recall that risk difference, which can also be called attributable risk, is the excess risk of the outcome in the exposed that is attributable to the exposure. (Recall our smoking example: "**80 heart attacks per 1000 population in a 10-year period are attributed to smoking**."), and then there is attributable risk percent, which is the percentage of the outcome, among those exposed, that is attributable to the outcome: **"Among smokers, 40% of the risk of heart attack is due to smoking."**

But now we might want to extend the argument, and ask, "What is the attributable risk of the outcome due to the exposure for the *entire population?* That is, we no longer care just about those who are exposed (i.e. just the smokers) we care about the entire population, (i.e. both smokers and nonsmokers). To demonstrate how we go about this, let's revisit *example E3.1,* which was our simple example of smoking and heart disease:

	Outcome occurred	Outcome did not occur
Exposed (n=1000)	200	800
Not exposed (n=1000)	120	880

We calculated the risk in the exposed group and the risk in the not-exposed group:

$$risk_{exposed} = \frac{200}{200+800} = 0.20$$

$$risk_{unexposed} = \frac{120}{120+880} = 0.12$$

Now we must calculate a new variable: the risk of the entire population. To do so, we must *weight* the risks of each group. We may know that the percentage of the population that are smokers, is say, 33%, and the percentage of the population that are nonsmokers, is say 67%. So the total risk of the outcome of heart disease in the total population is the sum of the weighted risks:

$$Risk_{pop} = (risk_{exposed})(portion\ of\ population\ that\ are\ smokers) + (risk_{unexposed})(portion\ of\ population\ that\ are\ nonsmokers)$$

$$Risk_{pop} = (0.20)(0.33) + (0.12)(0.67) = 0.15$$

And now our risk difference is

$$Population\ attributable\ risk = Risk\ difference = Risk_{population} - Risk_{unexposed}$$

$$PAR = 0.15 - 0.12 = 0.03$$

And remember when we talk about risk difference, we need units…per population per time period: 0.03 is the same as **30 heart attacks per 1000 people for a ten-year period.**

Interpretation: The risk of heart attack in the *total population* due to smoking is 30 heart attacks per 1000 people in a ten-year period. Recall the attributable risk (or just the "risk difference") was 80 heart attacks per 1000 people in a ten-year period. The population attributable risk is considerably less than the attributable risk, and this makes intuitive sense, since the attributable risk is measuring the increased risk of heart attack due to smoking among just among the smokers, and the population attributable risk is the increased risk of heart attack due to smoking among the entire population.

And, as with attributable risk, we can make this into a percentage:

$$Population\ attributbale\ risk\ percent = \frac{Risk_{population} - Risk_{unexposed}}{Risk_{population}}$$

$$PAR\% = \frac{0.15 - 0.12}{0.15} = 0.2 = 20\%$$

And the interpretation is that 20% of heart attacks in the entire population is due to smoking.

6. In general, the population attributable risk is less than the attributable risk (risk difference) because the attributable risk is the risk of the outcome due to the exposure among those with the _________________________, while the population attributable risk is the risk of the outcome due to the exposure among the __________________ population.

Section E3.4 The Element of Time (Introduction)

The element of time is an important concept in epidemiology, and will be explored in depth in future chapters, but a brief introduction is applicable here, as it presents another way to discuss the measures of association in cohort studies and randomized trials. This concept was already touched upon in this chapter when I talked about risk difference. I mentioned that risk difference only makes sense when it is described in *units,* and the units incorporated the element of time.

Let us bring back our illustrative study on smoking and heart attacks:

	Outcome occurred	**Outcome did not occur**
Exposed (n=1000)	200	800
Not exposed (n=1000)	120	880

Recall that the cumulative risk (I_c) in the exposed group was $\frac{200}{1000} = 0.2$ or 20%

And remember that this was a prospective cohort study in which the participants were followed for 10 years. So we can state that the risk is 0.2 for each person followed for 10 years. And that is the same as a risk of 0.02 *per person per one year*. "Per person per one year is called a "person-year" in epidemiology. And our risk is now 0.02 per person-year, or **0.02/p-y**. But by convention we don't like decimals in the numerator, so we multiply our 0.02 by 1000, and we now have **20/1000p-y.** We say the risk among smokers is "20 cases per 1000 person-years."

A "person-year" is just the number of persons multiplied by the total number of years of observation. So 1000 person-years could mean 1000 persons observed for 1 year, or 500 people observed for 2 years, or 100 people observed for 10 years.

Since the denominator of our risk now has a unit of time, it is now a *true rate*, and is called the ***person-time incidence rate*** (IR_{p-t}), and it gives us a measure of the *speed* at which a disease is occurring.

And so to repeat: The cumulative risk (I_c) for the exposed is 0.2, meaning that the risk for each individual person followed for 10 years is 0.2. The incidence rate (IR_{p-t}) is 0.02/p-y, meaning that the risk is 0.02 for each person each year. (or by convention, 20 cases per 1000 person-years.

7. The incidence rate is a more precise way of stating the risk, as it has the element of _____________ in the denominator, and so is a true rate.

The IR_c for the unexposed group is 0.012/p-y, or 12/1000p-y.

And then we can calculate our Incidence rate difference, which is

$$IR_{p-t}(exposed) - IR_{p-t}(unexposed)$$

Or: 20/1000p-y – 12 /1000p-y = 8/1000p-y

"The risk of heart attack *among smokers that is due to smoking is 8 cases per 1000 person-years.*"

And just like relative risk, we can calculate a ratio of incidence rates, which is called the "*Incidence rate ratio*" which is $\frac{IR_{p-t}(exposed)}{IR_{p-t}(unexposed)} = 1.67.$

(Just like relative risk, because the incidence rate ratio is a ratio, the units go away).

At this point, you may be asking yourself what is so great about the incidence rate? Afterall, an incidence rate of 0.02/p-y is exactly the same as a cumulative risk of 0.2 per person followed for 10 years. And you are right. They are telling us the exact same thing when we only know the total number of cases in a certain time period. But as will be discussed later, if we know *when* each case developed within that 10 year period, we can do more precise calculations of the incidence rates. But more on that later.

Summary thus far

The first four sections presented the measures of association for cohort studies and for experimental randomized trials. And those include the cumulative incidence (also called the "risk"), the relative risk, the risk difference (also called the "attributable risk"), the population attributable risk, the attributable risk percent, and the population attributable risk percent.

In the next section, I will discuss the unique measure of association that is used for case-control studies.

Section E3.5: Measure of Association for case-control studies: the Odds Ratio

Case-control studies (discussed in detail in section E1.2, differ from all other studies because they start with the outcome, and then work back to assess for exposure. Therefore, they require a unique measure of association. Once again I will bring up the previous fictitious prospective cohort study on cigarette smoking and heart attacks:

	Outcome occurred	**Outcome did not occur**	**Total**
Exposed (n=1000)	200	800	1000
Not exposed (n=1000)	120	880	1000

Notice that this time I added a third column on the right "total", which is the amount of people followed for 10 years who are "at risk" of the outcome occurring. If we were to run a similar study as a case-control study, we would start with the outcome, that is, we would take, say, 100 people who were recently diagnosed with a heart attack, and 100 people who were not, and then question them about the exposure in question (Do you smoke?). We might get results that look like this:

	Outcome occurred (n=100)	**Outcome did not occur (n=100)**	**Total**
Smokers	18	11	?
Nonsmokers	82	89	?

Notice the ?s in the last column. I put those there because the "total" column in a case-control study becomes irrelevant. We do not know how many people are "at risk" for heart attack because we *started* with an equal number or people who had heart attacks and did not. That is, we *invented* the number of participants on the third column (the "controls" in which heart attack did not occur). Since we have no idea, in our case-control study, of how many people are "at risk" for a heart attack, we cannot use the measures of association that I presented thus far: cumulative incidence (risk), relative risk, attributable risk, population attributable risk: they're all out in case-control studies!

We are left with one thing: the Odds Ratio.

To understand odds ratios, it is first necessary to discuss what "odds" are. And here is a description of odds, as opposed to probabilities:

Let's say that without looking I reach my hand into a bag containing 5 balls that are exactly the same except one is white and four are black. What is the probability that I will pull out a white ball? It is 20%. A "one out of 5 chance" that I will get a white ball. "Odds" is a little different. It is the probability of an event occurring *divided by the probability of the event not occurring.* In this example then, the probability of *not picking a white ball* (i.e. picking a black ball) is 80%. And so, the "odds" of picking a white ball is 0.2/0.8 = 0.25. (A shortcut way of thinking is ¼ (one white ball divided by 4 black balls). Remember a couple of things: 1. Odds is always greater than probability. (The probability of picking a white ball is 0.2). 2. Probability is always between 0 and 1 while odds can take on any value. (The odds of picking black ball is 4, while the probability of picking a black ball is 0.8). 3. If probability is very small, it is nearly equal to odds, but if the probability is high, then odds and probability are very different (4 and 0.8 respectively in our example.)

8. Odds is always ____________________ than probability, and odds is very similar to probability if the outcome has a _______ probability, but very different from probability if the outcome has a _________ probability.

We can say that:

$$Odds = \frac{probability}{1 - probability}$$

So looking back at our 2x2 table, in the "outcome occurred" column, we see that 18 of them were smokers and 82 of them were nonsmokers. What are the odds of being a smoker among these people?

$$Odds = \frac{18/_{100}}{1 - (18/_{100})} = 0.22$$

Or the shortcut, just divide

$$\frac{18}{82} = 0.22$$

So how do we interpret the odds? We say that among the people who had a heart attack, the odds of being a smoker is 0.22.

Then, among the controls (those who did not have the outcome), the odds of being a smoker is

$$\frac{11}{89} = 0.124$$

Now that we have the odds for each group, we can set up the odds ratio. The odds ratio is the odds of one group divided by the odds of the other group. By convention, we generally take the odds in the outcome group divided by the odds in the control group.

	Outcome occurred (n=100)	**Outcome did not occur (n=100)**
Smokers	a	b
Nonsmokers	c	d

The odds ratio is, by convention, $\frac{a/_c}{b/_d}$,

In our example, then, OR = $\frac{18/_{82}}{11/_{89}} = \mathbf{1.78}$

How do we interpret this odds ratio? We would say that the odds of being a smoker among people who have had a heart attack is 1.78 times the odds of being a smoker among those who have not had a heart attack. Or "you have a 78% higher odds of being a smoker if you had a heart attack than if you had not had a heart attack." Note that this is not really the question we are interested in. We are not, strictly speaking, interested in the odds of being a smoker if you've had a heart attack vs not; what we really care about (why we're doing the study) is the odds of having a heart attack if you are smoker compared to if you are not a smoker. So it appears as if our odds ratio is not really answering our question. However, with a little bit of algebraic manipulation, I will show you that through the "magic of the odds ratio," we actually can answer the question that we care about:

$$\frac{a/c}{b/d} \cdot \frac{d/b}{d/b} = \frac{ad}{cb} = \frac{ad}{bc} = \frac{a/b}{c/d}$$

It's magic! Our odds ratio is now $\frac{a/b}{c/d}$ which we can interpret as: The odds of having a heart attack if you are a smoker compared to the odds of having a heart attack if you are not a smoker. And we can say that the odds of having a heart attack is 78% higher if you are smoker than if you are a nonsmoker.

9. The odds ratio, by its exact definition, does not really answer the question we are interested in, which is the odds of an event if you are exposed vs nonexposed. Thankfully, though, with a bit of algebraic manipulation, we see that it actually ____________ answer the question!

Section E3.6 Prevalence

Before I conclude this chapter, there is one more measure of association to discuss, and that is Prevalence, which is used in cross-sectional studies. Recall section E1 in which I discussed a fictitious cross-sectional study on depression and Parkinson's disease.

A sample of 1250 people with depression and a sample of 1250 people without depression were surveyed and asked if they currently also carry a diagnosis of Parkinson's disease. They might find that the prevalence of Parkinson's among people with depression is 7 cases per 1250 people, and the prevalence of Parkinson's among people without depression is 3 cases per 1250 people.

The 2xs table would look like this:

	Disease (depression)	**No disease (no depression)**
Exposure (Parkinson's)	7	3
No exposure (no Parkinson's)	1243	1247

We would say that the prevalence of Parkinson's disease among people with depression is 7/1250 = 0.047, and we would say that the prevalence of Parkinson's disease among people without depression is 3/1243 = 0.0024. We can then define a **prevalence ratio**, which is

$$\frac{7/_{1250}}{3/_{1250}} = 2.33$$

The translation would be that you are 2.33 times as likely to have Parkinson's disease if you are depressed than if you are not. Recall that in cross-sectional studies, we can say nothing what is causing what, since it is a snapshot in time. We could just as easily asked what is the prevalence of depression among those with Parkinson's vs those without? In that case, the numbers would be:

$$\frac{7/_{10}}{1243/_{2490}} = 1.40$$

You are 1.4 times as likely to have depression if you have Parkinson's than if you do not have Parkinson's. I should point out, though, that if we were considering Parkinson's the disease, and depression the exposure, we would have started out with, say, 1250 people with Parkinson's and 1250 without, and might get results something like this:

	Disease (Parkinson's)	**No disease (no Parkinson's)**
Exposure (depression)	50	22
No exposure (no depression)	1200	1228

And our prevalence ratio would be:

$$\frac{50/_{1250}}{22/_{1250}} = 2.27$$

The relationship between incidence rate and prevalence

Prevalence and person-time incidence rates are related as such:

$$Prevalence = IR_{p-t} \times duration_{average}$$

As person-time incidence rate increases (more disease being infused into the population) we would certainly expect prevalence to increase. And also, as the average duration of the disease increases, the prevalence of disease will also increase. Note that increased duration can be a bad thing (no cures available) but can also be a good thing (people survive for longer with the disease).

Summary of Epidemiology 3

Measures of association for cohort studies and experimental trials include

Cumulative incidence (I_c) also called "risk" and is the probability of the outcome

Risk difference (also called attributable risk) is the risk of an outcome due to an exposure among those with the exposure. It is $risk_{exposed} - risk_{unexdposed}$

Population attributable risk is the risk of outcome due to an exposure for the entire population (both those with and without exposure). It is $Risk_{population} - Risk_{unexposed}$

Relative risk (risk of exposed/risk of unexposed)

Person-time Incidence rate (IR_{p-t}) is the rate that the disease is occurring in the population, and has units of person-time.

Prevalence is used in cross-sectional studies and is a snapshot measure of the number of cases among the exposed, or the number of cases among the not-exposed, and then we can calculate a prevalence ratio.

Biostats 3: Comparing Categorical Outcomes

In Biostats 2, I discussed how to compare results when the results are continuous, that is, something you can take the mean of. Of course, continuous outcomes are common in medicine—pretty much anything you can think of: height, weight, blood pressure, head circumference etc. But equally important (perhaps more important) in the world of medical research are *categorical* outcomes. And by far the most common of categorical outcomes, and therefore, the one that I will talk about most, is *binary* outcomes—that is, one of two things can happen. Either an event occurred, or it did not. "Yes or no": did an event occur? So you can imagine many scenarios in which we deal with binary outcomes. We may follow a group of people to see if, say, they had a heart attack or not (think lipid-lowering medication trials); or did they need to get admitted to the hospital or not? (think Covid vaccine or Covid treatment trials); or did they remain cancer free or not? (think chemotherapy trials), or did they develop a side effect of the drug or not? And the list goes on. The important point is that the outcome is not continuous, and nothing we can take the mean of, so it is a categorical outcome, and the reason I need to write this as a whole separate chapter is because the mathematics involved is entirely different. And now that you have a full review of all the measures of association in Epidemiology 3, we can really start to put all of this together.

Quick review

Biostats can get tricky if we don't periodically review what we already know and what we are about to learn, and how they are different etc. We often get "lost in the weeds" if we do not do this little exercise, so please hang with me for this!

In Biostats 1, I talked about the problem of having to interpret the data from one sample when what we really care about is the data from an entire population. I talked about the *standard error of the mean, or SE_{mean},* which mathematically is $\frac{s}{\sqrt{n}}$, and conceptually is the standard deviation of the distribution of a whole bunch of means—that is, if we took many many samples of the same size and graphed the distribution of all their means. But in Biostats 1, I only discussed samples of *continuous* outcomes—that is, something with a mean. But what about one sample that is not continuous, but rather a "yes/no" situation? Let's look at an example:

1. Binary outcomes are not continuous and therefore do not have a ____________________, so we can't use the standard error of the mean to describe one sample. We must use different mathematics.

A binary outcome study

JOURNAL ARTICLE

Seroconversion Following Nonoccupational Postexposure Prophylaxis against HIV FREE

Michelle E. Roland, Torsten B. Neilands, Melissa R. Krone, Mitchell H. Katz, Karena Franses, Robert M. Grant, Michael P. Busch, Frederick M. Hecht, Barbara L. Shacklett, James O. Kahn ... Show more

Author Notes

Clinical Infectious Diseases, Volume 41, Issue 10, 15 November 2005, Pages 1507–1513, https://doi.org/10.1086/497268

Published: 15 November 2005 **Article history ▾**

In this study, researchers studied the efficacy of postexposure prophylaxis in preventing HIV seroconversion by following people who had an exposure to HIV for about a year after they were given the therapy. Some converted to HIV-positive status, and some did not. So…"yes/no." The actual results were 7 out of 702 converted to HIV-positive, while 695 out of 702 did not convert. I will "fudge" their results a bit to the mathematics a bit easier. Let's say 27 out of 702 seroconverted and 675 out of 702 did not convert. How would this be reported? Most commonly, the researchers would report the *proportion* that seroconverted to be **27/702 = 0.038, or 3.8%.** In biostats, a proportion is often symbolized by $\hat{p}$ (called "p-hat"). Note that this $\hat{p}$ is not the same as the p-value that I talked about in the last chapter when discussing hypothesis testing. This "p-hat" refers to a proportion. So here we would say $\boldsymbol{\hat{p} = 0.038}$. And of course the $\hat{p}$ of those who did *not* seroconvert is **0.962**. Note that this is the same as "risk" or "cumulative incidence" that I discussed in section E3.2.

(Whenever a symbol has a "hat" over it in biostats, it indicates that it is only an *estimation* of that variable because it comes from our one sample, and not from the entire population that we are interested in.)

Section B3.1: The Binomial distribution

Recall that when we are dealing with a sample of continuous outcomes, the results of the sample tend to follow a normal distribution pattern. For example, a sample of 50 random people might have a systolic blood pressure distribution that looks like this:

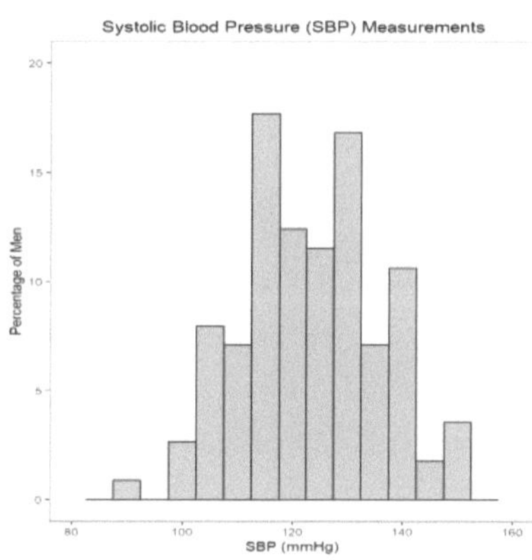

It looks indeed like a normal distribution, and as we increase the sample size, it will look even more like a normal distribution. But what of our binary "yes/no" study? What kind of distribution does one sample of this follow? Well, our (fudged) results showed that 96.2% of the people did not seroconvert, but 3.8% did seroconvert. So the new histogram distribution looks like this:

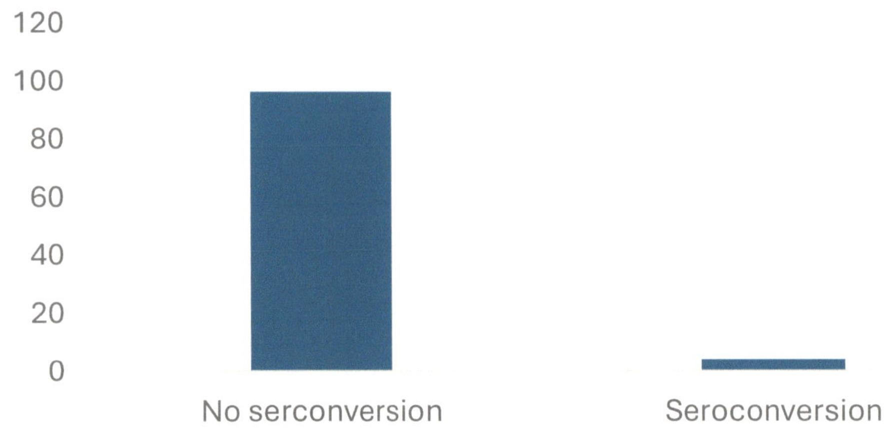

We really don't learn much from this, but this is what the binomial distribution of our one sample looks like. We can calculate the mean here, but it seems kind of silly. Ah, but let's do it anyway. For binary results, we assign a value of 1 to those who have a positive result (in general to those who had an event) in this case those who seroconverted, and we assign a value of 0 to those who did not have an event (in our case, those who did not seroconvert). So, there are 675 "0" values, and 27 "1" values. So the mean is $\frac{675(0)+27(1)}{702} = 0.038$. Notice that this number is the same as our proportion of 0.038. We can also think of this as our probability of seroconversion. And so our $\hat{p}$ is the proportion in question, and it also is the mean of the binomial distribution if we code "no event" as a 0 and "yes event" as a 1. And it also leads us to the expected number of events (or "successes" as it's known in the binomial distribution) by the formula:

$$x_{bi} = n\hat{p}$$

So in our one sample, the expected number of "successes" (that is, the number of seroconverts) is 702 x 0.038 = **27**.

Here is what a binomial distribution looks like. If we ran, say 40 trials, and the probability of "success" of each trial is 0.038, then we get the following distribution of successes:

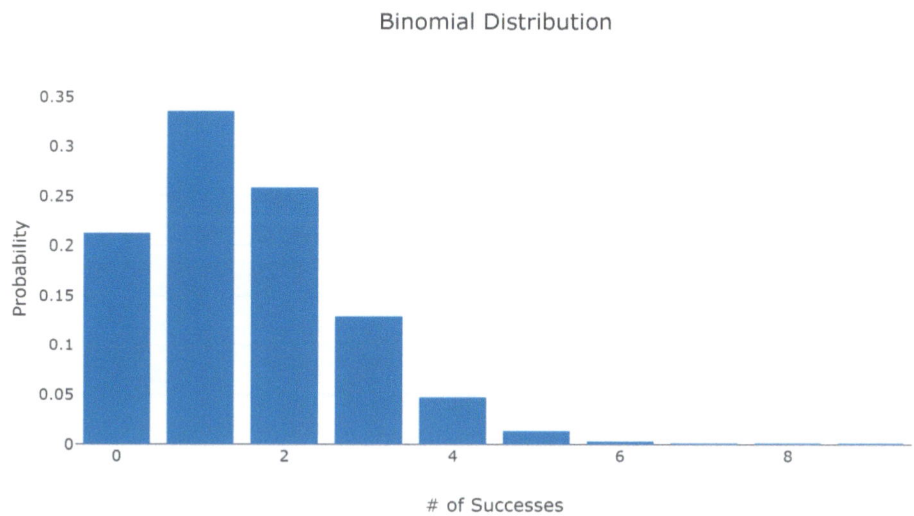

What is the value that comes out the most? It looks like around 1 or so by the graph. Mathematically this makes sense, because:

$$x = n\hat{p} = 40(0.038) = 1.5$$

In the binomial world, each person is one trial, with a probability of 0.038. So the above distribution could be one trial of 40 people, or 2 trials of 20 people, or 8 trials of 5 people etc. To see why these two n's are interchangeable in binomial distributions, think of a six-sided die. If we roll one die 6 times (we run six trials), we expect the number 2, say, to come up 1/6 of the time (that is, it should come up once). If we run one trial in which we roll 6 dice, we still expect the number 2 to come up once. If we roll 6 dice 6 times, that is the same as rolling one die 36 times, and we expect the number 2 to come up 1/6 of the time, or 6 times. So don't worry about the n in binomial: it can mean the number of participants or the number of trials, or a combination of the two. Remember that each person is his or her own trial. All that matters is the probability.

What if I ran 80 trials with a probability of "success" of 0.038?

Here is the distribution:

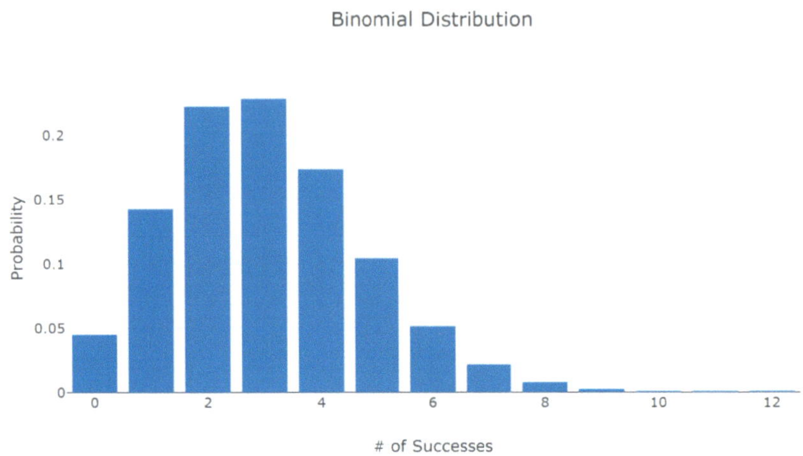

What is the expected number of "successes" given 80 trials? (Or, if you like, 20 trials each with 8 people, or 10 trials each with 8 people, or one trial with 80 people!). Looking at the graph, it is around 3 or so.

Mathematically?

$$x = n\hat{p} = 80(0.038) = 3.04$$

And in our study, (we're running it 702 times), here is the binomial distribution:

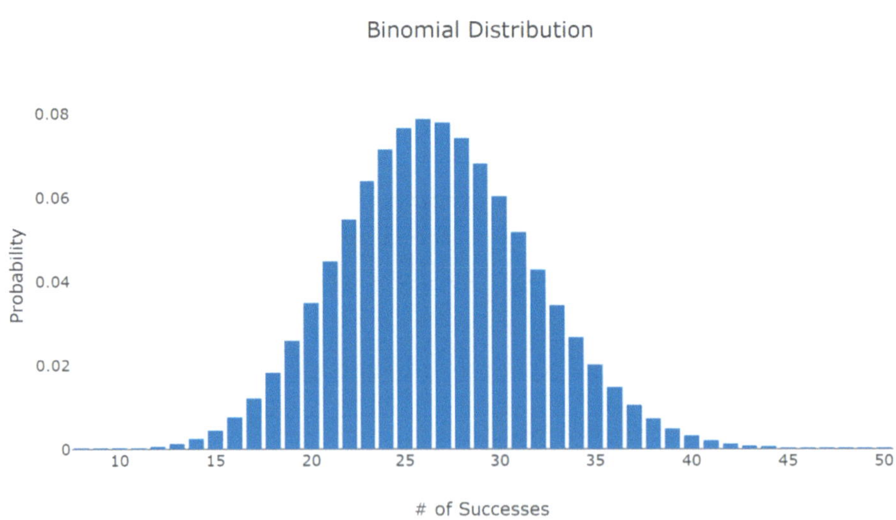

$$x = n\hat{p} = 702(0.038) = 27$$

2. The binomial distribution gives us the number of "successes," and depends only on the number of ____________________ and the probability of a "success."

Section B3.2: The Central Limit Theorem revisited

Remember the Central Limit theorem? No matter what the distribution of the sample, if we take many many samples, and graph the means of them, we get a normal distribution. Well, the same holds true for binary results. In our case, if we took many samples all of n = 702, we would get a proportion of somewhere around 0.038 for each of our samples, but surely it would vary around this value. Sometimes we get 0.034, sometimes 0.042, sometimes 0.039 etc. And so if we took, say 100 samples of size n = 702, we would get a normal distribution around the mean of 0.038. And the SD of this distribution is the "standard error" of the proportion. And that is the standard error of a proportion, and is given by the formula:

$$SE_p = \frac{\sqrt{p(1-p)}}{\sqrt{n}}$$

Just as in Biostats I when we proved that the SE of the mean is equal to the standard deviation of the distribution of the means of many samples, we can do the same for proportions:

Sample size	Mean of 5000 sample proportions	SD of 5000 sample proportions	Standard error
702	0.038	0.0072	$\frac{\sqrt{p(1-p)}}{\sqrt{n}} = 0.0072$
1000	0.038	0.0060	$\frac{\sqrt{p(1-p)}}{\sqrt{n}} = 0.0060$
10,000	0.038	0.0019	$\frac{\sqrt{p(1-p)}}{\sqrt{n}} = 0.0019$

So you see that the SD of the means of many many samples is equal to the SE of the proportion. And note, once again, that as the sample size increases, the SE becomes smaller. Back to our one sample: we said that $\hat{p} = 0.038$. But again that means nothing as it is just one sample. We hope that if we measure the entire population, the *true* proportion for the entire population will be the proportion we got from our single sample plus and minus two standard errors. That is our 95% confidence interval of our proportion.

0.038 ±2(0.0072) = **0.024 to 0.052**. Or we can say **3.8% (2.4% to 5.2%)**

Based on our sample of 702, we can be *reasonably* certain that the proportion of the entire population that would seroconvert would be somewhere between **2.4% and 5.2%.**

So I have shown you how to calculate the 95% confidence interval for one sample, when the outcome for that sample is a proportion (rather than a continuous outcome which was covered in chapter B1).

Section B3.3: Confidence interval of risk difference

In Biostats 2, I introduced comparing continuous outcomes, and so in this chapter I will introduce comparing categorical outcomes (especially binary "yes/no" outcomes). And most cohort studies and randomized trials, the results are in fact binary. Did a disease occur or did it not? Was the patient hospitalized or not? Did the cancer recur or not? Etc. Remember the standard error for the difference of two means? It was this:

$$SE_{(\bar{x}_1-\bar{x}_2)} = \sqrt{\frac{s_1^2}{n_1} + \frac{s_2^2}{n_2}}$$

Well, now I present to you the standard error of difference of proportions, which is:

$$\widehat{SE}_{\hat{p}_1-\hat{p}_2} = \sqrt{\frac{\hat{p}_1(1-\hat{p}_1)}{n_1} + \frac{\hat{p}_2(1-\hat{p}_2)}{n_2}}$$

Remember what we are doing: when conducting a cohort study or a randomized trial, the measure of association is cumulative incidence (risk). Cumulative incidence is the *proportion* of people at risk of the outcome who have the outcome. And since we are comparing two groups (one with the exposure or intervention, and one without), we have two different proportions, p_1 and p_2.

Let's look back at the simple cohort study I presented in E3.2. The exposure was smoking and the outcome was heart attack:

The cumulative incidence of heart attack among smokers is 200/1000 = 0.2. That is also the *proportion* of smokers at risk for heart attack who had a heart attack. And the cumulative incidence of heart attack among the nonsmokers is 120/1000 = 0.12. That is also the *proportion* of nonsmokers at risk for heart attack who had a heart attack.

3. The cumulative incidence is also known as the "risk" can also be thought of as the ______________________ of people at risk of the outcome who had the outcome.

The risk difference is 0.20 – 0.12 = **0.08**. But remember, like all things in biostats/epidemiology, we don't really care about the results in our one sample, we care about what the results would be for the entire population of smokers vs nonsmokers. We must present our results with its 95% confidence interval, so that we can be reasonably certain what the risk difference of the entire population would be. If we were able to run our experiment many many times, we would get a distribution of results, and that distribution would be…you guessed it…a normal distribution. And the standard deviation of the distribution of these differences of proportions is the standard error of our differences of proportions, and we need to identify 95% of these outcomes. So first, we calculate our standard error:

$$\widehat{SE}_{\hat{p}_1-\hat{p}_2} = \sqrt{\frac{\hat{p}_1(1-\hat{p}_1)}{n_1} + \frac{\hat{p}_2(1-\hat{p}_2)}{n_2}}$$

$$\widehat{SE}_{\hat{p}_1-\hat{p}_2} = \sqrt{\frac{0.2(1-0.2)}{1000} + \frac{0.12(1-0.12)}{1000}}$$

$$\widehat{SE}_{\hat{p}_1-\hat{p}_2} = 0.016$$

So our risk difference is now 0.08 ± 2(0.016). The 95% confidence interval is from (0.048 to 0.112).

Or we can say a risk difference of **8% (4.8% to 11.2%)**

Now we have a result that means something. We can be reasonably certain that in the entire universe of smokers vs nonsmokers, there is a risk difference for heart attack somewhere between 4.8% and 11.2%.

Section B3.4: Confidence interval for ratios (relative risk, odds ratio, incidence rate ratio)

In our example the RR is 0.2/0.12 = **1.67.** But, once again, that is meaningless because it is the result of one sample. We need to translate this to what we would expect from the entire universe of smokers vs nonsmokers. To do this, as before, we need our 95% confidence interval, and to get this, we need our standard error of the relative risk. If we ran our experiment many many times, we would get a whole bunch of relative risk, and the distribution of all these results, thanks to the Central Limit Theorem, would be…nope! Not a normal distribution! Fooled ya! It turns out that whenever we are dealing with a *ratio,* the results of many many experiments is not normally distributed because a ratio cannot be below 0. A ratio can go from 0 to positive infinity. But we can play a little mathematical trick to get the normal distribution that we need for standard errors. The natural log (ln) of the ratios *does* follow a normal distribution. I would like to convince you as to why this is the case. But it is OK if you don't need to be convinced of this; if you would just like to accept the fact that you must use the natural log of a ratio, then go ahead and skip to "**If you skipped the previous section, resume here!**"

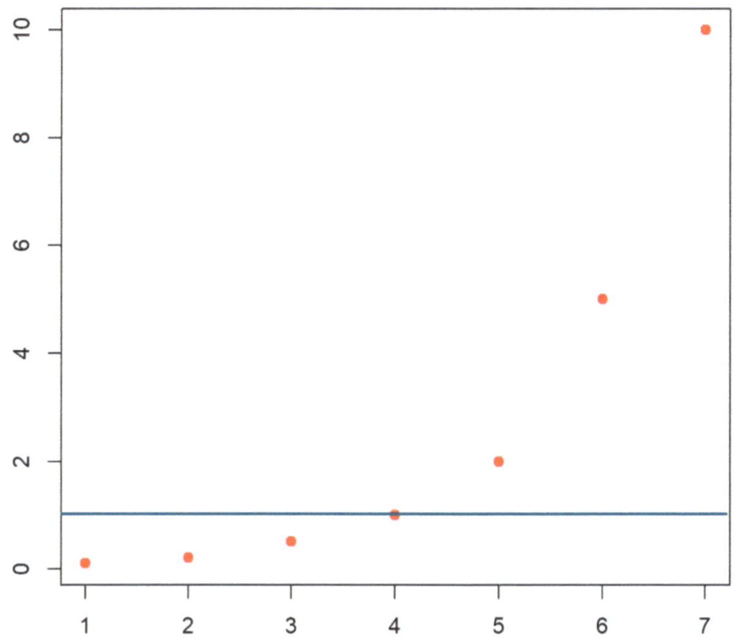

Each red point in the diagram is a ratio. Point 1 is ratio of 0.1. Point 2 is 0.2. Point 3 is 0.5. Point 4 is 1. Point 5 is 2. Point 6 is 5, and point 7 is 10. The horizontal line across is a ratio of 1. Look at point 1 and point 7. These are inverses of each other, so point 1 is $\frac{1}{10}$ while point 7 is $\frac{10}{1}$. But when graphed, point 1 is a lot closer to the horizontal line of 1 as compared to the graph of 10. But they should actually be equidistant from the horizontal line, because they are the same ratio, just flipped upside-down. The same is true of point 2, which is $\frac{2}{10}$, and point 6 which is $\frac{10}{2}$. Again, these two should be equidistant from the horizontal line of 1, and so on.

But, if we graph the natural log of the ratios, we get this:

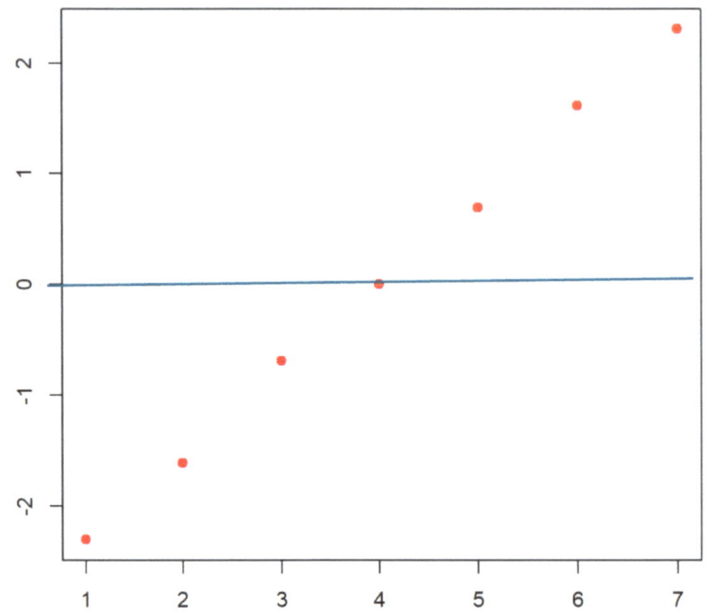

Point 1 is now the $ln(.1) = -2.3$, and point 7 is $ln(10) = 2.3$, etc. Now we see that the proportions are equidistant form the graph of $ln(1) = 0$.

So, when graphing ratios, we must always use the natural log of the ratios for it to make mathematical sense. You can see it goes from negative infinity to positive infinity, and you can see that inverse ratios are equidistant from the reference line.

One more example to drill the point home:

Let's say I have a bunch of ratios from repeated random experiments where the ratio of 1 comes up the most…so the ratio of $\frac{10}{10}$ comes up 8 times. Then the ratio to the left of $\frac{10}{10}$, which I'll pick to be $\frac{8}{10}$ comes up second most, say 6 times. Ties for second is the inverse of this ratio, or $\frac{10}{8}$, which also comes up 6 times. Then further to the left of $\frac{10}{10}$ comes a smaller ratio, that I will pick to be $\frac{5}{10}$, which comes up 4 times. Tied for third is the inverse of this ratio, which is $\frac{10}{5}$ and also comes up 4 times. Then further away from $\frac{10}{10}$ the next ratio is $\frac{2}{10}$, which comes up twice, and it's inverse of $\frac{10}{2}$ also comes up twice. And finally, a far away ratio of $\frac{1}{10}$ only comes up once, as does its inverse of $\frac{10}{1}$. I hope you can see that the ratios I picked and the frequencies would be what one might expect if random repeated experiments were conducted, and the most common result is $\frac{10}{10}$. But if I graph a histogram of the ratios, I get something like this:

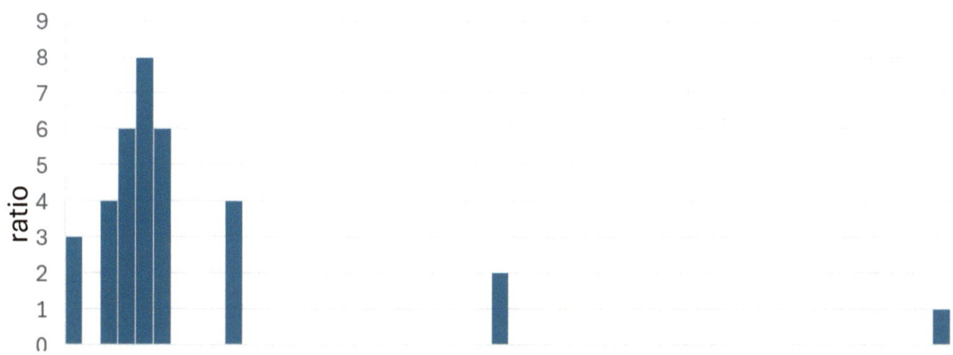

You can see that this is far from a normal distribution; it is heavily skewed to the right.

But now for the magic. If I graph a histogram of the natural log of the ratios, I get:

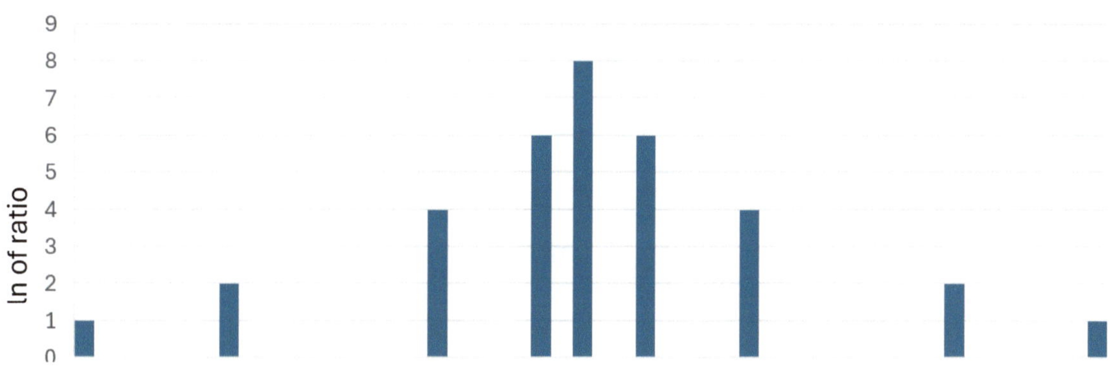

This is a normal distribution!!

(If you skipped the previous section, resume here!)

Our RR is 1.67. The formula for the standard error of natural log of the relative risk is:

The letters come from the "standard 2x2 table:

	Outcome occurred	Outcome did not occur
Exposed	a	b
Not exposed	c	d

So let's plug in our results!

	Outcome (heart attack) occurred	Outcome did not occur
Exposed (smoker)(n=1000)	200	800
Not exposed (nonsmoker) (n=1000)	120	880

$$\widehat{SE}(\ln(RR)) = \sqrt{\frac{1}{a} + \frac{1}{a+b} + \frac{1}{c} + \frac{1}{c+d}}$$

$$\widehat{SE}(\ln(1.67)) = \sqrt{\frac{1}{200} + \frac{1}{1000} + \frac{1}{120} + \frac{1}{1000}}$$

$$\widehat{SE}(\ln(RR)) = 0.124$$

The 95% confidence interval for the *ln*(RR) is $ln(RR) \pm 2(\widehat{SE}(\ln(RR))$

Our RR is 1.67. The *ln*(1.67) = 0.51. So we say the 95% CI = 0.51±2(0.124), or **(0.262 to 0.76)**

But, remember, that 95% confidence interval is the for the ln of the RR. To get the 95% CI for the actual RR, we take the *antilog* of our numbers (we "exponentiate") as follows:

95% CI = ($e^{0.262}$ to $e^{0.76}$), which is (1.30 to 2.14).

So, we say our **RR is 1.67 with 95% CI from (1.30 to 2.14)**

4. To get the SE of a ratio like the relative risk, we need to do everything on the ___________________ scale. And then when done we take the ___________________ of our results by exponentiating.

The process is similar for odds ratios and incidence rate ratios, with slight differences in the formulas.

For odds ratio:

Recall that the odds ratio is unique in that we only use it as a measure of association for our case-control studies.

95% CI of *ln*(OR) = $ln(\widehat{OR}) \pm 2(\widehat{SE}(ln(\widehat{OR}))$, in which $\widehat{SE}(ln(\widehat{OR})) = \sqrt{\frac{1}{a} + \frac{1}{b} + \frac{1}{c} + \frac{1}{d}}$

For incidence rate ratio:

95% CI of *ln*(IRR) = $ln(\widehat{IRR}) \pm 2(\widehat{SE}(ln(\widehat{IRR}))$, in which $\widehat{SE}(ln(\widehat{IRR})) = \sqrt{(\frac{1}{E_1} + \frac{1}{E_2})}$

Where E_1 and E_2 are the event counts in group 1 and 2. (That is, simply the total amount of outcomes that occurred in each group).

Summary thus far

I have explained how we calculate 95% confidence intervals for all the measures of association that are commonly used in cohort or experimental studies, specifically all those studies that have binary outcomes. I started with 95% CI for one sample, when that sample has a binary "yes/no" outcome, and then extended the demonstration to comparing two groups, when the outcome is binary "yes/no." I will next turn to hypothesis testing when comparing two groups that have categorical outcomes.

Section B3.5: Hypothesis testing for risk difference: Chi-square

Recall that a very important measure of association in cohort studies and randomized trials is *risk difference*, which is $risk_{exposed} - risk_{unexposed}$, and recall that risk is the same as *cumulative incidence* (I_c), which is just the *proportion* of people with the outcome, with the denominator being all those at risk for the outcome. So I will now discuss hypothesis testing for risk differences, which is sometimes referred to as hypothesis testing for difference of proportions. And recall in section B2.2 I introduced the concept of the null hypothesis, which, when comparing two means is:

$$H_0: \ \bar{x}_a - \bar{x}_b = 0$$

We assume the null hypothesis, which is that there is no difference between the means of two samples.

We do the same for difference of proportions:

$$H_0: \hat{p}_a - \hat{p}_b = 0$$

And as before, we run our study that sets out to reject the null hypothesis—to show that it is very unlikely that the null hypothesis is true.

For the difference of two means, we used the "student's t-test."

Chi-square test for independence

Now, for the difference of two proportions, we use **chi-square** testing, and specifically, the test in question is the "chi-square test for independence."

To explain what that means, I would like to go back to my fictitious study on smoking and heart attacks:

	Outcome (heart attack) occurred	**Outcome did not occur**
Exposed (smoker)(n=1000)	200 (a)	800 (b)
Not exposed (nonsmoker) (n=1000)	120 (c)	880 (d)

The goal of the chi-square test for independence is to see if the rows (exposure status) and columns (outcome) are *independent* of one another. We assume that they *are* independent of one another. That is, the null hypothesis in the chi-square test for independence is that the exposure status and outcomes have absolutely nothing to do with each other—one does not influence the other. They are "independent."

So here is how we go about it. The numbers in the cells: 200, 800, 120, and 880 are the "observed values." We first calculate "expected" values, which is the values that would occur in each cell if the rows and columns are indeed independent of one another. How do we determine "expected" frequency? For each cell, you do as follows:

Take the total in that row, multiply by the total in that column, then divide by the total number of all four cells. So, for cell a, we take (1000 x 320) / 2000 = 160. Do this for all the cells, and you can re-write your contingency table as follows, now with the "expected" in parentheses. I'll do one more, cell b: (1000 x 1680)/2000 =840. By the same process, we can write in all of our "expected" values in red:

	Outcome (heart attack) occurred	**Outcome did not occur**
Exposed (smoker)(n=1000)	200 (160)	800 (840)
Not exposed (nonsmoker) (n=1000)	120 (160)	880 (840)

And then we apply the chi-square formula, which is this:

$$\chi^2 = \Sigma \frac{(Observed - Expected)^2}{Expected}$$

The χ is the Greek letter "chi" and it's called "chi-square" because the difference in the numerator is squared.

So, we just sum up all the differences between the observed and expected to get our chi-square value:

$$\chi^2 = \frac{(200-160)^2}{160} + \frac{(800-840)^2}{840} + \frac{(120-160)^2}{160} + \frac{(880-840)^2}{840}$$

$$\chi^2 = 10 + 1.9 + 10 + 1.9$$

$$\chi^2 = 23.8$$

The higher the χ^2, the greater the differences between the observed and the expected values, and therefore the *less* likely that the rows and columns are independent of one another. In my example, considerably more smokers had the outcome than would have been expected if smoking had nothing to do with heart attacks.

(Of course, you do not have to calculate your chi-square value by hand these days, there are many calculators easily available on the internet that will calculate it for you. You just plug in the numbers in each cell, and the calculator gives you your chi-square value).

5. When χ^2 values are high, it is likely that there is indeed a connection between rows and columns; they are not ______________________ of one another.

Once we have our chi-square value, we need the p-value, which as you recall from Biostats 2, is the probability that the value in question (20.38) occurs just by chance alone. The further away from the null value of 0, the smaller the probability. And remember, if the p-value is less than 0.05, we say that it is just too unlikely to have occurred by chance, and therefore we can "reject the null hypothesis" and say that we have "statistically significant" results.

So once we have our χ^2 value, we need our probability of this occurring if the null hypothesis is true. And of course once again, the calculators will do that part for you. It will take the χ^2 value and then incorporate *degrees of freedom* to give you the probability. For chi-square testing, the degrees of freedom that we use are (# rows – one) x (# columns – one).

df = $(N_{rows} - 1)(N_{columns} - 1)$

So by far the most common scenario in chi-square testing, we use one degree of freedom. And here is the chi-square distribution:

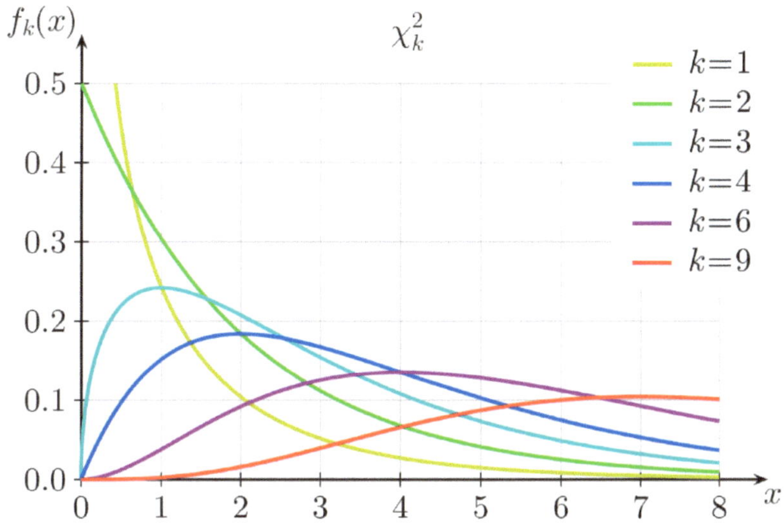

Notice that as degrees of freedom increases, the shape of the curve changes rather dramatically. This is in contrast to our distribution curves for the Student's t-test that I presented in section B2.3, where the curves only change slightly with increasing degrees of freedom.

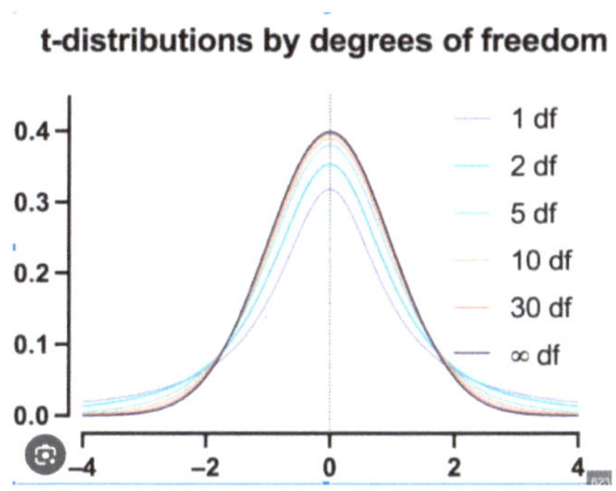

And notice that most of our chi-square curves are not normal distributions, but as we get to very high degrees of freedom, we do get a normal distribution. Here, for example is the chi-square distribution for 90 degrees of freedom (courtesy of Scribbr.com/statistics):

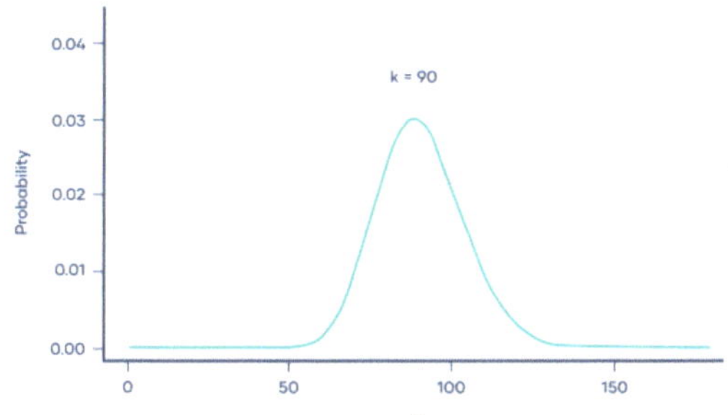

But back to our example—and the most common scenario when using chi-square—of one degree of freedom, so let's isolate the curve with 1 df:

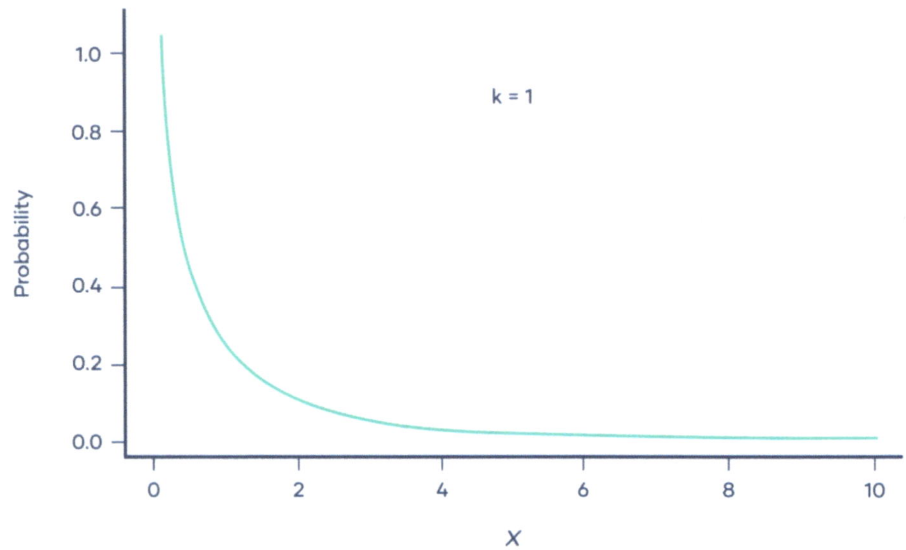

Remember that the important probability is 0.05 (or 5%), and I'll put a red dot on the distribution curve that approximately corresponds to a probability of 0.05:

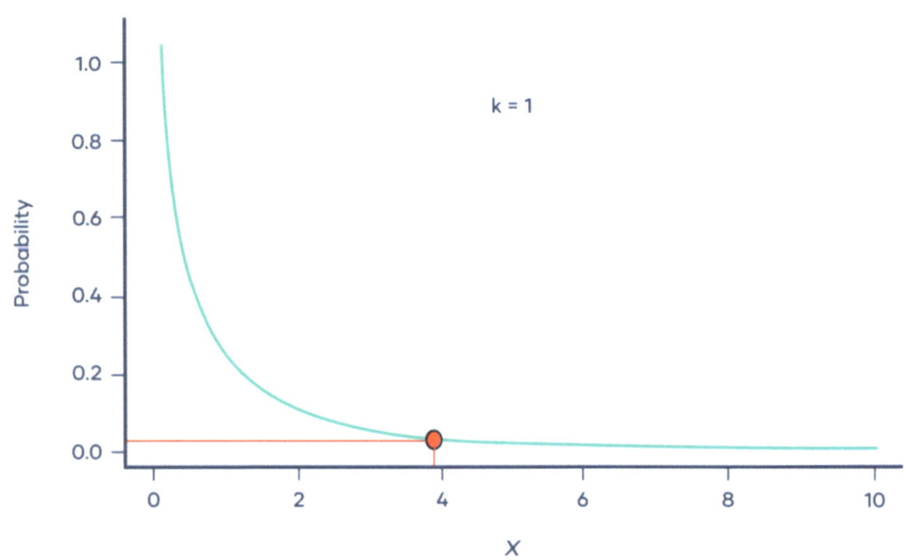

So somewhere around 3.8 is our cutoff…any χ^2 value greater than this has less than a 5% chance of occurring. We can look at the actual distribution table to see the precise value:

Degrees of freedom (*df*)	.99	.975	.95	.9	.1	.05	.025	.01
1	-------	0.001	0.004	0.016	2.706	3.841	5.024	6.635
2	0.020	0.051	0.103	0.211	4.605	5.991	7.378	9.210
3	0.115	0.216	0.352	0.584	6.251	7.815	9.348	11.345
4	0.297	0.484	0.711	1.064	7.779	9.488	11.143	13.277
5	0.554	0.831	1.145	1.610	9.236	11.070	12.833	15.086
6	0.872	1.237	1.635	2.204	10.645	12.592	14.449	16.812
7	1.239	1.690	2.167	2.833	12.017	14.067	16.013	18.475
8	1.646	2.180	2.733	3.490	13.362	15.507	17.535	20.090
9	2.088	2.700	3.325	4.168	14.684	16.919	19.023	21.666
10	2.558	3.247	3.940	4.865	15.987	18.307	20.483	23.209
11	3.053	3.816	4.575	5.578	17.275	19.675	21.920	24.725
12	3.571	4.404	5.226	6.304	18.549	21.026	23.337	26.217
13	4.107	5.009	5.892	7.042	19.812	22.362	24.736	27.688
14	4.660	5.629	6.571	7.790	21.064	23.685	26.119	29.141
15	5.229	6.262	7.261	8.547	22.307	24.996	27.488	30.578
16	5.812	6.908	7.962	9.312	23.542	26.296	28.845	32.000
17	6.408	7.564	8.672	10.085	24.769	27.587	30.191	33.409
18	7.015	8.231	9.390	10.865	25.989	28.869	31.526	34.805
19	7.633	8.907	10.117	11.651	27.204	30.144	32.852	36.191
20	8.260	9.591	10.851	12.443	28.412	31.410	34.170	37.566
21	8.897	10.283	11.591	13.240	29.615	32.671	35.479	38.932
22	9.542	10.982	12.338	14.041	30.813	33.924	36.781	40.289
23	10.196	11.689	13.091	14.848	32.007	35.172	38.076	41.638
24	10.856	12.401	13.848	15.659	33.196	36.415	39.364	42.980

And we see that the critical χ^2 value for one df is 3.841.

Our result was 23.8 which is way off the charts here! If we plug it into a chi-square calculator, we get: $p = 0.000027$.

This is an extremely small probability, meaning it is extremely unlikely that null hypothesis is true. We can conclude then, that the exposure *does* influence the outcome (they are not "independent"), and so we have a "statistically significant result."

More than one degree of freedom

But not all chi-square tests of independence have only one degree of freedom. Consider the following fictitious example:

Let's say we are studying men between the ages 40 and 60, and are trying to determine if there is an association between the relationship status of these men, and how much alcohol they drink. We identify four groups of men: currently single, currently in a monogamous relationship < 1 year, currently in a monogamous relationship 1-5 years, currently in a monogamous relationship > 5 years. And do they drink: 0-1 drink/day, 1-5 drinks/day, or >5 drinks/day.

We set up our contingency table: (the numbers in parentheses are the "expected", the calculation of which I will take you through).

	0-1 drinks/day	**2-4 drinks/day**	**>4 drinks/day**
Single	6 (16.5)	18 (12.5)	12 (7.0)
<1 year relationship	10 (13.8)	12 (10.4)	8 (5.8)
1-5 year relationship	18 (21.1)	16 (16.0)	12 (8.9)
>5 year relationship	56 (38.6)	22 (29.1)	6 (16.3)

In this study, there are three possible exposures (the relationship status), and three possible outcomes (drinks/day). Notice, by the way, that the outcome is no longer "binary" as there are three possible outcomes: 0-1 drinks, 2-4 drinks, or > 4 drinks. This is an example of a "categorical" outcome that is not "binary," but rather is an "ordinal-scale variable" (a value that can be ranked into one of several categories). We still use chi-square in this example, because the outcome is not continuous. That is, 10 people of the < 1 year relationship drank 0-1 drink/day. The "10" is not an average of anything!

6. We use chi-square hypothesis testing when the outcome is not __________________________. Chi-square testing is used even if the results are not binary "yes/no," but in general are __________________________________.

(If you're curious, by the way, go ahead and plug in the results of this study into a chi-square calculator and see what you get!...Or, better yet, do the calculation by hand and then plug in the actual χ^2 into the calculator and see what you get. If you get a χ^2 of 25.9, and a p-value of 0.00023, you did it right!)

Limitation of the chi-square test

We need to remember that chi-square is *only valid when each cell frequency is >5.* If any of the cell frequencies are <5, then the chi-square simply may not be valid. Therefore, if we have very small sample sizes and thus small cell frequencies, we have to use instead an *exact* test to determine our p-value.

Here is an example:

	DID WELL	DID POORLY
RECEIVED DRUG	8	1
CONTROL GROUP	4	5

For whatever reason, this is as very small study. Let's go ahead and make the mistake of using chi-square:

We first calculate the "expected" and put them in parentheses:

	DID WELL	DID POORLY
RECEIVED DRUG	8 (6)	1 (3)
CONTROL GROUP	4 (6)	5 (3)

$$\chi^2 = \Sigma \frac{(Observed - Expected)^2}{Expected}$$

$$\chi^2 = 4$$

Plug into a calculator, and you find that p = 0.046. The result is statistically significant. So, the groups and columns are NOT independent of each other.

OK. So now let's do this *exactly*. What do I mean by exactly? We look at *every possible* 2x2 contingency table that we may have, keeping our parameters, which is that there are 9 in each treatment group, and a total of 12 did well, and a total of 6 did poorly.

For example, the 2x2 table could have come out this way:

	DID WELL	DID POORLY	TOTAL
RECEIVED DRUG	9 (6)	0 (3)	9
CONTROL GROUP	3(6)	6 (3)	9
TOTAL	12	6	18

Or this way:

	DID WELL	DID POORLY	TOTAL
RECEIVED DRUG	5 (6)	4 (3)	9
CONTROL GROUP	7 (6)	5 (3)	9
TOTAL	12	6	18

Of course, there are others. We take the probability of *each* of these occurring, and then calculate the chance that our 2x2 contingency table would have occurred by chance, and add to the probabilities that all the other *less* likely contingency tables would have popped up. And we end up with a probability. And the p-value is 0.1312. This is > than 0.05, so now we see a NOT statistically significant result.

Again, this method is used when the numbers are small, and the Chi-square becomes inaccurate. This is an "exact test," and you may also see it referred to as "**Fisher's exact test**."

7. A chi-square test is inaccurate if any of the cells contain a number less than ____________. We must use an _______________ test instead.

Summary of Biostats 3

This chapter dealt with analyzing data from studies that have *categorical* outcomes. That is, outcomes that are not described by a mean value, but rather placed in certain mutually exclusive categories. While the most likely of these categorical outcomes is the binary "yes/no" outcome, there can be more than two categorical outcomes. I started by discussing 95% confidence intervals, first for one sample which has a binary outcome, and then extended the argument to the differences between groups with binary outcomes. There are 95% confidence intervals for risk differences, relative risks, odds ratios and incidence rate ratios. A key point is that for all ratios, one must use the logarithmic scale to make the results valid.

The second half of the chapter dealt with hypothesis testing for categorical outcomes, which is chi-square testing. Chi-square testing is a very useful and versatile test, so it was discussed in much detail.

Biostats 4: Power; Type I and Type II Errors

Section B4.1: Power

I would like to jump right in with an example. This is from an old study of 1979, when medical researchers were starting to investigate the benefit of aspirin for coronary artery disease.

Here is a quote from the abstract:

> *"A randomized controlled double-blind trial of aspirin in the prevention of death was conducted in 1682 patients who had had a confirmed myocardial infarction...Aspirin, 300 mg three times daily, was given for 1 yr. Total mortality was 12.3% in patients given aspirin and 14.8% in those given placebo, a reduction by aspirin of 17%, which was not statistically significant at p less than 0.05."*
>
> *Lancet. 1979 Dec;2(8156-8157):1313-5. doi: 10.1016/s0140-6736(79)92808-3.*

First, let's examine what they wrote in the abstract. I first noticed the reported reduction of "17%". What is this? This is the relative risk, which, to review, is the risk of the exposed divided by the risk of the unexposed. The actual reduction is the *risk difference,* which is, as we discussed, 14.8% minus 12.3% which is **2.5%.** OK, that aside, let us now check their work. What kind of a study is this? It's a randomized controlled trial in which one group received aspirin and the other received placebo. Are the results continuous or categorical? It's a "yes/no" binary result (did they die or not die?). So how would we do our hypothesis testing? Correct, we would use a chi-square test. So, we set up our 2x2 contingency table: (I added the raw numbers in parentheses)

	Died	**Did not die**
Received aspirin	12.3% (103)	87.7% (738)
Placebo	14.8% (124)	85.2% (717)

Now that you know how to this by hand, we can go ahead and use our calculator, courtesy of MedCalc:

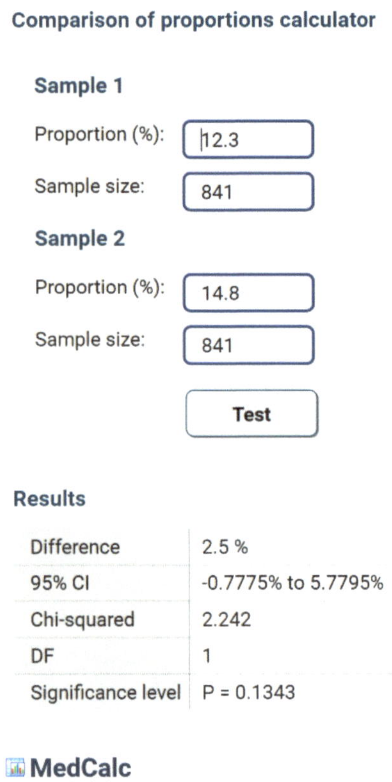

Our chi-square is only 2.42, which is less than the critical chi-square for one degree of freedom, which is around 3.8. And correspondingly, the p-value is 0.13, which is greater than 0.05, so we cannot reject the null hypothesis that aspirin and mortality have nothing to do with each other. This is not a "statistically significant" result, and we cannot conclude that aspirin benefits mortality.

But now, let's say, for the sake of argument, that the trial was a larger one, and 3000 people were in each group, but the results were *exactly the same: An ARR of 2.5%.* (I will refer to this study as "study B", while the first study is "study A.") Let's plug it in again:

Comparison of proportions calculator

Sample 1

Proportion (%): 12.3

Sample size: 3000

Sample 2

Proportion (%): 14.8

Sample size: 3000

Test

Results

Difference	2.5 %
95% CI	0.7680% to 4.2326%
Chi-squared	8.002
DF	1
Significance level	P = 0.0047

Now the p-value is statistically significant! What is going on? In the world of biostatistics, we say that study A was *underpowered* to detect the risk difference of 2.5. Study B, because it enrolled more people, had enough power to detect the difference. But note that there was nothing wrong with study A; the results were interpreted correctly…there is no statistical significance of a risk difference of 2.5 *when 841 people are in each group.*

1. In study A, the sample sizes were too ____________________ to detect a difference of 2.5%.

When researchers begin to think about a experimental trial in which they are testing a new drug or a new intervention, they think about two things: The first is that they hope to show a statistically significance result, because if they don't the new intervention is considered a failure. But they also need to think about the *clinical significance* of their result. Say, for example, they were testing out a new procedure to fix aortic stenosis which proved promising in animal models, but because it is a very expensive procedure to perform, there needs to be a *clinically* significant result for the new procedure to be "worth it." So before they start the trial, the researchers must consult with the appropriate expert cardiologists and surgeons etc, and agree on a certain cutoff value for the results. A difference below a certain cutoff value, *even if found to be statistically significant,* is just too small to be of clinical significance. No one would use it.

Then, once they decide on a cutoff value for a *clinically* significant difference, they then calculate the number of participants they need to enroll into the trial so that the trial has sufficient *power* to detect that difference. (In the aspirin trial that I presented, the researchers did not talk about clinical significance or power, but in recent times, this is considered standard protocol). If the authors of the aspirin trial had decided that a risk difference of 2.5% was indeed the cutoff of clinical significance, they would have known that they needed to recruit *more than* 841 people in each group. The exact calculation that they would have done would have told them that they needed to recruit at least 1442 people in each group to detect that difference.

So, two basic principles to start:

As we increase sample size, we increase the power to detect a difference in our measure of association.

The smaller the difference in the measure of association, the greater the sample size is needed to detect that difference.

To further explore this concept, I would like to present another fictitious example. Let's say I teach at a school with 1000 students, and my friend teaches at a different school with 1000 students. My friend and I have an ongoing feud as to whose students are smarter. Well, of course one thing leads to another, and I am *so sure* that my students are smarter than his that I offer a bet (which he happily accepts) that my students have an average IQ that is higher than that of his students. And off we go. We do not have the time or resources to do IQ testing on all 2000 of our students, so we decide to select a random sample of 20 students each, and test them. And here are the results:

My students' average IQ was **133**, and his students' average IQ was **128**

I of course start rejoicing and I tell my friend to pay up. He laughs at me, and tells me that the difference of 5 means that essentially the two groups have the same IQ.

So let us analyze the data to see who is right.

Our first task is to define the outcomes. Are they continuous or categorical? If you said continuous, you are correct. The results are the *means* of a continuous measure (IQ). And next question: What is the null hypothesis?

2. The null hypothesis in this example is that the average IQs of the two groups is ____________________________.

If you said that the null hypothesis states that average IQs of the two groups is the same, then you are correct!

Next question: what kind of test do we do to see if we can reject the null hypothesis, and hopefully win me the bet?

3. Since the outcomes are continuous, the appropriate hypothesis testing that we should do is the ____________________________ test.

If you said that we should do the Student's t-test, then you are right!

So let's use our MedCalc calculator, and plug in our values:

Comparison of means calculator

Sample 1

Mean:	133
Standard deviation:	8
Sample size:	20

Sample 2

Mean:	128
Standard deviation:	8
Sample size:	20

Test

Results

Difference	-5.000
Standard error	2.530
95% CI	-10.1214 to 0.1214
t-statistic	-1.976
DF	38
Significance level	P = 0.0554

Experiment #1

Of course my eyes go right to the p-value of 0.0554, which is every-so-slightly higher than 0.05, which means that I ever-so-slightly *cannot* reject the null hypothesis that the IQs are the same. And my friend not-so-slightly laughs at me and asks *me* to pay up!

But I just *know* that this was a result that was not due to chance. I just *know* that my students have an IQ that is on average 5 points higher than his students. I mean, I just know it. In fact, our experiment proved it! Since the p-value is 0.054, there is only a 5.4% chance that the 5 point difference in IQ occurred by chance alone! Here is our result presented graphically:

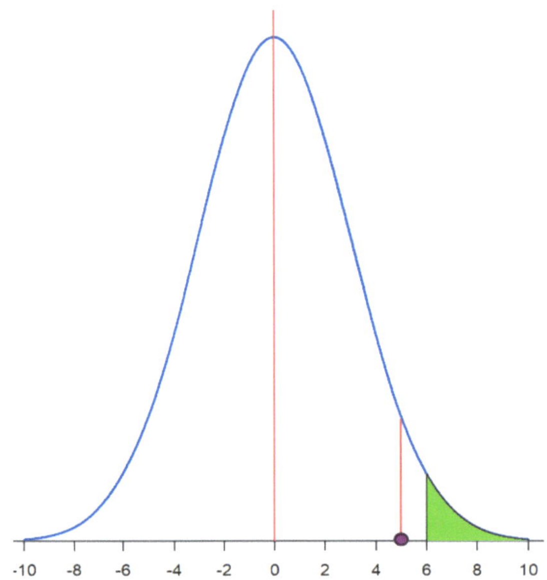

This is the distribution of results if we repeated our experiment many many times, and graphed the results, assuming as we always do, that the null hypothesis (no difference) is the reality. And so we have a normal distribution centered around 0. And the standard deviation is approximately 3. (It's actually 2.53, but I fudged it to 3 so we can see it better graphically). The green area is where I need the result to fall within in order to reject the null hypothesis. (The green area is more than 2 standard errors from the null). But our result of 5 is less than 2 standard errors away from the null. Even though there is only a 5.4% chance of these results occurring by random chance, my friend officially wins via the strict rules of biostats. What is there for me to do?

I amazingly was able to convince my friend to agree to a double-or-nothing on our bet, so that we run the experiment again, but his time with **50** random students from each group.

Our result for experiment #2 was exactly the same:

My students' average IQ was **133**, and his students' average IQ was **128**

Let's plug in these results:

Comparison of means calculator

Sample 1

Mean:	133
Standard deviation:	8
Sample size:	50

Sample 2

Mean:	128
Standard deviation:	8
Sample size:	50

Test

Results

Difference	-5.000
Standard error	1.600
95% CI	-8.1751 to -1.8249
t-statistic	-3.125
DF	98
Significance level	P = 0.0023

Experiment #2

So now our 5 point difference has only a 0.23% chance of occurring, and so we can reject the null hypothesis! Graphically, we are now here:

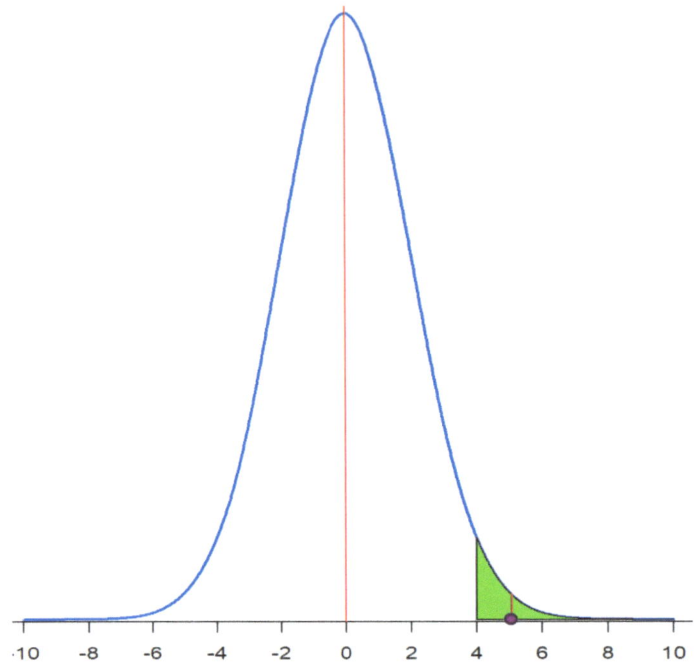

Figure B4.1

We are in the green zone. What has changed? The standard deviation has become smaller. It is now approximately 2. (Fudged up from 1.6 for demonstration purposes). And the standard deviation has become smaller only because we now have more people in our sample). And so our result of 5 is now outside of that 95% area, and we can reject the null hypothesis, and I win the bet!

4. As the sample size increases, standard deviation of the results of repeated experiments (the standard error) ________________________.

So it appears as if I was right all along; my students truly have a higher IQ than his. But the only way we could *really* find out for sure would be to test *every one* of my students and *every one* of my friend's students, If I was right all along, then the average IQ for *all* my students would be 5 points higher than the average IQ of all his students. And let us assume, for the teaching purposes, that we finally did test *all* the students, and that is indeed what we found. So we can see that in reality, my students score on average 5 points higher than students. So now let's look again at experiment #1. What happened here?

Remember that we always have to assume the null hypothesis in biostats, but understand that there is also a "reality curve." Here are the two curves when there were only 20 participants in each group:

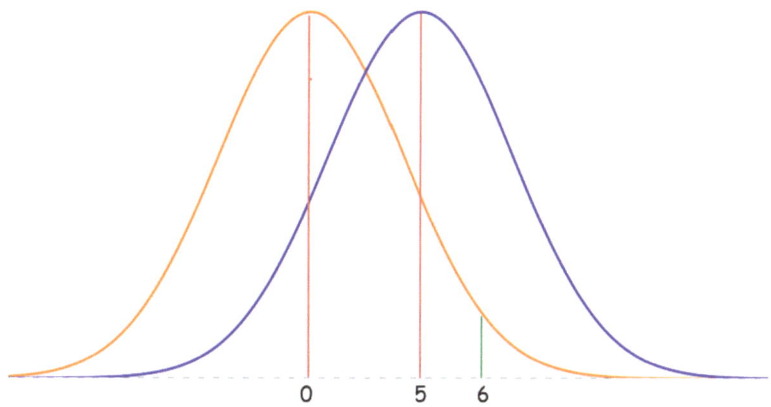

Concentrate first on the orange curve on the left. This is the "null hypothesis curve," which we *assume* is reality (because we don't know the reality when we conduct an experiment!). Note that the mean of the null curve is 0, and for demonstration purposes, the standard deviation is 3. Remember that we have to be to the right of 6 (or to the left of -6) to be in "reject the null" zone. (Why? Because 6 and -6 are 2 standard deviations away from the null value of 0). And now look at the blue curve on the right. This is the *real* "reality" curve. (Of course, we normally do not know what the real "reality" curve is, but in my little demonstration on IQ, we happen to actually know the *real* reality curve). Note that the mean of the reality curve is 5. That is because, in reality, the difference between IQs is 5, so if we run the experiment over and over and plotted our results, we would get the blue normal distribution. But focusing back on the orange curve again and see that a result of 5 is less than the 6 on the orange curve. So even if our result happens to be the most common mean of the reality situation, we have to conclude that it is not statistically significant.

Now let's look graphically at experiment #2, in which there were 50 participants in each group:

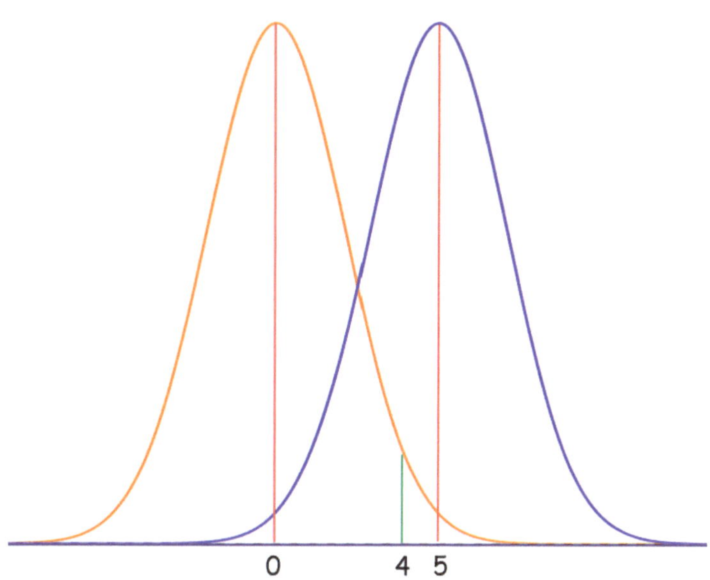

Since we have increased the sample size, you notice that the curves have become thinner because the standard deviations are now smaller (now approximately 2 instead of 3). And now a value of 5 is to the right of the green line, and so is now statistically significant.

So here is the main principle about power: as we increase sample size, it is easier to show statistical significance. With small samples, you need relatively large effect sizes (differences in means). The larger the sample size, the more likely you get a statistically significant result. Hopefully, this makes intuitive sense. If I only tested a small group of students, then a small difference in means is likely just due to chance. For example, if there were 5 students in each group, say, and the difference of means was 5, we would think that the difference of 5 was probably just a random phenomenon, and does not mean that my students on the whole score better. But if we had, say, 500 students in each group, and we got a mean difference of 5, we would think that it is extremely unlikely that a mean difference of 5 just occurred by chance…there really must be a difference in our groups! (But also…if I had just 5 students in each group, and I got a mean difference of say…20 points, I would start to think that there really is a difference!...smaller samples sizes can show statistical significance if the effect size is very large).

Section B4.2: Type II Error

Let's look back at experiment 1 and see what mistake my friend made:

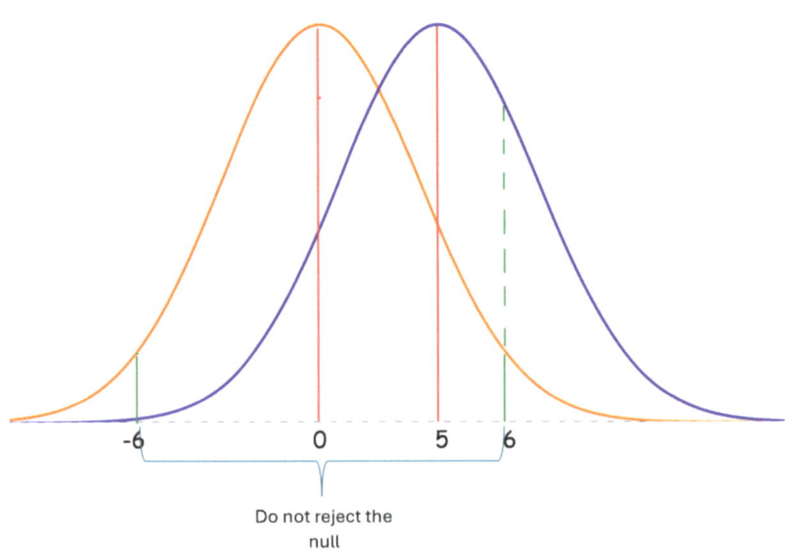

Figure B4.2

Remember we assume the orange curve (the null hypothesis). Our value of 5 was to the left of the green 6, and since the green 6 is two standard deviations away from the null, we had to say that our result of 5 was not statistically significant. So what my friend did, in essence, is he "failed to reject the null hypothesis when he should have." Look at the bracketed portion of the orange curve, which is the area of results in which we cannot reject the null. It goes from -6 to 6 (2 standard deviations below and above the mean of 0). But look at how much of the blue "reality" curve that area from -6 to 6 encompasses. I extended the green line up at 6 to demonstrate. You can see that the entire area under the blue curve that is to the left of the extended green line (all the way to -6) are results that are occurring in reality when we cannot reject the null hypothesis…it is most of our results! So, in reality we know that there is a difference of 5, but if our results in reality fall anywhere between -6 and 6, we have to *erroneously* reject the null hypothesis. We commit what's known as a "Type II error."

Type II error is the probability that we fail to reject the null hypothesis when we should have. You can think of it as a "false negative" error (you thought the result of the study was "negative" that is, no statistically significant difference between groups), but you were wrong!)

Type II error is known as β in the world of biostats.

And **power** is defined as $1 - \beta$, or the probability of *not* committing a type II error.

In the above figure, the β (the probability of failing to reject the null hypothesis when we should have) is the entire area under the blue curve to the left of the green line at value 6, and the power is the remaining area to the right of the green line at value 6. Just by looking at the graph, the power appears to be around 1/3 (or 33%), while the β appears to be about 2/3 (or 67%). So this study is *way* underpowered to detect a mean difference of 5. In fact, this study has only about a 33% chance of detecting a statistically significant result of 6 or greater.

5. Power is defined as 1 minus _____, which is the probability of committing a Type _____ error, which is when we fail to _________________ the null hypothesis when we should have.

Now experiment 2, in which there were 50 participants in each group:

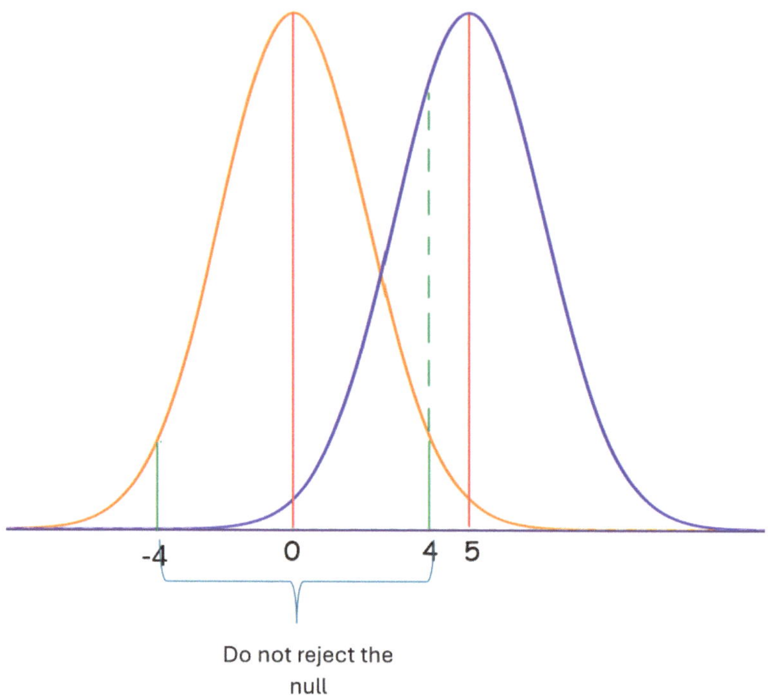

Figure B4.3

This is much better. The β, which is the area under the blue curve to the left of the extended green line is now much smaller, and the power $(1 - \beta)$, which is the area to the right of the extended green line is much larger. So because there are more participants, the power to detect a difference of 5 is much greater. By looking at the graph, it appears that we now have about a 60% chance of detecting a statistically significant difference of 4 or greater.

So far and away, the way to increase the power of a study is to simply increase the number of participants.

The second way to increase power is to increase the effect size. That is, perhaps my friend and I decided that an IQ difference of 7 is necessary to really say there is a difference. What happens if we conducted experiment 1, in which there were only 20 participants in each group, and we happened to show a difference of 7 points between the two groups. Here are results:

Comparison of means calculator

Sample 1

Mean:	134
Standard deviation:	8
Sample size:	20

Sample 2

Mean:	127
Standard deviation:	8
Sample size:	20

OK

Results

Difference	-7.000
Standard error	2.530
95% CI	-12.1214 to -1.8786
t-statistic	-2.767
DF	38
Significance level	P = 0.0087

This is a statistically significant result, even though there were only 20 participants in each group. This makes intuitive sense: A big difference between groups is less likely to be due to chance than is a small difference between groups.

To demonstrate graphically how power increases when one increases effect size, compare experiment 2:

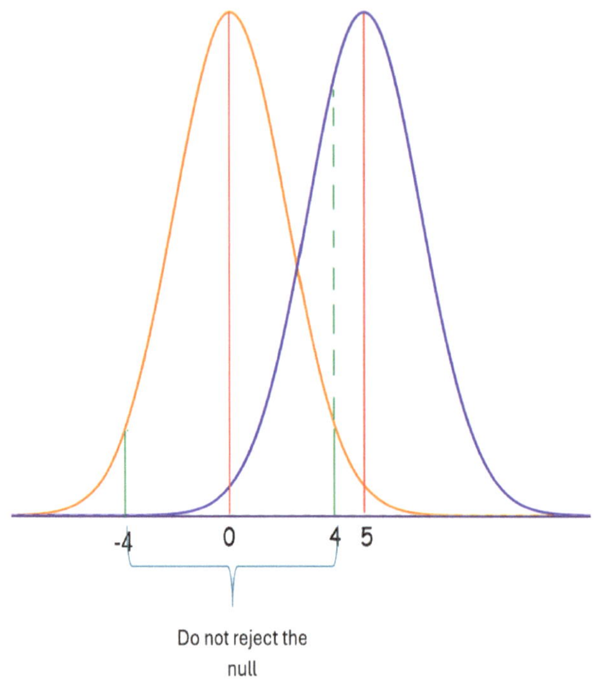

Figure B4.4

With experiment 3 in which we keep the number of participants the same (50 in each group), and therefore the standard deviations of these curves remain the same, but we increase the risk difference (the effect size) from 5 to 7:

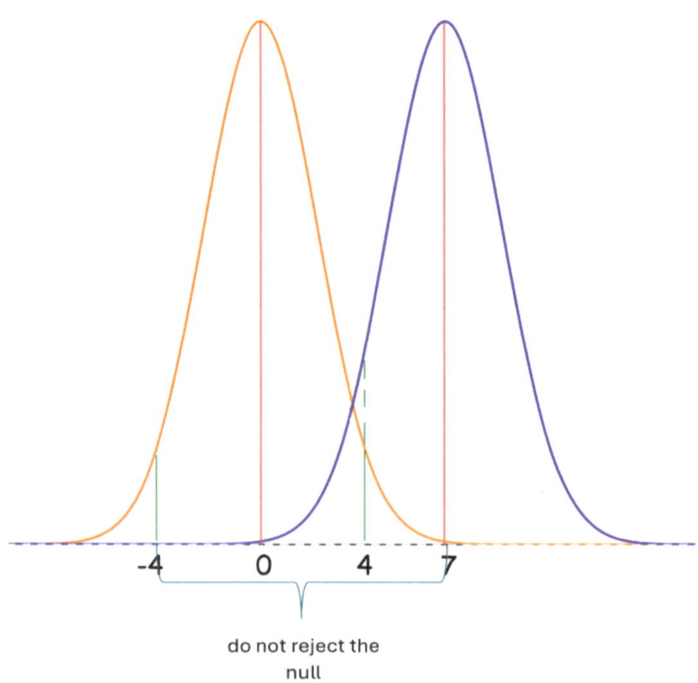

Now you see that the power (the area under the blue curve to the right of the extended green line) is even greater than it was in experiment 2 because we increased the effect size.

Summary thus far

The "power" of a study is the probability that a statistically significant effect size will be found given the *predetermined* effect size and the number of participants in the trial.

We increase power most commonly (by far) by increasing the number of participants.

We can also theoretically increase the power by increasing the effect size.

There is a third theoretical way to increase power, and that is by increasing the α of the study. And that leads me to the next topic.

Section B4.3: Type I Error

The concept of type I error is a bit silly, to be honest, but needs to be discussed as it does relate to power.

Recall that type II error is the probability of committing a "false negative" error—that is, the probability of failing to reject the null hypothesis when we should have rejected the null hypothesis. Or, stated in one more way: the probability of saying there is no statistically significant result when there actually is!

Well the converse also exists: we can make a type I error, which is the probability that we rejected the null hypothesis when we should *not* have.

Let's look again at Figure B4.2:

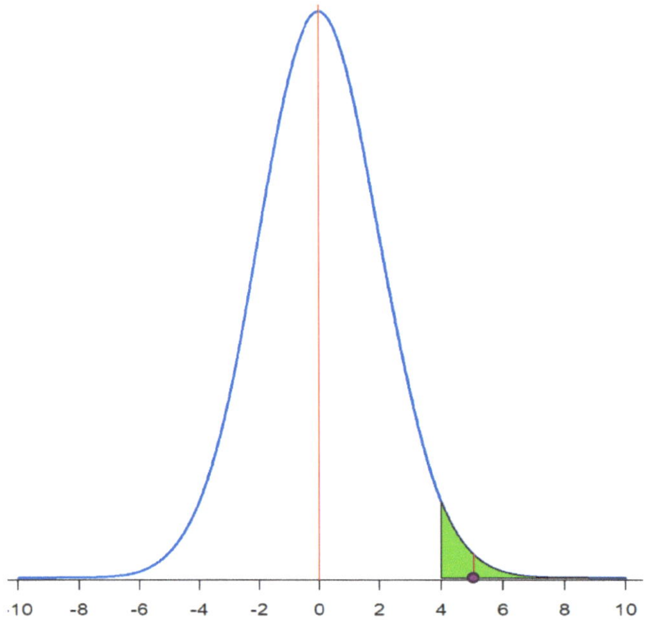

This was experiment 2 in which our result was as mean difference of 5, and we had 50 participants in each group, and our p-value was 0.0038. That means that the probability of a result of 5 occurring by chance is 0.38%. Since this is less than 5%, we reject the null hypothesis and declare a statistically significant result. But of course we could be wrong. Right? Yes of course. There is only a small chance that we are wrong in rejecting the null hypothesis, and that chance is…0.38%. So our Type I error probability is 0.38%. So the probability of committing a type I error is whatever our p-value is!

6. Type I error is the probability that we ______________________________ the null hypothesis when we should ____________ have.

The probability, then of committing a type I error is less than or equal to whatever we set our α to. (Recall that the α is what our cutoff is for rejecting the null hypothesis: by convention, this is almost always set at 0.05, or 5%). So it's indeed a bit silly to talk about Type I error, except to show how it's interrelated with Type II error.

Let's say we (for whatever reason) decided to increase our α. That is, we are accepting a larger possibility of rejecting that null hypothesis when we should not have. We increase this from the standard of 0.05 to, say 0.10. What would happen to our graph of figure B4.4?

Here is again figure B4.4:

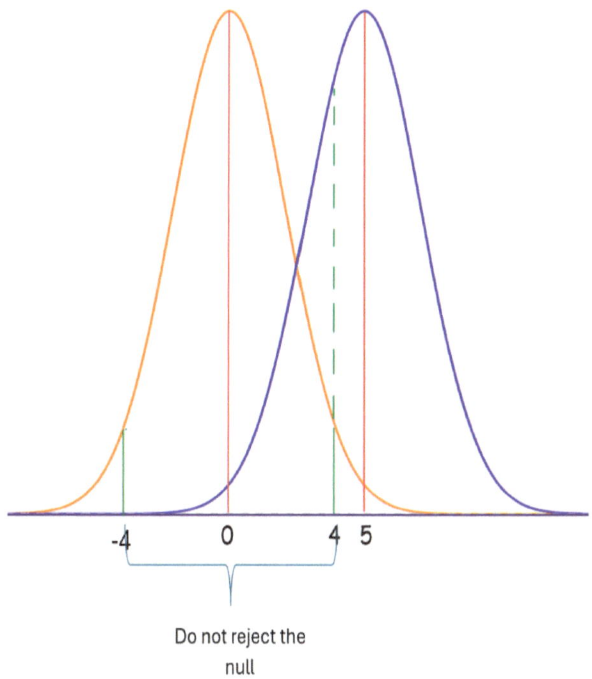

Remember that the β, which is the probability of making a Type II error, is everything under the blue curve to the left of the extended green line. But now we set our α to a higher value:

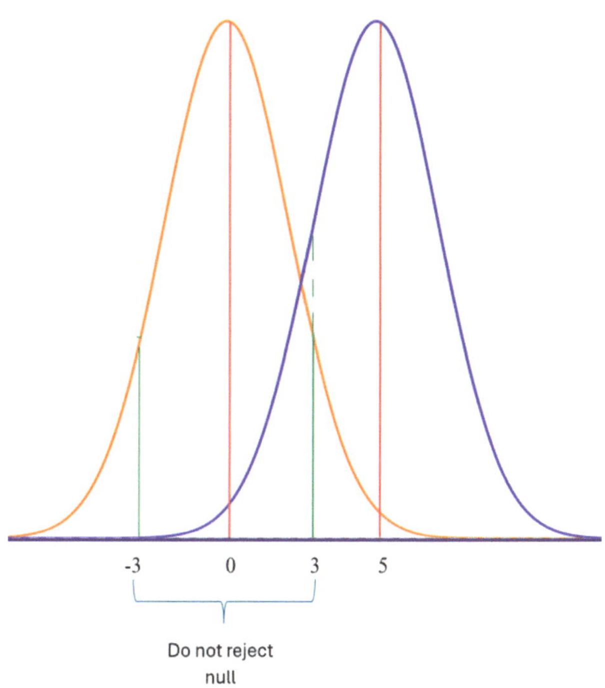

Now the "do not reject the null" area is narrowed, from -3 and so the extended green line has moved to the left, and so the β is less. And since power is $1 - \beta$, the power increases.

So that is the third way to increase power: by increasing the α. And this makes intuitive sense: Think back to our initial aspirin study from 1979, in which the p-value was 0.13, so the authors did not reject the null hypothesis. But what if, for whatever reason, the authors increased the industry standard of α from 0.05 to, say 0.15? Well then, the p-value of 0.13 would be considered statistically significant! So giving themselves a higher threshold for committing type-I error also *decreases* their chance of committing a type-II error. The two are very dependent on one another.

Summary and principles thus far

The "power" of a study is the probability that a statistically significant effect size will be found given the predetermined effect size and the number of participants in the trial.

A large sample size has more power to detect smaller effect sizes. Only relatively large effect sizes will show statistically significant results if sample sizes are small.

We increase power most commonly (by far) by increasing the number of participants.

We can also theoretically increase the power by increasing the effect size. (But this would be unusual, because normally the researchers first determine the "clinically significant" effect size before starting the experiment).

There is a third theoretical way to increase power, and that is by increasing the α of the study. But this would be highly unusual, because the industry standard of the α level is taken to be 0.05.

Section B4.4: Putting it all together

Power is a very important concept in contemporary medical literature, because researchers must first determine how many participants they need to enroll. Remember, as we enroll more participants in our trial, we incur greater expense and logistical difficulties, but we improve the quality of the study on many levels, not the least of which is that researchers are more likely to get a statistically significant result as shown above. So researchers must first decide on a clinically significant result, and then recruit enough people so that there will be enough power to detect that particular result. The industry standard usually sets power at 80%. That is, they want to enroll enough people so that they have an 80% chance of showing statistical significance for whatever *clinically significant* effect size they have decided on. And there is an equation for this, of course, which is worthwhile to examine a bit, but not to memorize, as there are calculators readily available!

Here is the formula:

$$n_1 = 2\left\{\frac{\left(Z_{1-\frac{\alpha}{2}} + Z_{1-\beta}\right)}{ES}\right\}^2$$

Let's discuss these things. n_i is the number in the sample of each group that is needed. The Z is our old friend the "z-score," or how many standard deviations away from the mean we need to be for statistical significance. The first Z is the Z we set our α value to… you know, 1.96 (I have been using 2 thus far). (Remember that 1.96 (or 2…close enough!...is the amount of standard deviations away from the mean (on either side) to get 95% of all the results included). The $Z_{1-\beta}$ thing: OK, well, 1− β is the "power" of the study. Usually, we want a Power of 80%. (That means there is a 20% chance we commit a Type II error). So, anyway, just as the Z for 0.05 is 1.96, I will tell you that the Z value for .2 is 0.84. And, if you get braver and choose a β of 90%, the Z value for this is 1.282. And what is ES? It is the "effect size, and is defined as:

$$ES = \frac{|p_1 - p_2|}{\sqrt{p(1-p)}}$$

And what is p? It is the "overall proportion." What is that? Well, what proportion might we expect will have an event? In the aspirin study, we might happen to know that approximately 15% of patients will die within a year of having a heart attack. How about p_1 and p_2? Well, these are what we are hoping to show in our experiment. Let's say (to be consistent with our current example) that we are hoping to show there is a 2.5% difference. So p_1 would be 15%, and p_2 would be 12.5% . Then, the p, or the "overall proportion" is the average of p_1 and p_2. So in our example it is 13.75%.

So,

$$ES = \frac{.025}{\sqrt{.1375(1-.1375)}} = 0.073 \quad \text{And } n_1 = 2\left(\frac{1.96+0.84}{0.073}\right)^2 = 2{,}942$$

So, we need 2942 people in each group to ensure that the experiment will have 80% power to detect a 2.5% difference in the proportions (with an α level of 0.05).

So then, once the clinically significant effect size is chosen, the researchers use the above formulas to come up with the number in each group that would be required to give them an 80% Power. 80% is generally accepted as a power cut off. With an 80% power, there is still a 20% chance that the experiment will result in a "false negative", in which it appears as if there is no significant difference in the groups, and the null hypothesis is proven. But again, just like an alpha level of 0.05, a beta level of 0.2 (Power of 80%) has generally been accepted in the world of statistics for many years. You may notice that it is less stringent then the alpha level. The reason for this is as follows: An accepted P value of 0.05 ensures that the researchers have to very aggressively prove that there is a significant difference between the two groups. And this overall is a good thing. In general, we are talking about some new experimental drug. Before we spend billions of dollars producing it, we really need to be sure that the difference in the two groups is truly statistically significant, and so we set the bar very high and we only allow a 5% chance that we are wrong. On the other hand, well, we are not so stringent on *negative* results. If we say there is no effect of the drug, then there is a 20% chance that we are wrong. But it seems best to err on this side, rather than declaring falsely that there is truly a significant result! (Of course, as you can imagine, the pharmaceutical industry would like to think otherwise!)

Biostats 5: Non-inferiority trials ("Me too!")

In this chapter, I will describe the ever-increasing phenomenon of "non-inferiority" studies/testing. In these studies, one drug (or treatment) is compared to another drug (or treatment) rather than the drug or treatment being compared to a placebo. Usually the purpose of these studies is to see if a new drug (a "me-too" drug) or treatment is as effective as an old established drug or treatment, thus allowing, of course, a whole new potential market for a pharmaceutical company. And so, as you can imagine, non-inferiority studies might be the most vulnerable to "fudging," as the profit-driven pharmaceutical industry is hyper-anxious about jumping on any existing money-making bandwagons.

In a way, non-inferiority testing is the opposite of the statistical analyses I have presented thus far, because with non-inferiority testing, the researchers are trying to prove that there is *no* difference between the two arms of the study, rather than all of the other types of studies, in which the researchers are trying to prove the opposite, that there *is* a statistically significant difference in the two treatment arms. The "null hypothesis," which the researchers hope to be able to reject with confidence, up until now has meant that there is "no difference in the treatment arms," now means that there "*is* a difference in the treatment arms."

1. The "null hypothesis" in non-inferiority trials is that there ________ a difference between the treatment arms.

The first thing that happens is that the researchers define an "non-inferiority margin," often referred to as δ (delta), and also often referred to as "M" for "margin" or "NI" for non-inferiority margin. The researchers take a well-known, established drug, which is the "active control," and the efficacy of which is referred to as C. And they have their new "me-too" drug, the efficacy of which is called T. They desire to show that the efficacy of their new drug, T, is similar in efficacy to the established control drug: that is, they want C minus T has to be small—specifically less than M. Thus, to prove non-inferiority, $C–T < M$.

2. To prove non-inferiority, researchers try to show that the efficacy of the old established treatment, C minus the efficacy of their new treatment, T is __________ than M.

Now the weird part is that M is chosen by the researchers somewhat randomly, and this is where all the controversy and difficulty and "fudgeability" etc. of non-inferiority trials arise. More on this later. At any rate, once the M is chosen, and the head-to-head experiment of new drug vs active control is concluded, the researchers conduct a statistical test. The statistical test is to determine if the C–T experimental results are close to M. For example, let's say the established cholesterol drug "Super-statin" has been shown in the past to lower cholesterol by 30%. The researchers are testing their new drug "Me-too-statin" and decide that if this drug lowers cholesterol by 25% or more, then (in their minds), it is "non-inferior." Thus, their "M" or "δ" or "NI" is 5%. Then they compare the two drugs head-to-head. They find that C was 31.3%. (That means, the active control drug lowered cholesterol by 31.3%), and they find that T was, say 28.2%. (That means that Me-too-statin lowered cholesterol by 28.2%). C–T then equals 3.1%. But of course, you know very well that only the 95% confidence intervals mean anything, so they would have to report the 95% confidence interval of this difference. They might report the difference (C–T) is 3.1% with a 95% confidence interval from 2.6% to 5.3%. With these results, then, the researchers have *not* proven non-inferiority. Because the 95% confidence interval crosses M, they have failed in their noble quest.

3. Since, in this example, the upper limit of the confidence interval was more than the pre-specified ______, the researchers could not conclude non-inferiority.

But if their results were: C–T is 3.1% with a 95% confidence interval of *2.6% to 4.8%,* then C–T is "truly" less than M, and they *have* proved non-inferiority, and they laugh all the way to the bank.

4. Now the upper limit of the confidence interval is _________ than the pre-specified value of M, and so the researchers happily conclude ________________________.

So here is the wiggly reality of M, the difference in the two efficacies. The researchers themselves determine what this value should be. In this study, they could theoretically pick an M as high as 30%. That would of course be the largest possible value they could pick, and I know it seems silly, but important to talk about for reasons that will shortly become clear. If M is chosen to be 30%, then all the study has to show is that T is greater than 0, and you would have non-inferiority. For example, the C in the new study ends up being, say 32% (it lowered cholesterol by 32%), and the T in the study was, say 4% (it lowered cholesterol by only 4%). Well, C–T = 28%, which is less than the M of 30%, and so, non-inferiority is proven! And so that is an extreme example of choosing the largest M possible (the same as the known efficacy of the control drug). In that case, all the new drug has to do is show some efficacy (even lowering cholesterol by a little bit), and we have non-inferiority.

The established efficacy of the control drug or treatment is referred to as M_1. Any researcher worth his or her weight should know that *just proving efficacy* is not at all the same as proving non-inferiority, *so they would be crazy to choose an M equal to M_1.* Indeed, declaring that that Me-too-statin was non-inferior to Super-statin just because Me-too-statin lowers cholesterol by only 4% would be to nearly wipe out the effect of Super-statin! (That is, if the market would "accept" the new drug Me-too-statin, then the market would have to accept that a 4% reduction is just as good as a 30% reduction!)

So a good researcher chooses an M that is considerably smaller than M_1, and this is referred to as M_2. In our above example, M_2 was chosen to be 5%. That is quite reasonable. The researchers state that if C–T is < M_2, then we have established non-inferiority, as described above.

> M_1 is the effect of the active control drug as proven in past placebo-controlled studies
>
> M_2 is the largest clinically acceptable difference between the new test drug and the known active control drug (the NI margin, or the δ)

In our example, we picked an M_2 of 5%, which was actually commendable. In general, if an M_2 is about *half* of M_1, it is considered pretty good (at least in the cardiovascular studies).

You can imagine that the choosing of M_2 is truly the linchpin of these studies. And while the researchers are free to choose whatever value for this they would like, there certainly are standards and methods that are described by the FDA (which has done a good job guiding the industry on this, in their attempt to prevent the potential unfettered nature of these "Me-too" studies) that guide the choices.

Analyzing data from NI studies

There are two accepted methods to analyze the data from non-inferiority studies: "fixed margin" and "synthesis." In the fixed margin method, M_1 is chosen based on prior studies of the control drug compared to placebo, usually by applying meta-analysis to those studies. The end of the 95% confidence interval that is closest to the null hypothesis is chosen as the M_1. For example, in our example of Super-statin vs Me-too-stain, we know from the literature that Super-statin lowered cholesterol by 30% vs placebo. We arrived at that 30% by doing a meta-analysis on the five trials that compared Super-statin with placebo. And that gave us 30%, with a 95% confidence interval from 27.2% to 33.5%. Therefore, we would choose 27.2% as our M_1, as it is closer to the null hypothesis (i.e. closer to no difference between Super-statin and placebo).

5. We get our M_1 by combining all the results from previous trials that compared the old standby treatment with ______________. We specifically use the end of the confidence interval that is closest to the ________ _____________________, that is, closest to no difference between the two.

And then the M_2 is chosen usually at around 50% of the M_1 for cardiovascular studies. (But always remember that the criteria and guidelines for the choosing of M_2 are *very* controversial). A great example from the medical literature was from the 1990s when the makers of a new thrombolytic agent, reteplase, decided to compare it head-to-head with the existing standard-of-care thrombolytic agent, streptokinase, in the treatment of acute myocardial infarction.

(Randomized double-blind comparison of reteplase double-bolus administration with streptokinase in acute myocardial infarction. (INJECT): trial to investigate equivalence. *Lancet* 1995: 346; 329-36)

I remember practicing Emergency Medicine at the time. Streptokinase and Alteplase were two thrombolytics that were commonly used. Streptokinase was not patented and therefore very inexpensive, and Alteplase was patented and very expensive. The Reteplase makers wanted in, too. Well so in this study, the researchers commented on a meta-analysis comparing thrombolytics with placebo in the treatment of acute myocardial infarction, and found that compared with placebo, thrombolytics offered a benefit of 2.7% (fewer deaths with thrombolytics). The lower boundary of the 95% confidence interval was 2.1%. So the researchers considered 2.1% their M_1.

6. The researchers chose 2.1% as their M_1 because it is the end of the confidence interval closest to the null hypothesis, meaning ___ _____________ between thrombolytics and placebo.

They then took 50% of that and declared 1.05% to be their M_2, or their non-inferiority margin. So, they declared that in their head-to-head matchup, if reteplase performed within 1.05% of streptokinase, it is non-inferior. (Or more precisely stated, the *upper boundary* of the 95% confidence interval had to be less than 1.05%.) Indeed, the results showed that there was a difference of –0.51% with a 95% confidence interval from –1.74% to 0.73%. Since the upper limit, 0.73%, is less than 1.05%, non-inferiority was successfully proven, and the product was approved by the FDA, and the makers of reteplase laughed all the way to the bank. (But we never used it much in the ED because we were too used to using either streptokinase or alteplase. haha.)

In 2005, AstraZeneca tried really hard to have their new anticoagulant medication ximelagatran approved for use to help prevent stroke in patients with atrial fibrillation. And so they conducted a non-inferiority trial of ximelagatran vs the old standby, warfarin. Here is a quote from their statistical analysis section:

(Albers, et al. Ximelagatran vs warfarin for stroke prevention in patients with nonvalvular atrial fibrillation: a randomized trial. JAMA. 2005 Feb 9;293(6):690-8. doi: 10.1001/jama.293.6.690.)

"The objective was to establish whether ximelagatran was noninferior[23] to warfarin within an absolute margin of 2.0% per year for the difference in rates of primary events.[14,24] This margin was based on the expected rate during warfarin therapy and a prespecified judgment about

clinically meaningful difference. The criteria required that the upper bound of the 1-sided 97.5% confidence interval (CI) for the difference in event rates not exceed 2.0% per year

And so you see they chose as their M_2 a value of 2.0%. That is, if the endpoint of the study (stroke or systemic thromboembolic disease) in patients taking ximelgatran was within 2.0% of those events that occurred in patients taking warfarin, then the researchers would claim non-inferiority. At first glance, this does not seem unreasonable. If you review the studies done in the late 80's and early 90's that compared warfarin with placebo, you find that there is a difference of about, say 2% to 5%. That is, say 6% of those on placebo might experience a stroke while, say 2% of those on warfarin would. And then they ran the NI study, head-to-head vs warfarin, and came up with the following results:

"primary events occurred in 37 patients assigned to receive warfarin and 51 patients assigned to receive ximelagatran, corresponding to incidence rates of 1.16% and 1.61% per year, respectively (p = .13 for a difference between treatments)"

OK, so the difference between the two groups was 1.61–1.16 = .45%. But of course, as in all studies, a particular number is meaningless unless it is accompanied by a 95% confidence interval. And here it is:

Table 2. Rates of Primary and Secondary Events According to Assigned Treatment*

	No. (%) of Patients (Event Rate, % per Patient-Year)			
	Ximelagatran (n = 1960)	Warfarin (n = 1962)	Difference (95% CI)	P Value
Intention to treat				
Primary events	51 (1.6)	37 (1.2)	0.45 (−0.13 to 1.0)	.13
Ischemic stroke	45 (1.4)	36 (1.1)†		
Hemorrhagic stroke	2 (0.1)	2 (0.1)		
Systemic embolism	6 (0.2)	1 (0.03)		
Primary event or death	153 (4.8)	151 (4.7)	0.10 (−0.97 to 1.2)	.86
Mortality	116 (3.6)	123 (3.8)		
Fatal stroke or fatal systemic embolism	10 (0.3)	3 (0.1)		
Fatal stroke	10 (0.3)	3 (0.1)		
Fatal hemorrhagic stroke	2 (0.1)	0		
Fatal or disabling stroke	16 (0.5)	10 (0.3)	0.19 (−0.12 to 0.50)	.25
Nonfatal disabling stroke	6 (0.2)	7 (0.2)		
On-treatment model				
Primary events	41 (1.6)	28 (1.0)	0.55 (−0.06 to 1.2)	.09
Transient ischemic attack	30 (1.2)	24 (0.9)		
Myocardial infarction	26 (1.0)	37 (1.4)		
Composite of mortality, stroke, systemic embolism, and myocardial infarction	110 (4.2)	119 (4.3)	−0.13 (−1.2 to 0.98)	.84
Composite of ischemic stroke, systemic embolism, and transient ischemic attack	67 (2.6)	52 (1.9)	0.66 (−0.14 to 1.5)	.12
Major extracerebral bleeding	63 (2.4)	84 (3.1)	−0.66 (−1.6 to 0.23)	.15
Subdural hematoma	5 (0.19)	7 (0.25)	−0.06 (−0.32 to 0.19)	.78
Minor bleeding	715 (36)	854 (44)	−8.4 (−12.4 to −4.4)	<.001
Major or minor bleeding	737 (37)	903 (47)	−10 (−14 to −6.0)	<.001

Abbreviation: CI, confidence interval.
*Differences calculated only for prespecified end points. No patient was counted more than once for each composite end point.
†One patient who had 2 ischemic stroke events is counted once in this table.

Top line: you see the difference of .45% with 95% confidence interval from –.13 to 1.0. The authors therefore state:

"The upper bound of the 95% confidence interval (CI) surrounding the difference of 0.45% per year was 1.03, well below the specified margin of 2.0% per year."

So they seemed to do the proper thing and take the upper limits of the confidence interval (1.03) and report happily that that is below their chosen M_2 of 2.0%. They have (in their minds) achieved non-inferiority.

"Not so fast," said the FDA, who actually used this particular study to demonstrate to researchers how to properly conduct a non-inferiority trial. This document was published in November of 2016, titled:

Non-inferiority Clinical Trials to Establish Effectiveness Guidance for Industry.

I would like to go through in some detail what the FDA taught us, as it incorporates the main gist of this chapter, as well as some other statistical techniques touched upon earlier in this book.

The first and probably the most important step in a non-inferiority study is establishing the M_1, and from it, the M_2. The researchers must review all the studies that had been done that established how well warfarin did compared to placebo. (Or they could use a well-designed meta-analysis if one were available. In this case a meta-analysis was not available). And so the researchers chose, somewhat randomly I might add, around 4% as their M_1. They did not specifically say this, but since their M_2 was 2%, and assuming they are using the 50% rule (that M_2 is normally considered about half of M_1) then we can guess that M_1 was assumed to be around 4%. But the FDA article points out to them the exact method by which they *should have* arrived at their M_1 and M_2. As no meta-analysis was available, they should have done their own, based on the six studies that were already out there comparing warfarin with placebo. Had they done that, as the FDA did, they would have discovered that the Relative Risk of warfarin vs placebo in preventing stroke or thromboembolic disease was .361 (thus favoring warfarin), with a 95% confidence interval spanning from .248 to .527. The proper thing then to do would have been to take the upper limit of the 95% confidence interval (the limit that is closest to the null hypothesis) in this case .527, and should have been their M_1.

7. Sorry, researchers: no cheating on picking your M_1. Look at all pre-existing literature, and do a ____________ ______________ of the results!

And their M_2 should have been half of this. But a little bit of math first. Remember that relative risk is a ratio, and whenever we are dealing with ratios, we must use the logarithm scale. So, first we take $ln(0.527) = -0.64$. Then $-0.64/2 = -0.32$. Then the antilog of $-0.32 =$ **0.726**. This is the M_2, or the non-inferiority margin that the researchers *should* have chosen if they were good researchers.

Now let's look at the numbers in the trial, as portrayed in table 2 above. 51 events occurred in the ximelagatran group, while 37 events occurred in the warfarin group. So let's first calculate the relative risk of warfarin vs. ximelagatran.

$$RR = \frac{37/_{1962}}{51/_{1960}} = \mathbf{0.72}.$$

Then, we can calculate the 95% confidence interval of this, because we know that in statistics, one value means nothing without its confidence interval. How do we do that? (Refer to section B3.4). The SE for a relative risk is give by:

$$\widehat{SE}(\ln(RR)) = \sqrt{\frac{1}{a} + \frac{1}{a+b} + \frac{1}{c} + \frac{1}{c+d}}$$

$$\widehat{SE}(\ln(0.72)) = \sqrt{\frac{1}{37} + \frac{1}{37+1925} + \frac{1}{51} + \frac{1}{51+1909}} = 0.218$$

So, $SE(-0.33) = 0.218$. And so the 95% CI is $-0.33 \pm 2(0.218)$

and this is –0.77 to 0.11. But remember, we are in "natural log world" so we have to take the *antilog* of these, by raising e to these exponents:

$$e^{-0.77}\ to\ e^{.0.11} = 0.\mathbf{46\ to\ 1.12.}$$

So, our Risk ratio is **0.72 with 95% confidence interval from 0.46 to 1.12**. This means that warfarin performed better than ximelagatran by a factor of anywhere from 0.46 to 1.12, with the point estimate of 0.72. Remember that you always have to take the worse end of your confidence interval, in this case 1.12. In order for them to demonstrate non-inferiority, that number, the 1.12, would have to be less than the correct M_2 of 0.726, which it clearly is not.

The researchers continued their guise by including this nice Kaplan-Meier curve, worth taking a peak at. (I will discuss Kaplan-Meier curves in great detail in chapter B8, but for now just know that if the p-value of the curves is > 0.05, it means that there is no statistical difference between the two arms, even though the curves visually appear to be different). As you can see, ximelagatran does not do as well as warfarin, but the p = .13 here means that although the curves appear to be different, they are actually the same, statistically speaking.

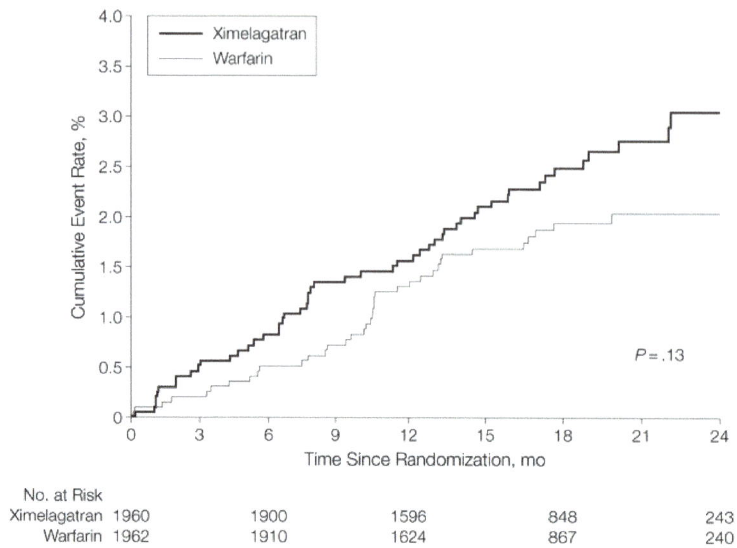

So, ximelagatran has to be non-inferior, right? **Wrong**. And that is the great deception of non-inferiority trials. The p-value of .13 here just tells that that warfarin is *not superior* to ximelagatran in a statistically significant way. Although that was our thinking in all the conventional statistical methods that I have discussed thus far, when you are living in the world of non-inferiority, you have to turn your brain upside-down a bit, and remember that proving that A is not superior to B is *not the same* as proving that B is non-inferior to A. It's just not. And so the Kaplan-Meier curves they included were meaningless and misleading.

8. The log-rank test of Kaplan-Meier curves tells us if one thing is statistically-significantly ______________ to the other thing, but does not tell us anything about non- ______________.

There is another method that the FDA likes even more than their "fixed margin" method, and it is referred to as the "synthesis" method. In the synthesis method, the confidence interval that was derived in the NI study itself is adjusted to account for the variability of the efficacy of the control drug. It is a bit fancy and somewhat complex, but worth discussing. The synthesis method does not use the separate 95% confidence intervals (one from the old studies that compared the control drug vs placebo, and one from the new NI study), and so it does not specifically state an M_1. But it does tell us if the new drug succeeds in being at least 50% effective as the old stand-by, while also telling us if the new drug is superior to placebo, had there been a placebo arm in the new NI study. What?? Yes, I know. The synthesis method is elegant, and rather esoteric in that it combines the data from the placebo-controlled trials of the old stand-by drug (warfarin in our case) with the data in the new NI study in such a way that a p-value can be calculated that gives us the significance level of whether or not the new drug retained 50% of the effectiveness of the old stand-by.

9. The FDA also likes the "synthesis method," which is probably even better than the "fixed margin" method because it takes into account the ______________ in data from all the studies.

The formula used for the z-score for this is as follows:

$$\frac{RR_{NI} + (RR_P)\frac{1}{2}}{\sqrt{\left([SE_{NI}]^2 + \frac{1}{2}[SE_P]^2\right)}}$$

Don't freak over this; the basic idea is that the bottom half of the fraction takes into account the standard errors of the data from the studies, so this is the "adjustment" made for the differences in the data from all the studies. The top half is sort of like the null hypothesis…recall that we need to prove that the Relative risk of the new NI trial is greater than half the RR of the established placebo-controlled trials (RR_P). We can actually plug all the numbers in: The RR_{NI} was 0.72. (But remember, RR only works when dealing with log scale, so we need to take the ln of everything! *ln*(0.72) = -0.33. RR_p we said was .361 (from the meta-analysis of the prior studies), and *ln*(0.361) = -1.019. The Standard errors we can calculate. SE_{NI} = .216, and SE_P = 0.154.

Plug everything into the crazy z-score equation above and you end up with **–0.58**. Now that we have the z-score, we can just plug it into a calculator to get the p-value. You will see that $p >$ 0.05, meaning we *cannot reject the null hypothesis.* And remember that in non-inferiority studies, the null hypothesis states that there *is* a difference. So if we cannot reject this; we have not established non-inferiority.

Well the point of these two exercises is that with either method that the FDA likes, the fixed margin method or the synthesis method, the researchers in the ximelagatran vs. warfarin trial did not prove non-inferiority despite their claim, and so the product was not approved for the prevention of stroke for patients in atrial fibrillation. Sorry, guys. Nice try.

Number of participants

Recall that in all "normal" studies (not these crazy non-inferiority studies), the researchers want the studies to include as many participants as possible. That is so they can avoid the Type II error of failing to see a difference between their drug, and say, placebo, because the study was "underpowered" to detect a difference. Well, the opposite is true with non-inferiority trials. The fewer the participants, the more likely the researchers will be able to show non-inferiority when there truly is *not* non-inferiority. And, of course, the larger they set the non-inferiority margin, the easier it is for them to prove non-inferiority. As they increase the M (or δ), they decrease the number of patients needed…but as they increase M they also weaken the strength of the study itself.

10. In non-inferiority trials, if the researchers do not include enough participants, it will be _______________ to demonstrate non-inferiority.

And so the researchers must take all this into account when calculating sample size, and they are tempted to have a smaller sample size (less money, and easier to prove non-inferiority) at the risk of weaker evidence. There are statistical formulas that guide the researchers in picking the number of participants for the trial, just like for "normal" i.e. superiority studies, and I encourage you to review Biostats 4 which described Type I and II errors, and Power. In superiority trials, a power of 80% was considered acceptable, in general, allowing for a 20% chance of a "falsely negative" result, i.e. that their experiment appears to show no benefit of the treatment, when there actually is a benefit. In non-inferiority trials a type I error is falsely concluding non-inferiority when in fact the new treatment is actually inferior, and Power is the probability of correctly concluding non-inferiority when the new treatment is indeed non-inferior. And so when you read a non-inferiority trial, be sure to look for words along these lines:

Assuming that 5% of patients would discontinue the trial, we calculated that the enrollment of 425 patients in each group would provide the trial with 85% power to show noninferiority of the new treatment at a one-sided alpha level of 0.025.

"Intention-to-Treat"

I discussed this in detail in chapter E2, but it is an especially big deal in non-inferiority trials. Recall that in experimental trials, participants often drop out of their treatment protocols. In Intention-to-treat analyses, these people are analyzed as if they remained in their assigned group, while in "per-protocol" analyses, they are analyzed depending on what treatment they actually received. In intention-to treat-analyses, as more and more participants drop out of their treatment protocols, the difference of results in the two arms is diminished. For the normal superiority trials, like say drug vs placebo, this is usually not too much of a big deal (for the general public, that is!) because non-adherence only means a diminished positive effect of the drug compared to placebo, and the researchers will be less likely to conclude that their new drug is superior to placebo. But in non-inferiority trials, this reality is more problematic because as the effect size difference diminishes and as the two treatment arms approach each other, non-inferiority becomes easier to prove!

11. Be careful with ___________________ ____ _________ trials; they can problematic in non-inferiority trials.

But as I discussed in Epidemiology 2, the per-protocol approach is also far from perfect as considerable bias is introduced with this analysis. And I mentioned that in general the FDA favors intention-to-treat analyses over per-protocol analyses, but in non-inferiority studies they tend to lean more in favor of the per-protocol approach. Suffice it to say, I think, that if the researchers predict that there will be a greater than 5% dropout, they should include *both* results in their analysis. And even better would be if the researchers, when reporting their per-protocol results, adjust their results based on some of the new methods, such as "inverse probability weighting," which estimates an individual's probability of adhering to a particular arm given observed confounders, and uses the predicted probability as a weight to inflate or deflate the individual's influence on the overall treatment effect in the group.

> *(Mansournia MA, Altman DG. Inverse probability weighting. BMJ2016;352:i189. doi:10.1136/bmj.i189 pmid:26773001)*

Summary of Biostats 5

Non-inferiority trials are becoming more and more commonplace, and are probably the least trustworthy of all the trial methods. We must be careful when reading and analyzing them. We must make sure the researchers have chosen a valid non-inferiority margin and explained how they arrived at it. We must make sure they didn't "cheat" by having too few patients; we must make sure they used both "intention-to-treat" and "per-protocol" numbers (at the very least), and we must make sure they use the proper "fixed-margin" or "synthesis" method to do their calculations. In general, we must remember to look at every non-inferiority trial in a somewhat jaded way, as there are often grotesquely huge amounts of money for the pharmaceutical company riding on just a little bit of fudging here and there.

Epidemiology 4: Bias

One of the main goals of epidemiologic research is to explore the association between an exposure and an outcome. Mainly, of course, we are interested in the possibility that the exposure may be a *cause* of the outcome. Or, if the exposure happens to be a preventive measure, like for example an exercise program to prevent heart disease, we are interested in the possibility that the exposure actually *causes a reduction* in the outcome. If we observe a significant association between the exposure and the outcome, it is possible that the exposure is *causing* (or at least part of a causal mechanism) of the outcome. (Or, if we are conducting a cross-sectional study, the outcome may be causing the exposure). Here are the four possibilities that might be explaining an apparent association between an exposure and an outcome:

THE EXPOSURE ACTUALLY **CAUSES** THE OUTCOME

CHANCE

CONFOUNDING

BIAS

Chance

As discussed in previous chapters, we need to rule out chance as the explanation for the apparent association. This is what all of our hypothesis testing is for…we need first to be able to say that our association, although it may have occurred by chance, was *very unlikely* to have occurred by chance.

Confounding

As discussed in previous chapters, the apparent association between an exposure and an outcome may be false if the association was actually due to the presence of other factors known as confounders that are messing up our results.

And then there's **BIAS**, which is the subject of this chapter.

Bias basically refers to errors in the inherent design of the study, or of the collection of the data, that leads to a systemic deviation from the truth. That is, even if chance has been essentially ruled out, and confounding has been eliminated (or at least minimized), there is still something *inherently* wrong about our study that prevents us from drawing our desired conclusion of a true association. Because bias is much more of an issue in *observational* studies than it is in experimental studies, this chapter is written with attention to observational studies.

There are basically 2 broad classifications of bias: *information bias* and *selection bias*

Section E4.1: Information Bias: Introduction

Information bias simply means that our methods of obtaining data about our participants are flawed, so that the information about exposure and/or outcome is inaccurate. Measurement techniques in medicine are never perfect. We may, for example, be researching the possible relationship between the percentage of body fat and the development of heart disease. Unfortunately, the methods used to measure body fat are notoriously inaccurate. Indeed, the only way to *accurately* measure body fat is to dissect a cadaver, take out the fat, and weigh it! Since we hope that we are not doing that in our research, we are limited by indirect measurement methods (calipers etc.) that are far from perfect, and we may be left with false criteria for deciding who is in the "low body fat" group and who is in the "high body fat" group. Or, we may have inaccuracies in measuring the outcome: again, short of cadaver dissection, we are left with indirect measures such exercise stress testing, which is far from perfect in determining the presence of cardiac disease.

It is important to understand that information bias can work in either direction: it can create an apparent association when no such association actually exists, or it can create a lack of apparent association when one actually exists.

1. Although we tend to think of "bias" meaning a systemic error that creates an apparent association when there really is none, information bias can actually do the opposite: it can make an actual ______________________________ disappear.

So since information bias occurs by erroneous methods of measurement, we often see the term "measurement bias" used interchangeably with "information bias." And (in case that is not confusing enough), we also see the terms "misclassification bias" used…since ultimately our measurement error causes us to misclassify participants, either with respect to their exposure status, or with respect to their outcomes. And if *that* is not confusing enough, the misclassification of participants can either occur *randomly,* in which case it affects both groups approximately equally, or it can affect one group more than the other. The former case is referred to **"non-differential misclassification**," and the latter case is referred to as **"differential misclassification."** Although differential misclassification appears to more strictly meet the definition of bias (because one group is affected more than the other), non-differential misclassification is also a bias, because it affects our association, as will be shown below).

So, to review:

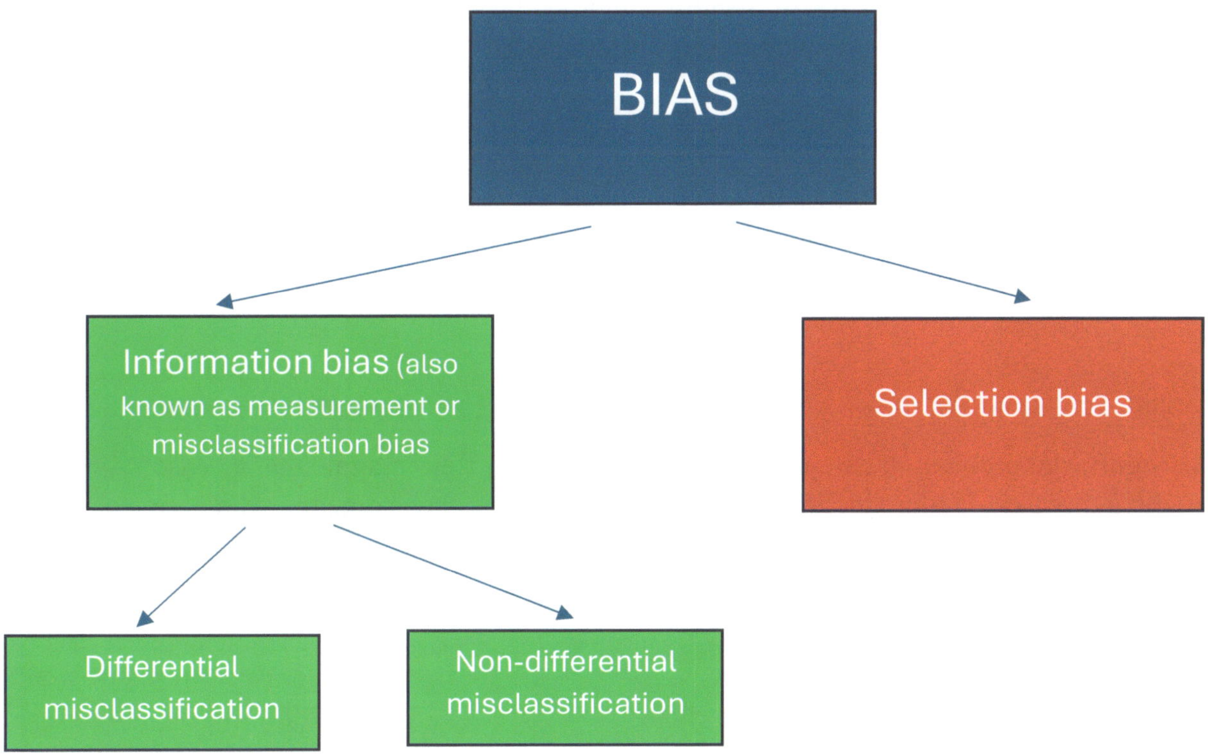

Section E4.2: Differential misclassification bias

I would first like to explore *why* differential misclassification bias might occur, first in case-control studies, and then in cohort studies.

Recall that in **case-control studies,** participants are identified by outcome status…that is, "cases" (those who have the outcome in question) are recruited, and then "controls" (those who do not have the outcome in question) are recruited. In both groups, the researchers look back in time to see who had the exposure of interest and who did not. So in these types of studies, the problem of misclassification usually occurs when researchers look back in time to identify the exposure status.

Interviewer bias:

Let's say the "cases" are those with cancer and the "exposure" in question is exposure to toxic chemicals. If the interviewer knows, for example, that the person she is interviewing has cancer (is a case), the interviewer (being human) may be more likely to "press" the participant. You know: "Are you *sure* you never had an exposure?" This not uncommon, and not the "fault" of the interviewer; the researchers, being human are "hoping" to prove their hypothesis. Afterall, they have already done a lot of research and spent a lot of money on their hypothesis. If they end up with a negative study, they are disappointed on many grounds, not the least of which is that negative studies (studies that show no association) are considerably less likely to be accepted for publication in the journals.

Recall bias:

This is a significant problem in case-control studies. You can well imagine that a "case"—a person with a disease—is more inclined to "recall" an exposure than someone who is free of disease. It is human nature to seek a possible cause of one's disease. A particularly clear example is the mother of a child with birth defects questioned about possible exposures she might have experienced while pregnant.

Reporting biases

Simply stated, participants are often not accurate in their reporting of a possible exposure, for a variety of reasons. There may be a "social desirability bias," in which the participant may be not forthcoming on an exposure if it is of a sensitive nature (for example, sexual habits, drug use, violent and unlawful behavior etc.), and it is quite conceivable that one group would be more inclined to be less than truthful about their exposures than the other group. An interesting type of reporting bias is known as "obsequiousness bias," in which participants are not entirely truthful because they are telling the interviewer what they (the participant) thinks they (the interviewer) wants to hear.

Recall that in **cohort** studies, subjects are identified based on their exposure status, and then followed to see if an outcome occurs. In these types of studies, most of the misclassifications occur at identifying the outcome.

Diagnostic biases

Researchers may be more likely to "go the extra mile" to identify a possible outcome if they know that the participant had the exposure in question: they might examine the medical record a bit more thoroughly or question the participant in a more aggressive manner. This type of bias occurs if the researchers are not blinded to the exposure status of the participants.

Detection bias

Let's say researchers are exploring the relationship between cigarette smoking and heart disease in New London County, CT. They identify, say 5000 smokers and 5000 nonsmokers in New London County and follow them for ten years. Because cigarette smoking is associated with many diseases that may require hospitalization, and because hospitalized people may be more likely to be diagnosed with heart disease than non-hospitalized people, then a detection bias may occur. (More smokers are diagnosed with heart disease only because they are hospitalized).

The effect of differential misclassification bias

I will not examine how differential misclassification bias can affect the results. Let's take a case-control study, and say we have the following results:

	cases	**controls**
exposure	100	80
No exposure	50	70

2. As this is a case-control study, the measure of association is an _______ _____________ .

That's right! The measure of association is indeed an odds ratio!

3. And odds ratio is calculated by the fraction ______ / ________ .

That's right! The odds ratio is indeed calculated by $\frac{a/c}{b/d}$

The odds ratio here is **1.75.**

Now, let's say there is a differential misclassification happening, so that 20% of the exposed cases are misclassified as not exposed, while only 10% of the exposed controls are misclassified as unexposed. Our misclassified 2x2 table now looks like this:

	cases	controls
exposed	80	72
Not exposed	70	78

Our biased ratio is now **1.24.**

So you can see the rather dramatic effect that differential information bias can have on the results.

In our case, the bias caused the odds ratio to decrease (move toward the null). But please understand that a differential measurement bias can also cause the measure of association to head away from the null, and create more of an association than actually exits. This bias direction would occur if more of the unexposed controls were misclassified as exposed. Here is an example of that: Let's say 20% of the non-exposed cases were misclassified as exposed, while only 10% of the non-exposed controls were misclassified as exposed:

	cases	controls
exposure	110	87
No exposure	40	63

Our biased OR is now **2.0** (away from the null)

The same would hold true if our study was a cohort study:

	outcome	No outcome	total
Exposed	100	50	150
Not exposed	60	90	150

4. Since this is a cohort study, the measure of association is the _________ _______________.

That's right! Since this is a cohort study, the measure of association is indeed the relative risk!

5. And the relative risk is the _______________ in the exposed divided the _______________ in the exposed.

The RR here is: **1.67**

In cohort studies, we tend to think of the misclassification occurring in the outcome classification (but it can occur in either: that is, subjects can be misclassified based on their exposure *or* on their outcome.)

Let's say that 20% of the exposed people who had an outcome were misclassified as not having had an outcome, while only 10% of the unexposed people who had an outcome were misclassified as not having had an outcome.

	outcome	No outcome	total
Exposed	80	70	150
Not exposed	54	96	150

The biased RR is now **1.48** (toward the null)

A differential misclassification bias can cause the measure of association to go in ___________ direction from the null.

Section E4.3: Non-differential measurement bias

In non-differential measurement bias, there are errors in measurement that are random—that is, they do *not* affect one group more than the other. (Of course, by random chance, it *may* affect one group more than the other, but there is no reason to think, other than by random chance, that it would).

For example, in a case-control study in which the exposure is blood pressures of the participants, and if there is some error in blood pressure measurement (the wrong size cuff, examiner experience, problem with calibration, etc.) then errors in measurement can occur. We would expect that these errors would occur more or less equally in both groups. Let's see what happens when there is a non-differential misclassification in a case-control study:

	Cases	**Controls**
Exposure	100	80
No exposure	50	70

So in our example, the actual OR = **1.75.**

Now let's see what happens if 20 % of all cases who were exposed *and* 20% of all controls who were exposed were misclassified as not having an exposure. Now we see:

	Cases	**Controls**
Exposure	80	64
No exposure	70	86

The biased OR = **1.54**

As opposed to differential misclassification, in non-differential misclassification, the falsely-biased result *always* goes toward the null. Don't believe me? Let's say that 20% of all cases who were *unexposed and* 20% of all the controls who were *unexposed* were misclassified as being exposed:

	Cases	**Controls**
Exposure	110	94
No exposure	40	56

The biased OR = **1.64** (toward the null)

And now let's look at cohort studies.

Here again is the actual unbiased results:

	outcome	No outcome	total
Exposed	100	50	150
Not exposed	60	90	150

The actual RR is **1.67**

Let's say that 20% of the exposed people who had the outcome were misclassified as not having had the outcome, *and* 20% of the unexposed people who had an outcome were misclassified as not having had an outcome.

	outcome	No outcome	total
Exposed	80	70	150
Not exposed	48	102	150

The biased RR is **1.67** (no change!)

Fooled you on that one!

But remember that in cohort studies the misclassification can also occur by exposure status. So let's say that 20% of the exposed people who had an outcome were misclassified as not having had an exposure, *and* 20% of the exposed people who did not have an outcome were misclassified as not having an exposure:

	outcome	No outcome	total
Exposed	80	40	120
Not exposed	80	100	180

The biased RR is **1.5** (towards the null)

What is the bottom line of all this? In non-differential misclassification, the measure of association is always erroneously *closer to the null* (except in one case: cohort studies in which the misclassification occurred by outcome status: in this case the measure of association does not change. But in general our true association diminishes with non-differential misclassification.

7. Unlike differential misclassification, in which the measure of association can move either ____________ or ________________ from the null, in non-differential misclassification, the measure of association never moves _______________ from the null.

Section E4.4: Selection bias

Selection bias is a very important problem in observational studies. Selection bias refers to the fact that the results we get from our one sample that we studied may not be the same as the result that we would have gotten if we had studied the entire target population, and that difference is due to the nature of the participants that were selected.

Researchers in general are trying to answer questions applicable to a group of people. That group can be anything. For example, researchers might be wondering if vitamin D intake is associated with decreased incidence of osteoporosis among American postmenopausal women. They unfortunately cannot include *every* postmenopausal American woman into the study, but they hope that the results of their study can be generalized to all American postmenopausal women. In this case, the group consisting of all American postmenopausal women is referred to as the *target* population. Or another example would be when researchers were exploring possible causes of AIDS in the early 1980's. In this example the *target* population might have been all homosexual men. Or if researchers are studying the effects of malnourishment in children living in Somalia in the present day, the target population is all children currently living in Somalia. The target population is in general defined by *person, place and time,* and is the large group that researchers are hoping to make conclusions about in their research project.

In the case of AIDS research in the 1980s, the *target* population—the population that researchers want to make inferences about—is all homosexual men. But researchers of course could not include all homosexual men into their studies, so they then select a subset of the target population referred to as the *source population:*

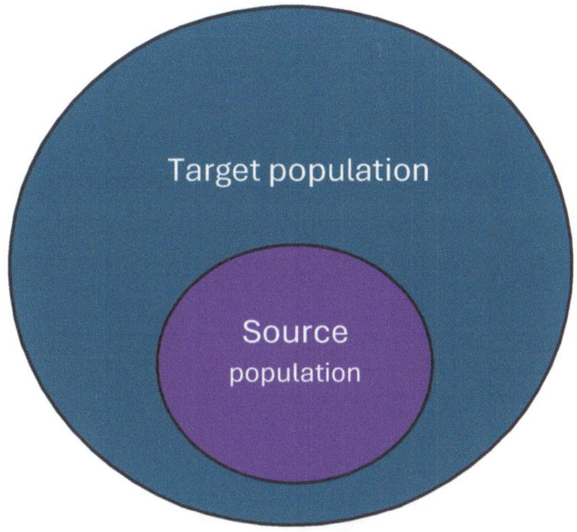

The researchers may have chosen as their source population homosexual men living in New York and San Francisco in the early 80s who attended health care clinics. This is a manageable number of people to study and is a group that they assumed would be well representative of the entire target population.

But the reality of epidemiologic research is that many of the people in the source population would not, for a variety of reasons, actually be eligible or be able to participate in a particular study, and so yet another subset is identified, and that is the subset of the source population who actually take part in the study. And this group is referred to as the *study population:*

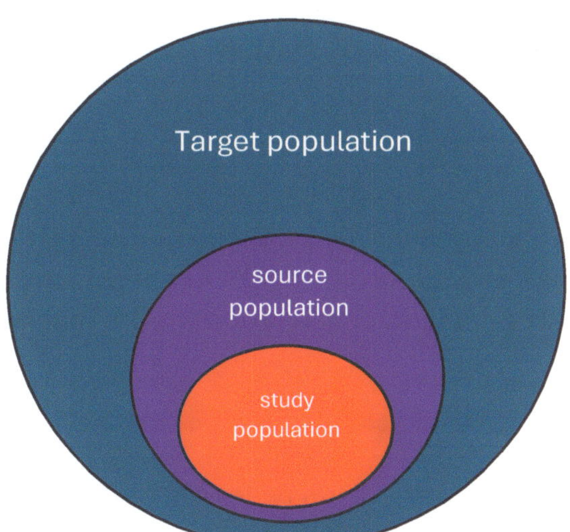

Selection bias can occur either when the source population is chosen from the target population, or when the study population is chosen from the source population, or both.

We hope that the measure of association in the study population is the same as (or close to) the measure of association of the target population.

But when selection bias occurs, the measures of association are not the same because as we move from target population to source population, and then from source population to study population, the relative weights of the 2x2 tables change.

But what if because of selection as we move from target to source, and then from source to study, that there is not an equal representation of the 2x2 table?

That is:

TARGET POP

Exposed + outcome	Exposed No outcome
Not exposed + outcome	Not exposed No outcome

=

SOURCE POP

Exposed + outcome	Exposed No outcome
Not Exposed + outcome	Not Exposed No outcome

=

STUDY POP

Exposed + outcome	Exposed No outcome
Not Exposed + outcome	Not Exposed No outcome

The *ratios* of each cell must be the same for the subgroups. That is, if 1/10 of all participants in the target population are exposed + outcome, then 1/10 of the source population must be exposed + outcome, and 1/10 of the study population must be exposed + outcome. If not, then we have selection bias.

8. If the ratios of the cells in the study population is not the same as the ratio of the cells in the target population, then ______________________ ____________ might occur.

To help clarify this, I would like to jump to a real example from the literature. It goes way back to 1979, and it is the classic example of selection bias. Interestingly it was authored by one of the leaders of epidemiology at that time, and by goofing on this study he has taught many students over the years about selection bias, so it is definitely worth taking a look at.

MacMahon et al: Coffee and Cancer of the Pancreas *N Engl J Med* 1981;304:630-633

The association he was interested in was the exposure of coffee consumption and the outcome of pancreatic cancer. So they did a case-control study in which the cases were the patients with pancreatic cancer, and the controls did not have pancreatic cancer. Here is the actual wording:

> We conducted a case–control interview study. The cases were patients with histologic diagnoses of cancer of the exocrine pancreas who were in any of 11 large hospitals in the Boston metropolitan area and Rhode Island between October 1974 and August 1979

And importantly, here is how they chose the controls:

> To assemble a control series, the interviewers also attempted to question all other patients who were under the care of the same physician in the same hospital at the time of an interview with a patient with pancreatic cancer. Either before the interview (if the information was known) or afterward, patients with diseases of the pancreas or hepatobiliary tract or diseases known to be associated with smoking or alcohol consumption were excluded.

Note "under the care of the same physician in the same hospital at the time…" and note "patients…with diseases known to be associated with smoking or alcohol consumption were excluded."

And more about the controls is noteworthy:

> because of the nature of the practices of many of the physicians who were responsible for patients with cancer of the pancreas, patients with gastroenterologic conditions were probably overrepresented in relation to a general hospital population.

Here are there results (I put them in a 2x2 table):

	Pancreatic cancer	No pancreatic cancer
Coffee consumption	347	555
No coffee consumption	20	88

The odds ratio is $\frac{347/20}{555/88} = \mathbf{2.75}$

That certainly appears to be a very strong association. The odds of having pancreatic cancer if you are a coffee drinker appears to be 2.75 times the odds of having pancreatic cancer if you are not a coffee drinker.

I will spill the beans at this point, and tell you that ever since this study came out, many subsequent studies and meta-analyses have shown no association between coffee consumption and pancreatic cancer. So where did they go wrong?

Selection bias almost always occurs because of the way the *controls* are selected. In this study, how were the controls chosen? The controls were other patients admitted to the hospital by the same group of physicians (gastroenterologists) who admitted the pancreatic cancer cases, and they (the controls) were admitted with a variety of other gastrointestinal conditions. And one thing we know about patients who are treated by gastroenterologists, they are likely to suffer from chronic GI complaints, and were likely advised to cut down or eliminate their coffee consumption. So the controls in the *source* population (and thus the study population) may well have had less coffee consumption than the controls of the *target* population. By the way, what is the target population in this study? That is, who are the researchers hoping to generalize their results for? Well, probably all adults, right? At any rate, we would guess that the vast majority of the target population (all adults) are not being treated by a gastroenterologist and therefore the target population would consist of a higher percentage of coffee drinkers. To make matters worse, they also excluded people who were admitted with diseases thought to be due to alcohol or tobacco intake. Well, especially back then, cigarette smoking was associated with coffee consumption, so if you eliminate cigarette smokers, you also eliminate coffee drinkers. Bottom line, the "b" of the 2x2 table of our study population is likely to be *underestimated* compared to the target population:

Exposed case	Exposed control
Not exposed case	Not exposed control

Under-represented

We can calculate the ratios of the cells in our study group:

STUDY POPULATION

34.3%	**55%**
2 %	**8.7%**

But in the target population, the ratios might actually be something like this:

TARGET POPULATION

18.8%	**75%**
1.2%	**5%**

Since the total number of participants in the study population was 1010, we can fill in the cells with the raw numbers *if* the ratios in the study population were the same as the ratios in the target population:

STUDY POPULATION with corrected ratios

	Pancreatic cancer	**No pancreatic cancer**
Coffee consumption	190	757
No coffee consumption	12	52

And now what is our odds ratio?

$OR = \frac{190/12}{757/52} = \mathbf{1.09},$ and the apparent association between coffee consumption and pancreatic cancer vanishes.

And this is selection bias. Selection bias occurs when the controls in the study population are not representative of the controls in the target population. (One of the four cells in our study population 2x2 table is over- or under-represented as compared to that of the target population).

The above case is a demonstration of how selection bias is a big problem when selecting our source population (and then our study population) from our target population, and how we must be very careful to make sure that the controls in our source population are the same as the controls in our target population. But we can also have a form of selection bias when we go from the source population to the study population. To review: when we have identified our source population (the people we plan on studying) we often are forced to whittle that down for a variety of reasons. But a problem is created when the participation rate is low (that is, the percentage of people in the source population that go on to become the study population is low). Take a look at this paper:

> De-Kun et al. Hot Tub Use during Pregnancy and the Risk of Miscarriage. *American Journal of Epidemiology,* Volume 158, Issue 10, 15 November 2003, Pages 931–937,

The researchers were wondering about a possible association between hot tub use and miscarriage. Here are their results:

TABLE 2. Association of use of a hot tub or Jacuzzi* during pregnancy with the risk of miscarriage, Kaiser Permanente Medical Care Program, Oakland, California, 1996–1998

	Miscarriage					
	Yes (*n* = 170)		No (*n* = 888)‡		Hazard ratio†	95% confidence interval
	No.	%	No.	%		
Hot tub or Jacuzzi use						
No	144	15.1	809	84.9	1.0	Referent
Yes	26	24.8	79	75.2	2.0	1.3, 3.1

Their measure of association is the Hazard ratio, which I will talk about in an upcoming chapter, but for now, you can consider it to be the same as an incidence rate ratio. So a hazard ratio of 2 basically means that the risk of miscarriage among those who used a hot tub was twice the risk compared to those who did not.

But take a look at this from the study:

> Of 2,729 eligible women, 164 (6 percent) were contacted too far along in their pregnancy (>15 weeks) for interview; 317 initially agreed to participate but were unable to schedule an interview; 1,185 (43.4 percent) refused to participate; and, ultimately, 1,063 (39 percent) completed the interview.

So only 39% of the *source population* became the *study population.* At first glance, this may not seem like a problem. We would not expect that the 61% who chose not to participate were inherently different than the 39% who chose to participate…but they *might* be different in some way, who knows? Maybe, *for whatever reason,* cell "a" of the 2x2 table in the study population is over-represented compared to the source population. For example, look at this from the study:

> Because we recruited pregnant women during early gestation (median, 40 days), 103 of the 170 women who experienced miscarriages had already miscarried before the in-person interview was conducted. Those women were still included in the study although the information on their exposures, including use of hot tubs or Jacuzzis, was ascertained up to the time of miscarriage only.

So most of the women were interviewed *after* their miscarriages occurred. Is certainly conceivable that women who miscarried were more inclined to be interviewed than women who did not miscarry. The potential problems of a low participation rate was analyzed beautifully by Irva Hertz-Picciotto and Penelope P. Howards in their commentary soon after the study was published. In their analysis, they presented a fictitious scenario about those who chose *not* to participate. (Colored boxes were my addition)

TABLE 1. Hypothetical scenarios for exposure of nonparticipants in a study of hot tub or Jacuzzi* use and the risk of miscarriage†

	Cases		Noncases		Total no.	Risk ratio
	No.	Proportion	No.	Proportion		
Participants					1,058	1.64
Unexposed	144	0.85	809	0.91		
Exposed	26	0.15	79	0.09		
Scenario 1						
Nonparticipants					1,671	1.00
Unexposed	235	0.88	1,236	0.88		
Exposed	32	0.12	168	0.12		
Total population					2,729	1.21
Unexposed	379	0.87	2,045	0.89		
Exposed	58	0.13	247	0.11		
Scenario 2						
Nonparticipants					1,671	0.78
Unexposed	240	0.90	1,221	0.87		
Exposed	27	0.10	183	0.13		
Total population					2,729	1.05
Unexposed	384	0.88	2,030	0.89		
Exposed	53	0.12	262	0.11		

* Any type of whirlpool bath; Jacuzzi Brands, Inc., West Palm Beach, Florida.

† These scenarios demonstrate how small differences between those persons who self-select to participate and those who do not could have produced the observed data even if *no* association exists between exposure and outcome in the total population.

First, look at the top box in red. This is the actual results of the study. (They calculated risk ratio instead of hazard ratio and that is why their result was 1.64 instead of 2). Now look at the blue box "scenario 1". In this scenario, they took the 1671 women were did not agree to participate, and assumed that their results, had they participated, were similar to the results of the actual participants, but *a little different.* You see that in the nonparticipants, 12% of the exposed were cases, which is a little bit less than the 15% among the actual participants; and among nonparticipants, 12% of the exposed were noncases, which is a little bit more than the 9% among the actual participants. That is really just a small difference between the participants and nonparticipants that one might even expect could occur by random chance. So then in the green box, they added the raw numbers of these nonparticipants to the raw numbers of the participants, and came up with final results of what would have happened if all the nonparticipants were also in the study. You see that the relative risk is now 1.21, which is considerably less of an association! In fact, let's do a little review and check to see if a relative risk of 1.21 is statistically significant or not. If you need a review on this, go back to chapter Biostats 3: Comparing categorical outcomes. In general, you recall that the null hypothesis for a risk ratio is a risk ratio of 1. So we can check for statistical significance by calculating the 95% confidence interval, and then seeing if the confidence interval includes 1.

9. If the 95% confidence interval of the relative risk includes _____, then the results are not ____________________ ______________________________.

And how do we calculate the 95% confidence interval?

10. The 95% confidence interval is 2 ________________ _________________ away from our result in either direction.

That's right! The 95% confidence interval is 2 standard errors below our result, and 2 standard errors above our result. And how do we get the standard error of a relative risk? Well, the formula is given in section B3.4, and is this:

$$\widehat{SE}(\ln(RR)) = \sqrt{\frac{1}{a} + \frac{1}{a+b} + \frac{1}{c} + \frac{1}{c+d}}$$

It is certainly not expected that you knew that by heart. So if you like, go ahead and calculate the standard error and then the 95% confidence interval using this formula; or, it is perfectly acceptable to just use a calculator that you can find online (like MedCalc) and let them do the work.

So hopefully you ended up with a 95% confidence interval of (0.95 to 1.56). That includes 1, and so indeed the association between the exposure of hot tub use and outcome of miscarriage is gone (statistically speaking).

(And the calculator will also tell you that the p-value is 0.12, which is greater than 0.05)

Bottom line here: As the authors point out, if those who had not agreed to participate in the study actually did participate, and their (the nonparticipants) results were just *a little* different than the participants, the results of the experiment change dramatically. And so we see a form of selection bias: even though we may not be able to identify for certain why those who are in the study population are inherently different from those who are in the source population, if there are significantly fewer people in the study population, then the results just may not be reliable.

Summary of Epidemiology 4

Bias is a systemic deviation from the truth that is a big problem in observational studies. It is due to either errors in measurement (information bias), or errors in selection of the controls (selection bias).

Measurement bias can be either differential misclassification bias, in which the error is occurring in one group more than the other group, and this kind of bias results in a measure of association that is either away from the null (more of an association) or toward the null (less of an association), or non-differential misclassification, in which the measure of association always toward the null.

Selection bias occurs when the controls chosen from the study population are inherently different than the controls from the target population. It is always a concern in observational studies, and the authors are obligated to explain how they managed and accounted for possible selection bias.

Epidemiology 5: Confounding and Effect Measure Modification

Section E5.1: What is Confounding?

Confounding is a very important topic in epidemiology and biostatistics. I mentioned it briefly in my discussion on randomization in Epidemiology 2 and would like to expand on it here. A confounder is basically a factor that messes up an apparent association, and is a big problem in all kinds of studies, but mostly in observational studies. For example, we might be exploring the possible association between physical inactivity and cancer. That is, is physical inactivity (the exposure) associated with the development of cancer (the outcome)? Might it even be a *cause* of cancer? To show the association, we might propose an observational study in which one group has the exposure (they are "physically inactive" according to a certain set of parameters), and the other group does not have the exposure (they are not "physically inactive"). Both groups are followed for some time in the future and watched for the outcome (whether or not they are diagnosed with cancer).

Of course, there are many other factors that are known to be associated with, or cause cancer. One of course is cigarette smoking. The problem is that if we compare an inactive group with an active group, you can bet that there would be more cigarette smokers in the inactive group. So if we found in our experiment that more people in the inactive group developed cancer, we would not know how much of that difference was due to the physical inactivity, or the cigarette smoking, or both. We say that cigarette smoking is a *confounder* as it is messing up the results that show an association of the exposure with the outcome, and so we must account for it in our results.

For something to be a confounder, it has to be associated with the exposure *and* it has to be a risk factor for the outcome.

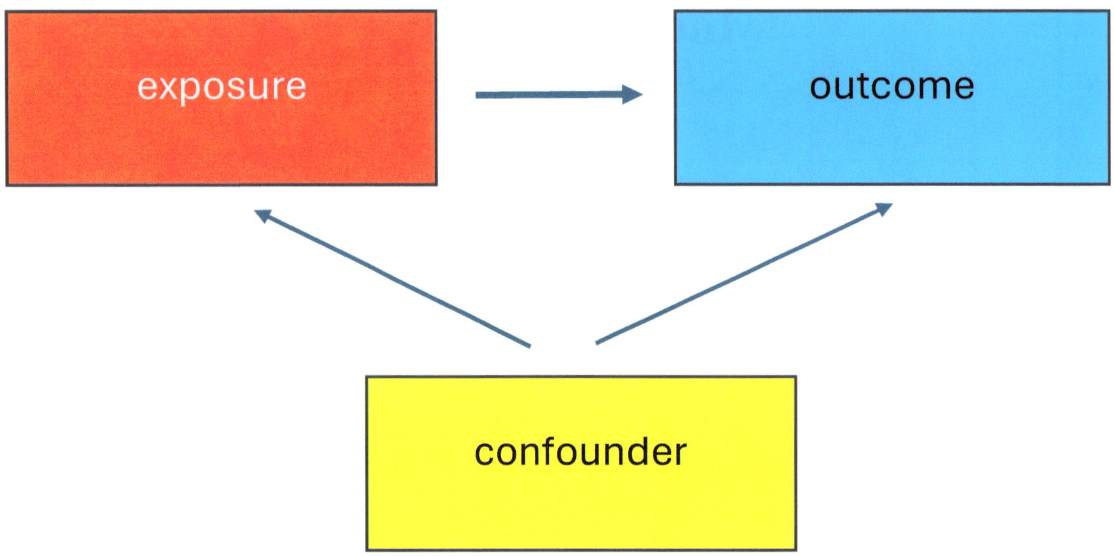

The reason that it has to be related to the exposure in order to be a confounder is as follows: If it is associated with the exposure then we would expect more people in the exposed group to also have the confounder. If the amount of people with the possible confounder is the same in each group, then it wouldn't affect the results, right? So for example, what about family history of cancer? Well there is no doubt that family history of cancer is a risk factor (associated with) the outcome of cancer. But it is not associated with inactivity, so we would not expect more people in the physical inactivity group to have a family history of cancer than those in the unexposed group.

1. If a factor is associated with the outcome but not with the exposure, then it likely will _________ be a confounder because it should not be ____________________________ distributed.

Here's a little exercise: what other factors may be confounders for this study? Can you think of anything else that is associated with the exposure, and is a risk factor for the outcome? The first one that comes to my mind is age. Age is associated with the exposure, because as people age they become less physically active. And age is certainly a risk factor for cancer.

How about asbestos exposure? Is that likely to be a confounder? It certainly is associated with the outcome but is not associated with inactivity. Therefore, even though asbestos exposure can certainly cause many cases of cancer, it should not be more prevalent in the exposed group, so should not "mess up" our results.

How about hours watching television? Is that expected to be a confounder? Well it is certainly associated with the exposure; but, as far as we know is not directly associated with cancer, so we would not expect it to be a confounder.

What about being overweight? What do you think? I would say it certainly *could* be a confounder: it is surely associated with physical activity, and has been linked to certain forms of cancer.

What about alcohol intake? It is certainly associated with cancer. Is it associated with the exposure? Hard to say for sure…it might be!

Oh, there is another "rule" about confounding that you should know: if a third factor is on the *causal pathway* between exposure and outcome, then it would not be expected to be a confounder. An example that comes to mind: We are analyzing the association between alcohol intake and liver cancer, and we wonder about cirrhosis of the liver as possible confounder. Well, cirrhosis is an intermediate in the causal pathway between alcohol intake and liver cancer, so it would *not* be expected to be a confounder.

The 3 "rules"of confounders

1. They must be associated with the exposure
2. They must be associated with (considered a risk factor for) the outcome
3. They must not be an intermediate in the causal pathway between exposure and outcome.

Section E5.2: Can we prevent confounding?

The short answer is…no. Confounding is ubiquitous in epidemiologic studies. It is always there, whether we are aware of it or not.

Randomization

Confounding is generally considered an issue in observational studies, rather than experimental studies. And that is because, as discussed in detail in Epidemiology 2, in experimental studies the two groups are *randomized.* That is, the researchers themselves choose the groups, and can (should) be very careful to pick the two groups entirely randomly, so that all possible confounders will be more or less evenly distributed among the groups. In observational studies on the other hand, the participants themselves are choosing their groups. They determine if they are physically inactive or not. (The researchers would of course give them guidelines, but it is ultimately up to each participant to determine his or her own classification), and so obviously there are likely to be many confounding factors present.

But even in experimental studies confounding can be present because of simple luck. After randomization, it is still quite possible that some potential confounders ended up being unevenly distributed among the groups. And so, even in experimental trials, good researchers will also report on possible confounding, and account for it when they analyze their data.

In observational studies, there are things the researchers can do to *minimize* the presence of confounding.

Enrollment restriction

If we know for certain that one or more factors are strong confounders, we can *restrict* our enrollment to include only those who have the confounder, or only those who *don't* have the confounder, or only those who have a certain level of the confounder. For example, in our study, we might have just enrolled overweight smokers between the ages of 50 and 60. That certainly eliminates the three major confounders that we were concerned about. But remember of course, there are still other confounders present that we would still need to account for!

Matching

This is often used in case-control studies. Recall that in case-control studies we start with a group of people who are cases (that is, they have the disease or the outcome in question), and then we look to see how many of each group had the exposure in question. So if we pick, say 1000 people with cancer, we would match them with controls who have the same confounder in question. If smoking is the confounder, and we see that 200 of the 1000 people with cancer are smokers, we would make sure that when we choose our controls (those without cancer) so that 200 of *them* are nonsmokers. It is best to do this carefully on a one-to-one basis. For example, take each case and identify the confounders present: let's say case 1 is a smoker age 55 and not overweight. We would choose control 1 to also be 55, a smoker and not overweight. We would then do the same for all the other cases!

While we can also use this method for cohort studies, in which each participant with the exposure is matched one-to-one with each control in by the confounders in present, in practice this is generally not done, simply because in most cohort studies we try to recruit as many people as possible, and deal with the confounding in the analysis.

2. A useful method of minimizing confounding in case-control studies is by __________________, and is ideally done on a _______ to ________ basis.

Section E5.3: How we deal with confounding in the analysis

When researchers analyze the results of their study, they must take into consider the confounding that is likely present. (If it wasn't *eliminated* as described in the previous section). When something is expected to be a possible confounder, the researchers must take it into account by "controlling" for it. (This is also sometimes referred to as "adjusting.").

Here are some fictitious results from our fictitious observational study on inactivity and cancer:

	Cancer	**No cancer**
Inactive	120	880
active	70	930

What is the measure of association that we should use? The result is binary ("yes/no") and so one measure of association that we can use is the relative risk.

3. Since the measure of association is the relative risk, this must be a ______________ study.

$$\text{Relative Risk} = \frac{120/1000}{70/1000} = \mathbf{1.71}$$

This looks like a pretty strong association; we would interpret it as follows: the risk of cancer if you are inactive is 1.71 times the risk if you are not inactive. Or, those who are physically inactive have a 71% higher risk of cancer than those who are not physically inactive. That is quite a strong apparent association. But the researchers would recognize that a very likely confounder of the results would be cigarette smoking. So they need to see how much cigarette smoking is “messing up” their results, and one way they could do this is by “stratifying” the results as follows. They divide the results by the confounder as follows:

Cigarette smokers				Non-smokers			
	Cancer	No cancer	total		Cancer	No cancer	total
Inactive	67	133	200	Inactive	53	747	800
active	25	75	100	active	45	855	900
total	92	208	300	total	98	1602	1700

Then we just do the side-by-side RR:

For cigarette smokers, RR = $\frac{67/200}{25/100}$ = **1.34** For non-smokers: RR = $\frac{53/800}{45/900}$ = **1.33**

The first thing to notice is that among the 1000 inactive people, 200 were smokers, and among the 1000 active people, only 100 were smokers. And so it is not surprising that more of the inactive people developed cancer. And we now see that among the smokers, there was a 34% higher risk of cancer if they were inactive, and among the nonsmokers, there was a 33% higher risk of cancer. We would then average these two values (using a formula for weighted average) and end up with an **RR = 1.33.**

We would say that the **“relative risk of developing cancer if you are inactive *adjusted for cigarette smoking status* is 1.33”**

The “unadjusted” relative risk was 1.71, and the relative risk *adjusted for cigarette smoking* is 1.33. What does this mean? It means that cigarette smoking contributed a good amount of the apparent connection between inactivity and cancer (but inactivity still had an effect!).

4. The relative risk adjusted for cigarette smoking is less than the unadjusted risk. So this means that a good amount of the apparent association between ________________ and ____________ is actually due to ____________ ________________.

In general, if the measure of association adjusted for one another factor differs by 10% or more from the unadjusted measure, we say that indeed that other factor is a confounder.

5. Since relative risk adjusted for cigarette smoking is more than ________ % different than the unadjusted relative risk, we say that cigarette smoking is a ________________.

And one epidemiologic definition here: note that in our example the presence of the confounder makes the measure of association appear higher than it actually is. (We thought it was 1.71, but it was actually 1.33). So, the presence of the confounder causes a spuriously high measure of association, and by "high" I mean *away from the null*. When it goes in that direction, we say that the confounder is a "positive confounder." (I know it's a bit confusing because the word "positive" has a positive connotation, but hey…I don't make the rules!). Positive confounding is the most common type of confounding, but negative confounding can also occur! What if the measure of association is less than 1? For example, picture an observational study that measured the effect of fish oil intake and the development of heart disease. The exposure is fish oil intake, and so the researchers may find a protective effect, with a relative risk of perhaps 0.72. But then they realize that physical fitness may be a confounder, and when they adjust for high levels of physical fitness, they find that the RR is now 0.88. So…more people in the high fish oil group were also physically fit, and so a good portion of the reduction of the RR in the fish oil group was due to the fact that they were more physically fit. So, in this case, physical fitness is acting as a confounder. It is also considered a *positive* confounder. Why? Because the confounder's presence makes it look like the measure of association is further away from the null than it actually is. We thought it was 0.72, but it was actually 0.88.

Back to our example:

OK then, if the researchers are doing a good job, they would take this to the next level, and say, well…what about being overweight? That is a confounder…we better try to adjust for this as well. And so they could again stratify…so they end up with four groups: Cigarette smokers who are overweight, cigarette smokers who are not overweight, nonsmokers who are overweight, and nonsmokers who are not overweight. After averaging all 4 groups, they might find that the relative risk is now **1.25.**

The researchers would now say: **"The relative risk of developing cancer if you are inactive *adjusted for cigarette smoking status, and overweight status"* is 1.25.**

So now the relative risk is going further down; that is, heading toward 1. Remember what is so significant about a relative risk of 1? That means there is no association between the exposure and the outcome; it is the *null hypothesis.*

6. As we add more positive confounders into the mix, we see that the relative risk gets ____________ ________ the null hypothesis.

Oh but then the researchers continue their careful analysis, and realize that age is a very possible confounder, and should be factored in. And when they factor age in (along with the other confounders), they find that the relative risk is now **1.03.** (Obviously we cannot stratify for every single age, as the numbers would be too small to analyze, but fortunately there is a mathematical way of doing this that I will discuss in a later chapter!)

The researchers would now say: **"The relative risk of developing cancer if you are inactive *adjusted for smoking, weigh status, and age is 1.03."***

Well, 1.03 is pretty much the same as 1, and so the researchers would likely conclude that there is *no significant association between physical activity status and the development of cancer.* They would conclude this because after adjusting for three possible confounders, the relative risk is just about 1.

7. Pretty much all of the apparent association between physical inactivity and cancer was actually due to three ____________________________.

And so you can see why confounders are such a problem in medical research. When researchers are looking for a possible association between an exposure and an outcome, it is their job to identify as many possible confounders as they can and then adjust their results for all of them. Even if they are not sure if a factor is a confounder or not, they should consider that possibility. For example, in this study, alcohol *may or may not* be a confounder and should be adjusted for *just in case it is.* Even factors that one would not think is a confounder because it is not associated with the exposure—for example we said that family history of cancer is not associated with inactivity. Although this is correct, it is strongly associated with the outcome. Even though it is not associated with the exposure and therefore should not be unevenly distributed among the groups, there is always a chance that we got unlucky and by chance alone there were significantly more people with a family history of cancer in the inactive group than the active group. Therefore, careful researchers will still take into account *possible* confounders that are strongly associated with the outcome...*just in case* they are confounders "by mistake."

Section E5.4: What is Effect Measure Modification?

It is unfortunate that effect modification and confounding are so often confused with one another. They are actually completely different phenomena, and the only reason I have including them in the same chapter is really to point out the differences. Unlike confounding, in which a third factor causes a spurious association between an exposure and an outcome, effect measure modification is an actual biological phenomenon that causes a real change in the association. For example, let's say we are exploring the association between the exposure being cigarette smoking and the outcome being the disease mesothelioma. We might find a relative risk of say

4.0, meaning that cigarette smokers have 4 times the risk of developing mesothelioma than do nonsmokers.

	+mesothelioma	**No mesothelioma**
smokers	40	60
nonsmokers	10	90

Relative risk = **4.0**

But now let's add in the third factor, which is exposure to asbestos. Let's say we were very careful at the start of our study to match asbestos exposure status in each group equally. That is, the number of smokers with asbestos exposure was exactly the same as the number of nonsmokers with asbestos. We then stratify our results by asbestos exposure status:

Now we stratify our results by asbestos exposure:

asbestos exposure		
	+mesothelioma	No meso
smokers	32	18
nonsmokers	4	41

Relative risk = **8.0**

No asbestos exposure		
	+mesothelioma	No meso
smokers	8	42
nonsmokers	6	49

Relative risk = **1.33**

What is going on here? We see a *very* large difference in the relative risks when stratified by asbestos exposure. This is a classic example of effect measure modification. We know for sure asbestos is not a confounder. Why? Because 50% of the smokers had asbestos exposure, and 50% of the nonsmokers had asbestos exposure. When the third factor (asbestos exposure) is equally distributed among the groups, it cannot be a confounder. (It is not associated with the exposure). Furthermore, when something is a confounder, the stratified relative risks, although different than the unstratified, are very similar to each other. (they both would have been about 1.33 if it were a confounder). So there is some kind of *biological interaction* going on between cigarette smoking and asbestos exposure that makes the measure of association skyrocket when both are present. And that is why "effect measure modification," is also sometimes called "interaction," meaning there is something going on between the factor (asbestos) and the exposure (smoking) that affects the outcome.

Unlike confounding, which is a nuisance to researchers as it is messing up their apparent associations, and must be fixed (adjusted), effect measure modification is a true and interesting biological effect that must be noted and hopefully studied in the future by the researchers. It does not need to be "fixed" or adjusted for, but rather pointed out and studied.

8. When results are stratified by a third factor, and the resulting measures of association are very different from one another, then an ____________________, also called _______________ ________________________ __________________________, is occurring between that third factor and the exposure being studied.

This is not at all the same as ____________________________.

Section E5.5: Examples from the literature

Because the differences between confounding and effect measure modification continue to be confusing to many students, I would like to provide some examples from the literature to help clarify.

> Loeb et al. Do Environmental Factors Modify the Genetic Risk of Prostate Cancer? *Cancer Epidemiol Biomarkers Prev* (2015) 24 (1): 213–220.

In this study, the researchers analyzed the effect measure modification of the presence of alleles that increase the risk of prostate cancer, and an array of environmental/medicinal factors. Here is a portion of their results table:

	OR (95% CI) of higher genetic risk (≥12 risk alleles)			
	Total	**Nonadvanced stage**	**Advanced stage**	**Aggressive (advanced stage or Gleason s**
Overall	1.98 (1.67–2.34)	1.91 (1.54–2.36)	2.04 (1.67–2.49)	1.73 (1.33–2.25)
BMI at age 20				
Normal	2.11 (1.73–2.57)	2.09 (1.62–2.68)	2.13 (1.69–2.70)	1.93 (1.42–2.63)
Overweight	1.78 (1.23–2.58)	1.59 (0.98–2.57)	1.93 (1.24–3.00)	1.58 (0.89–2.79)
Obese	0.69 (0.19–2.57)	0.59 (0.10–3.56)	0.90 (0.18–4.55)	0.52 (0.06–4.35)
Aspirin				
Nonuser	**2.25 (1.80–2.83)**	**2.25 (1.68–3.00)**	2.26 (1.73–2.95)	1.89 (1.34–2.67)
User	**1.67 (1.30–2.15)**	**1.54 (1.12–2.13)**	1.79 (1.32–2.42)	1.54 (1.03–2.30)

Take a look at the upper box highlighted in red. That is the overall odds ratio of 1.98, meaning that the odds of developing prostate cancer if you have the alleles (genetic risk factors) is 1.98 times the odds if you don't have the alleles.

9. By the way, odds ratio is used here as a measure of association because this was a ________________ - ____________________ study.

Now let's look down to aspirin. When they calculated the stratified odds ratio for aspirin use, they found among nonusers the risk went up, but among aspirin users the risk went down. What is going on here?

To answer the question, I would like to first present the wrong assumption that aspirin is simply acting as a confounder. That is not at all the case; but if it were, please follow along on this little mental exercise of what we would expect the odds ratios of nonusers and users to be if it *were* a confounder. If it were a confounder, the stratified odds ratio would *both* be lower, say both around 1.67. And what would *that* mean? That would mean that aspirin is acting as a positive confounder. The increased odds ratio of 1.98 was falsely high due to the presence of the confounder, aspirin. Somehow aspirin intake must also be causing prostate cancer, and once it's controlled for, the actual result decreased down to 1.67. It's a positive confounder in this theoretical case because its presence made the odd ratio *appear* higher (away from the null) than it actually is. And if aspirin was a *negative* confounder, what would we see? We would see the stratified odds ratios to both be higher than 1.98, say 2.25. But again, the odds ratio for the aspirin users would be 2.25 *and* the odds ratio for the nonusers would be 2.25. And let's think what *that* would mean: it would mean that the presence of aspirin is making the odds ratio smaller (closer to the null) than it actually is. That is, the presence of aspirin is protecting against cancer, so it appears that the odds ratio is 1.98 when it is actually 2.25. Aspirin is a negative confounder in this scenario because it falsely makes the odds ratio appear *closer* to null than it actually is.

Now, the right answer. Aspirin is not a confounder because the odds ratios of the stratified results go in opposite directions: one goes up and one goes down. So we have to switch off our brain in the way it thinks about confounding…we now see that there is something going on between the presence of aspirin and the presence of the alleles that makes aspirin protective against the development of prostate cancer. So there is a huge difference. If it were a confounder, either positive or negative, the researchers would have to adjust for it in their results, and would no doubt find it interesting that aspirin was either causing (if positive confounder) or protecting against (if negative confounder) prostate cancer. But instead there is an interaction between the presence of the alleles and the aspirin. Something is going on so that aspirin is protective against cancer *only in the presence of the alleles.*

10. Again, if the stratified results are the same as each other but different than the unadjusted, the factor is a ____________________. But if the stratified results are different from one another, it means that there is ____________________ ____________________ ____________________ is present. (Or that there is an ____________________ between the two factors.)

The second paper I would like to present examined effect measure modification between the presence of an allele that increases the likelihood of developing Parkinson's disease, and the exposure to pesticides.

> Rhodes, et al. Pesticides that inhibit the ubiquitin–proteasome system: Effect measure modification by genetic variation in SKP1 in Parkinson's disease. *Environmental Research* Volume 126, October 2013, Pages 1-8

And here is a portion of their results table:

Genetic variant pesticide exposure level	Homozygous wildtype		Variant carriers		Interaction	
	Cases/Controls[a]	OR[b] (95%CI)	Cases/Controls[a]	OR[b] (95%CI)	OR (95%CI)	*p*-value
SKP1 rs2284312						
No/low exposure to all UPS-inhibiting pesticide[c]	79/148	1.00 (Reference)	29/52	1.01 (0.59, 1.73)	n.c.	n.c.
High exposure at either residence or workplace	68/103	1.25 (0.83, 1.90)	33/37	1.65 (0.95, 2.85)	1.30 (0.60, 2.83)	0.506
High exposure at both residence and workplace	43/50	1.62 (0.98, 2.66)	29/7	7.57 (3.14, 18.3)	4.63 (1.59, 13.5)	0.005

(The "homozygous wildtype" are those without the gene that is a risk factor for Parkinson's, and the "variant carriers" are those with the gene). In red you see the two stratified odds ratios, stratified by presence or absence of the gene. The authors did not give the total (unadjusted) odds ratio, so I will add this:

	+ Parkinson's	No Parkinsons's
High exposure at both home and work	72	57
No exposure	108	200

You can calculate the odds ratio (which would be the unadjusted odds ratio), and if you do, hopefully you get **2.34.**

The odds ratios stratified by the presence or absence of the gene is:

Gene not present: OR = **1.62**. Gene present: OR = **7.57**

Is this confounding? Clearly not, and I hope this is very obvious at this point in my discussion! There is a powerful interaction going in between the presence of the risk factor gene and exposure to the pesticides so that the presence of both results in a dramatically increased risk of Parkinson's.

Here is an exercise for you: Let's assume that the presence of the risk factor gene was acting as a confounder instead of an effect modifier. And the presence of the gene increases your likelihood of developing Parkinson's. We know that the crude (unadjusted) OR for the pesticide exposure is 2.34. So what would you expect would be the OR for pesticide exposure *adjusted for the presence of the risk factor gene* to be? Would it be less than 2.34, or greater than 2.34?

11. If the presence of the risk factor gene were a confounder, we would expect the adjusted odds ratio to be __________ than 2.34.

If you said less than 2.34, you are right! It would be a positive confounder. The gene presence is also contributing to the increased incidence of Parkinson's, and so the 2.34 is falsely high (away from the null). If you adjust for its presence, the result would be smaller (closer to the null).

So I hope that these two examples for the literature help you to understand the very important differences between confounding and effect measure modification!

Summary of Epidemiology 5

Confounding is when a third factor is also contributing to the outcome, and so it is causing a falsely high or low measure of association. The authors must carefully seek out all possible confounders that might be messing up their measure of association between the exposure they are interested in and the outcome, and they must adjust their results to account for all the confounders. As often happens, the crude measure of association goes away when taking into account significant confounders. Confounders are a statistical nuisance that are not addressed in detail in the papers, but rather simply "fixed" by adjusting for them. When one stratifies the results by the presence of absence of a confounder, the resulting measures of association differ from the unadjusted by 10% or more, but are roughly *equal to each other.*

Effect measure modification is quite different. Here, a third factor is interacting with the exposure in some biological way that results in a dramatically different measure of association when it is present vs when it is not. This is important and needs to be discussed and analyzed and hopefully studied in more detail by the researchers. When one stratifies the results by presence or absence of an effect modifier, the resulting measures of association are *very different from one another.*

Biostats 6: Regression

Now that you have a basic understanding of confounding, I will present how confounders are usually dealt with in the analyses of modern epidemiologic studies. Regression is an extremely useful and widespread tool for the analysis of the relationship between two or more variables, It allows researchers to detect, analyze and control for confounders, to detect interactions between variables, and to quantify the strength of association between variables. Therefore a thorough understanding of regression is required in the study of biostatistics.

Section B6.1: Correlation

I will start my discussion with “correlation,” which is slightly different than regression, but the two are very much related, and an understanding of correlation is necessary as a basis to the understanding of regression.

“Correlation” simply refers to how two factors are related to one another. That is, as one factor increases, does the other factor also increase? Or are they totally “independent” of one another?

Take a look at the following:

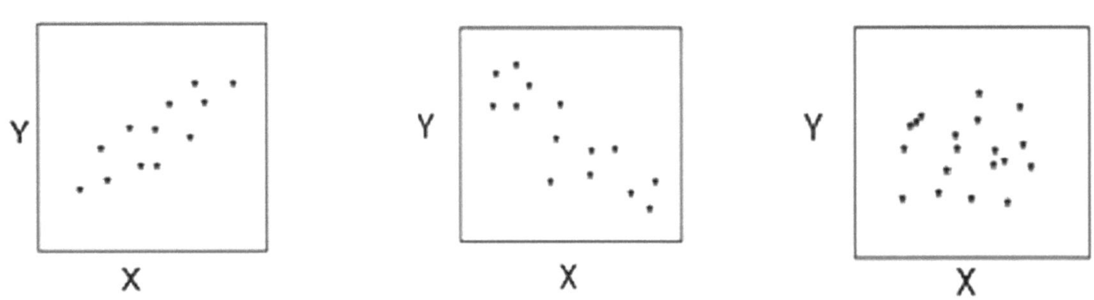

The graph on the left illustrates a "positive correlation," perhaps for example between grade-point average and hours spent studying. As one factor increases, in general so does the other. The graph in the middle shows a "negative correlation" perhaps for example between grade-point average and hours of video games played. As one factor increases, in general the other factor decreases. The graph on the right shows no obvious correlation, perhaps between the size of the TV and the average time spent watching it. Notice that in the first two graphs that do show a correlation that the correlation is not "perfect." There is some variability…as one increases, the other does not necessarily increase *as much* for all points. If it were a "perfect" positive correlation, all the points would fall on a straight line as shown here.

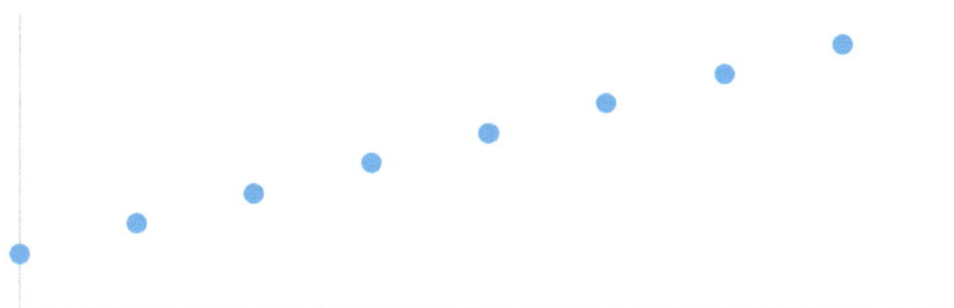

And so we define a "correlation coefficient," denoted by the variable r, to describe how well the two things are correlated. The r value can go from -1 to +1. Values of -1 and +1 mean perfect correlation, and of course you never see that in real life situations. Here are some examples:

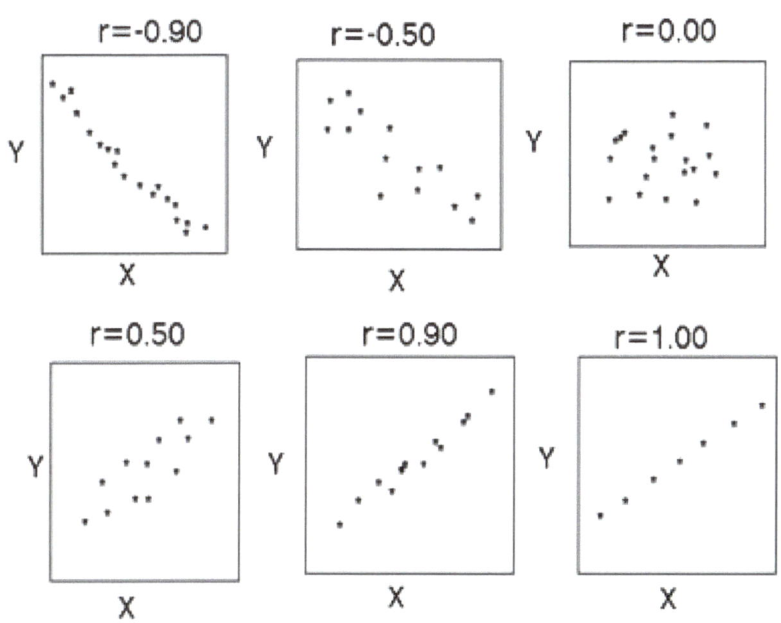

The actual equation for calculating r is a bit complex, and of course you do not need to memorize it, but a bit of familiarity is helpful:

$$r = \frac{Cov(x.y)}{\sqrt{(s_x{}^2)(s_y{}^2)}} \qquad \textbf{\textit{equationB6.1}}$$

"Cov(x.y)" is the "covariance of x and y and is defined by $\frac{\Sigma[(X-\bar{X})(Y-\bar{Y})]}{n-1}$

$s_x{}^2 = \frac{\Sigma(X-\bar{X})^2}{n-1}$ and $s_y{}^2 = \frac{\Sigma(Y-\bar{Y})^2}{n-1}$ (These are the variances of the of the x and y values).

So it's basically a sum of all the distances between each value and the mean x and y values.

1. The correlation coefficient, r, is a measure of how closely ____________________ two things are. If they are exactly perfectly correlated, the r is ____________. If there is absolutely no correlation between the two, the r is ______________. The coefficient r can go from ________ to ____________.

An important point about correlation is that the *slope* of the line has nothing to do with the magnitude of the correlation. The magnitude of the correlation is a measurement of how close the points are to the "best line." For example, if I were showing the correlation between height and weight, you can imagine that the slope of the line would change quite a bit depending on the units of height and weight.

Now of course, like all things in biostats, correlation of a sample means nothing; we care about the entire population. Therefore, to discuss the entire population we can generate a 95% confidence interval for our correlation.

Here is an example of a scatter plot showing the relationship between weight (in pounds) and systolic blood pressure (in mmHg). It was from a sample of 67 people:

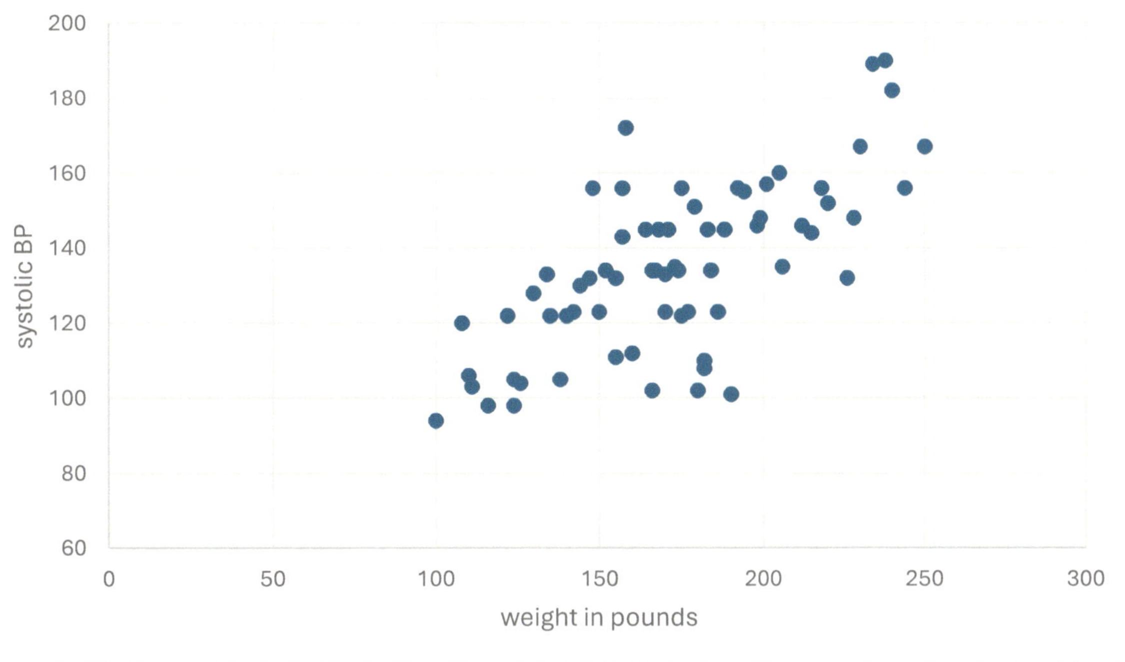

By looking at the graph, there appears to be a correlation between the two variables. Indeed, the computer tells us that

r = 0.70

That is a pretty strong correlation. But of course we would like to know what the correlation is for the entire population (whatever that population might be…all Americans, etc.). So, we need a 95% confidence interval. And how do we get that? Just as in previous chapters, we need the standard error, which is the standard deviation of the results if we ran our experiment over and over.

And the formula for the standard error of the correlation is:

$SE = \sqrt{\frac{1-r^2}{n-2}} = \sqrt{\frac{1-0.7^2}{67-2}} = 0.09.$ And, as before, the 95% confidence interval goes from 2 standard errors below to 2 standard errors above our value. OR (0.52 to 0.88). And so we can conclude that we have a statistically significant correlation, because if it were not statistically significant, the 95% confidence interval would include 0.

For hypothesis testing, we need to see how many standard errors away from the null our result is, (the t-score), so, that is 0.70/0.09 = 7.8.

7.8 standard errors is very far way from the null, so we certainly expect our probability (p-value) to be quite low. In fact when we plug in our t-score of 7.8 into our calculator, we get a p value of < 0.00001.

2. If the 95% CI of a correlation coefficient, r, includes 0, then we ____________________ reject the null hypothesis.

Section B6.2: Simple Linear Regression

So now that we know that there is a *correlation* between these two factors, we now go to the next level, which is analyzing a regression analysis between the two. Regression is a bit different than correlation. In regression, we are concerned about how one factor *influences* another factor. We designate one factor as the "independent variable," and the other as the "dependent variable," and our goal is to see how if and by how much the independent variable influences (causes change in) the dependent variable. By convention, we put the independent variable on the x-axis, and the dependent variable on the y-axis.

Our example again:

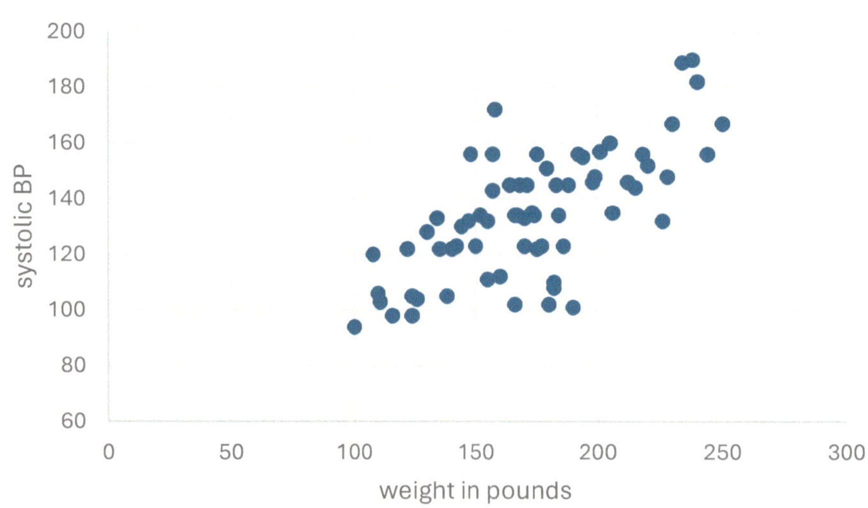

We now say that weight is the independent variable, and we want to see how much a change in weight causes a change in systolic blood pressure, which is the dependent variable. And this is one major difference between regression and correlation. In correlation, it does not matter which variable is put on which axis, the correlation will always be the same…it's how closely related to one another they are. In regression, axis *does* matter: we only care about the relationship in *one* direction, and that is how much the independent variable is influencing the dependent variable.

3. In regression, we put the independent variable on the _____ axis, and the dependent variable on the _______ axis, and we want to know how much the ________________________ variable influences the ________________________ variable.

We start by constructing a regression line through the points:

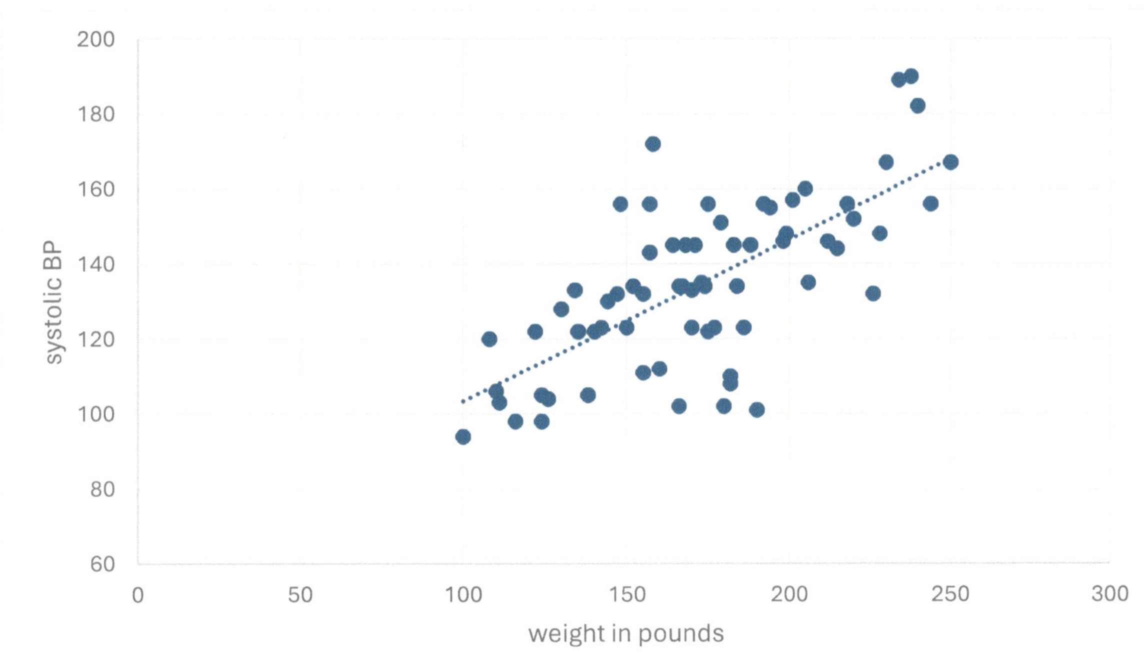

The regression line can be thought of as the "line of best fit" through the points that balances the differences between all the data points and the line. And it is the *slope* of this line that is very important to us. The slope of the line is calculated by a "least squares" method that's a bit complex, but if you're interested is given by:

$$Slope = r(\frac{s_y}{s_x})$$

s_y and s_x are the standard deviations of the y values and x values, and if you recall the formula for r (equation 9.1), you will see how complex the formula is!

Once we have the slope (the computer tells me that the slope is **0.43),** then write the equation for the line. I'm sure you remember your 8th grade algebra, when you learned that the equation for a line is $y = mx + b$, in which m is the slope, and b is the y-intercept.

In the world of biostats, the equation of the regression line is written like this:

$$y = \beta_0 + \beta_1 x$$

β_0 is our y-intercept, and β_1 is the slope of the line, also called the *regression coefficient.*

The computer also tells me that the y-intercept is **60.3**.

So the equation of the line is: $y = 60.3 + 0.43x$

Or, $$\boldsymbol{Systolic\ BP = 60.3 + 0.43(weight)}$$

Now that we have our regression equation we know how much systolic blood pressure is influenced by weight, and we can predict the outcome. For example, we could predict that someone who weighs 200 pounds would have a systolic BP of:

$$Systolic\ BP = 60.3 + 0.43(200) = 146.3\ mmHg$$

We can also say that since the slope is 0.43, for every one pound increase in weight, we expect a 0.43 point increase in systolic blood pressure. (For every 10 pounds increase in weight, we expect a 4.3 point increase in blood pressure).

Please note that β_0, the y-intercept, has no real practical meaning. Recall that the y-intercept is the y value when x is 0. Obviously in real life situations our x (weight here) cannot be 0! It is only used for the mathematics.

4. In regression, β_1 is the _______ of the "best line" and tells us how much the dependent variable changes with a change in the independent variable.

Residuals

Let's look at one particular person on the scatter plot:

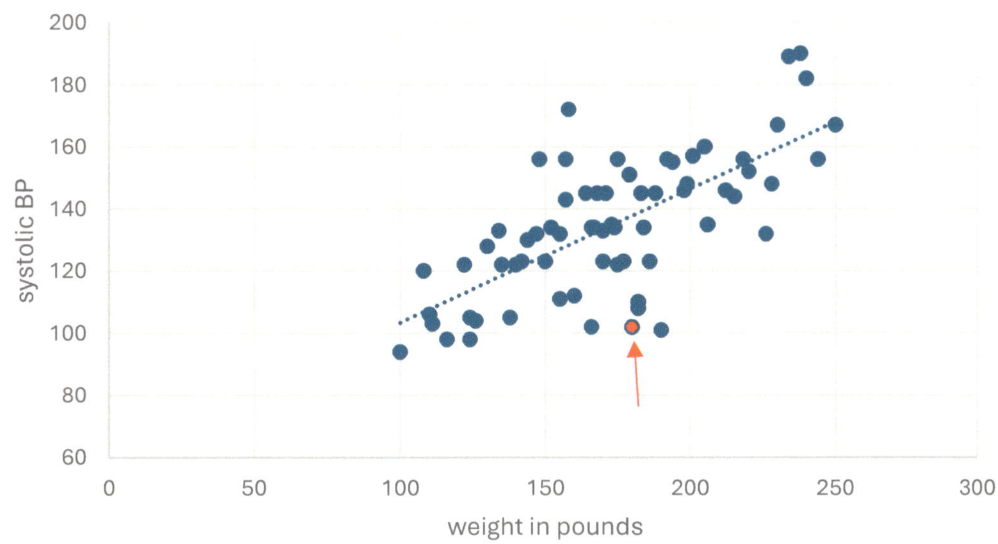

The data point in red is a person who weighs 178 pounds. What would we expect his systolic blood pressure to be?

$$Systolic\ BP = 60.3 + 0.43(178) = 136.8\ mmHg$$

But as you can see by the plot, his actual blood pressure is 102 mmHg. Most of the people have readings that do not fall right on the "best line," and the difference between one's actual output and one's expect output is called the "residual."

By convention, $\boldsymbol{residual = observed - expected}$, so here residual is $102 - 136.8 = -34.8$

Populations

I know I sound like a broken record, but again, the scatter plot shows a *sample* of 67 people. And as usual, we do not care about our one sample, we care about the entire population. So if we took many many samples of 67 people, we would get many many slopes of the regression line, and if we averaged all the resulting regression slopes and plotted them, we would get, you guessed it…a normal distribution! So, the standard deviation of that distribution is…the standard error of the slope.

And of course there's a fancy formula for this.

$$SE_{\beta_1} = \frac{\sqrt{\frac{\Sigma(y_i - \hat{y}_i)}{n-2}}}{\sqrt{\Sigma(x_i - \bar{x})}}$$

But of course, we can just ask our computer or calculator to give us the standard error, and in this case, $SE_{\beta_1} = 0.055$.

So then for the entire population, we would say that the regression coefficient for the independent variable x (which is weight in pounds), is:

$$\beta_1 = \mathbf{0.43 \pm 2(0.055) = (0.32 \text{ to } 0.54)}$$

And of course, we can then do hypothesis testing. You know the drill: how many standard errors away from the null is our result?

By the way, what is the null value of a regression coefficient? The null value is 0, meaning that there is no influence of one variable on the other.

The t-score would be $\frac{0.43}{0.055} = 7.8$, and as you can imagine, the p-value is very very small.

5. When we calculate our regression coefficient, β_1, we learn how much our y-value is influenced by our x-value, but that is only for one small sample. Since we really care about the entire ____________________, we must calculate a ____________________ interval.

Coefficient of Determination

Look again at our scatter plot:

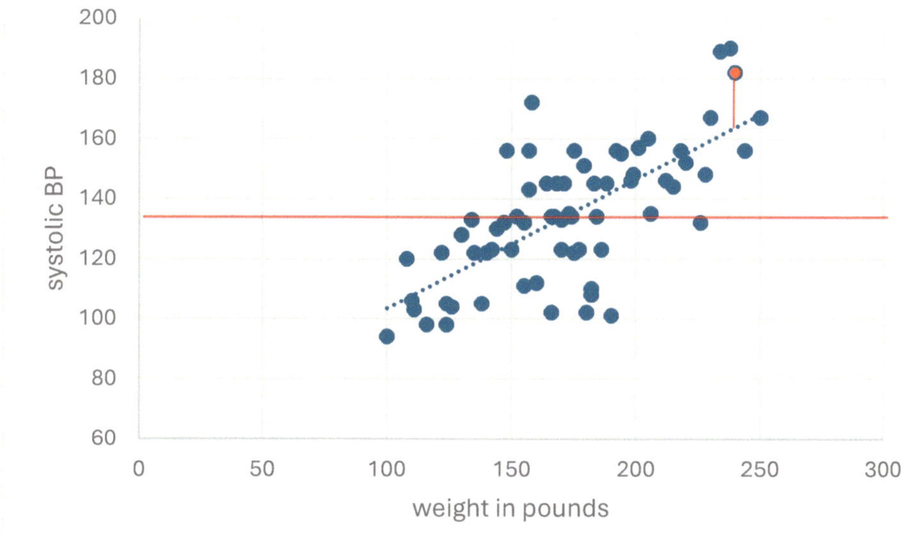

Although a few of the points lie on right on the regression line, most do not. And that is because there are other factors other than weight that are influencing blood pressure. For example, genetic factors, physical activity, cigarette smoking, etc. If weight were the *only* factor that was making blood pressure change, then all the points would like directly on the regression line. So, the "residuals" are due to all the other factors. In the graph above, I have drawn one such residual as the red line going down from the point in red to the regression line. That distance is referred to as $y - \hat{y}$, where $\hat{y}$ is the expected value (if there were no other factors).

Now I will draw a different line:

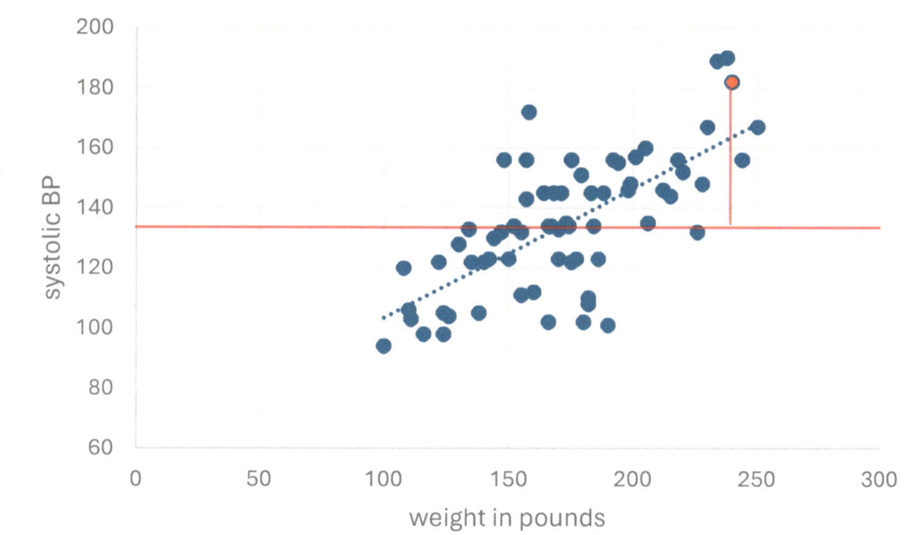

Here the line goes from y to the mean of all y values. This is referred to as $y - \bar{y}$, and is the difference that is due to the regression itself. What do I mean by "due to the regression itself?" Well, our value in red, the systolic blood pressure is not 136.4 (the mean) because it's influenced by weight…because the weight causes changes in blood pressure. (And this particular point is also influenced by other factors or else it would be right on the blue regression line!)

So what the coefficient of determination tells us is what proportion of the total differences is due to the regression itself vs due to the error, and by "error" I mean due to all the other factors that may be influencing blood pressure.

The coefficient of determination is called R^2, and is given by $\frac{variation\ due\ to\ regression\ itself}{total\ variation}$

And it is called "R^2" because it is, in fact, the square of the correlation coefficient, r.

And so if R^2 is 1, then all of the variation is due to the factor in question, and there are no other factors that are influencing our outcome. If R^2 is 0.5, then 50% of the variation of the output (the dependent variable) is due to the variation of the independent variable. And if R^2 close to 0, then all the variation in the points is due to other variable, and our independent variable of interest is not influencing the outcome at all.

6. The coefficient of determination is labeled as __________, and is the square of the ______________________________ ______________________________. It tells us what percent of the total ______________________ of the y-value is due to variation in the x-value.

Section B6.3: Simple Logistic regression

Everything I have talked about thus far in this chapter was ***linear*** **regression**, because outcome was continuous: blood pressure is a continuous measure. But there are three other kinds of regressions, two of which I will discuss in this chapter, and one I will save for a later chapter.

Here are the three regression types that are discussed in this chapter:

Regression	Outcome	Predictor(s)
Linear	Continuous	Continuous, binary, categorical
Logistic	Binary	Continuous, binary, categorical
Poisson	Incidence	Continuous, binary, categorical

In **logistic regression**, the outcome is not continuous, but rather is binary—that is, did an event occur or not? In **Poisson regression**, the outcome is an incidence rate. Note that in all types of regression, the predictor (the independent variable) can be any type at all: continuous, binary or categorical. (If you need to review continuous vs categorical variables, I covered them in Biostats 2 and 3.

I believe that **logistic regression** is the most prevalent (and relevant) type of regression that we see in modern medical research. So much of research deals with outcomes—did an event occur or did it not—and use logistic regression to analyze their data. Therefore, the majority of the remaining chapter focuses on this type of regression.

Often in epidemiologic studies, the outcome is not continuous, it is categorical, and by far the most common categorical outcome is *binary*: did an event occur, yes or no? And one of the ways that we describe yes/no outcomes is with *odds*. What are the odds of an event occurring? (We also of course often use "risk" or cumulative incidence, but in the world of multiple regression we almost always talk about odds). So when the outcome (the dependent variable) is the odds of an event occurring we use *logistic regression.* Logistic regression can be "simple" if only one independent variable:

$$(Odds\ of\ event) = \beta_0 + \beta_1 x_1$$

Remember that odds is a *ratio*, and whenever we are dealing with a ratio, we have to convert it into the logarithmic scale. I explained why this is so in detail in Section B3.4, so feel free to review this if you like!

So the actual logistic regression equation becomes:

$$ln(Odds\ of\ event) = \beta_0 + \beta_1 x_1$$

To help with the deep dive into logistic regression, I would like to present another fictitious study:

Investigators sought to examine the relationship between climate and hospital admissions for congestive heart failure.

They performed a case-control study by identifying 2152 patients who were admitted to the hospital due to CHF exacerbation in the month of July of one year across the continental 48 states.

The predictor of interest was whether the patient lived in a "warm" state (average yearly temperature > 55ºF), or in a "cool" state (average yearly temperature ≤ 55ºF).

The 3795 controls were people with a prior diagnosis of CHF who were not admitted into the hospital during that time period.

And here are the results

State climate	Cases (hospital admission)	Controls (no admission)
Warm state	1253	1803
Cool state	899	1892

Table B5.1

The regression equation is this:

$$ln(Odds\ of\ event) = \beta_0 + \beta_1 x_1,$$

where x_1 is the predictor "did the patient live in a warm state? It is coded as a 1 if they did, and as a 0 if they did not.

The computer tells us that the regression equation results is:

$$ln(odds\ of\ being\ admitted) = -0.74 + 0.\mathbf{38}x_1$$

equation B6.1

0.38 is our *regression coefficient*. What does this mean?

Well let's say a person does not live in a warm state. Then,

$$\ln(odds\ of being\ admitted) = -0.74 + (0.38)0 = -0.74$$

To get the actual odds (to convert back from the logarithmic scale) we *exponentiate* the coefficient. Thus,

$$odds\ of\ being\ admitted(cool\ state) = e^{-0.74} = 0.48$$

And of course you can calculate this directly from the 2x2 table. The odds of being admitted in in a cool state is just

$$\frac{899}{1892} = 0.48$$

Now, what if a person lives in a warm state?

$$ln(odds\ of\ being\ admitted) = -0.74 + 0.\mathbf{38}(1) = -0.36$$

And so,

$$odds\ of\ being\ admitted(cool\ state) = e^{-0.36} = 0.70$$

Recall that the measure of association between the two groups is the odds ratio.

The magic of logistic regression:

Follow me along with a bit of algebra do demonstrate the magic of the logistic regression: We are comparing two groups. In one group, x_1 is coded as 1 (i.e. that particular factor is present), and in the other group, x_1 is coded as 0 because the factor is not present.

So, in group a, $x_1 = 1$:

$$ln(odds\ of\ event) = \beta_0 + \beta_1$$

And in group b, $x_1 = 0$:

$$ln(odds\ of\ event) = \beta_0$$

Following me so far? So,

$$ln\left(odds_{group\ a}\right) - ln\left(odds_{group\ b}\right) = \boldsymbol{\beta_1}$$

Do you see that?

Ok, now just reverse this so easier to see:

$$\boldsymbol{\beta_1} = ln\left(odds_{group\ a}\right) - ln\left(odds_{group\ b}\right)$$

Now, remember a property of logarithms that says that:

$$ln(a) - ln(b) = ln\left(\frac{a}{b}\right)$$

Therefore,

$$\beta_1 = ln \frac{(odds_{group\ a})}{(odds_{group\ b})}$$

And what is $\frac{(odds_{group\ a})}{(odds_{group\ b})}$? It is the ODDS RATIO!!

So our regression coefficient β_1 is the ln of the odds ratio of being admitted if in a warm state compared with living in a not warm state!

(And that is the magic of logistic regression)

So since our regression coefficient is 0.38, then the odds ratio is $e^{0.38} = \mathbf{1.46}$

The odds of being admitted if living in a warm state is 1.46 times greater than the odds of being admitted if not living in a warm state.

And of course you can confirm this by directly calculating the odds ratio from the 2x2 table (table B5.1):

$$OR = \frac{a/c}{b/d} = \frac{1253/899}{1803/1892} = 1.46$$

7. In logistic regression, the regression coefficient is the ln of the ________ ____________.

More magic of logistic regression

So magic #1 of logistic regression is that the regression coefficient is equal to the *odds ratio*.

Magic #2 of logistic regression is that it can handle independent variables that are *continuous.* And that is something we cannot do with a 2x2 table! Remember, our output is binary (yes/no), and in the above example, the independent variable, (yes/no warm state) was also binary. And so we can set up our 2x2 table. But what if our independent variable is continuous? For example, the researchers might be curious if a person's weight influences whether or not they were admitted into the hospital. Weight is a continuous variable, so we cannot calculate our odds ratio via a 2x2 table. Now we really need our computer to give us a regression equation.

So, here is the scenario: the outcome is binary—was the person admitted to the hospital, yes or no?

The input (the independent variable) is now continuous (weight in kilograms). Again, the logistic regression equation is:

$$\ln(Odds\ of\ event) = \beta_0 + \beta_1 x_1$$

Now, our x_1 is weight in kilograms.

$$\ln(being\ admitted) = \beta_0 + \beta_1(weight)$$

And the computer gives us this result:

$$ln(odds\ of\ admitted) = -1.2 + \mathbf{0.034}x_1$$

Our regression coefficient is now **0.034.** This means that for every one kilogram increase in weight, the *ln* of the odds of being admitted increases by 0.034.

And just as before, the regression coefficient gives us the odds ratio.

$$OR = e^{0.034} = 1.035$$

Take a second to translate this into words:

For every one kilogram of weight increase, the odds of being admitted is 1.035 times higher. Or, for every kilogram increase in weight, there is a 3.5% higher odds of being admitted.

To repeat: we are using a *logistic* regression. Why? Because the *output* (the y-value, or the dependent variable) is binary.

8. The different kinds of regression that we use only depends on the ____________________ variable; it does not matter what kind of variable the _________________ variable is.

The output is binary; the input is now continuous, and the only way to mathematically analyze the continuous input is with logistic regression; we cannot do it "by hand."

Populations

Well of course, the β_0 and β_1 we obtain in our logistic regression are based on one sample. As usual, in biostats we are not concerned about are one sample, we are concerned about how it relates to the entire "universe." As such, we must again define a 95% confidence interval which, as before is based on the standard error. The good news is that in logistic regression, the standard error cannot be calculated by hand; it has to be done by the computer, which uses a "maximum likelihood" method for calculating β_0 and β_1. You do not need to know the details, but essentially the computer comes up with values for β_0 and β_1 for the sample that is the "most likely" of all possible values for β_0 and β_1 given the data in our sample, and when it gives us these values, it also gives us the standard errors associated with them.

In equation B5.1, the regression coefficient, β_1 was 0.38. The computer would also give us the standard error SE_{β_1}= 0.11.

So, $$\beta_1 = 0.38 \pm 2(0.11) = (0.16, 0.60)$$

But remember that we are on a logarithmic scale, so we have to convert back:

$$odds\ ratio = e^{0.38}\ , 95\%CI\ (e^{0.16}\ to\ e^{0.60})$$

$$odds\ ratio = 1.46\ (1.17, 1.82)$$

Section B6.4: Simple Poisson regression

Although I won't go into too much detail about Poisson regression, it is important for you to be somewhat familiar with it. In Poisson regression, the output is an incidence rate, and the measure of association when comparing two groups is the incidence rate ratio. (If you need a refresher, I discussed person-time incidence rates and ratios in section E3.4

Like logistic regression, the output in Poisson regression is a ratio, and so we need to be in the logarithmic scale. The basic equation is:

$$\ln(incidence\ rate\ of\ event) = \beta_0 + \beta_1 x_1$$

And recall the incidence rate is the number of cases (or events) per person-year. Here is an example from the literature:

Marcus et al. HIV infection and incidence of ischemic stroke. *AIDS* 28(13): 1911-1919, August 2014.

The purpose of the study was to determine if there is an association of HIV infection with incidence of ischemic stroke.

Here is a portion from their results section:

Results:

Among 24 768 HIV-positive and 257 600 HIV-negative individuals, the ischemic stroke rate per 100 000 person-years was 125 (*n* = 151 events) for HIV-positive and 74 (*n* = 1128 events) for HIV-negative individuals, with an adjusted rate ratio of 1.4 [95% confidence interval (CI) 1.2–1.7). Compared with

Notice that the results are incidence rates and incidence rate ratios, and therefore the regression that they use is Poisson. Here is a portion of their methods section:

Methods:

We used Poisson models to obtain rate ratios for incident ischemic stroke associated with HIV infection, both overall and stratified by $CD4^{+}$ cell counts (cells/µl) and HIV RNA copies (copies/ml), with HIV-negative individuals as the reference group. We also obtained rate ratios for risk factors in the HIV-positive subset.

By the same algebraic argument that I presented for logistic regression, in Poisson regression the exponentiated version of the regression coefficient is the *incidence rate ratio.*

And also, as with all types of regression, we must calculate a 95% confidence interval of the regression coefficient, so that we can give a reasonable estimate for the entire population. And similar to logistic regression, the computer gives us the values of β_1 and β_0 by the "maximum likelihood" method, and also gives us the corresponding standard errors. Then, you know the drill: it's 2 x the SE above and 2 x the SE below the results that gives us the 95% CI.

And that is all I'll mention about Poisson regression; there will be a bit more on it in Biostats 6.

Summary of Biostats 6

First I discussed *correlation,* which is a measure of how closely two factors are associated with one another.

I then discussed *regression* which is how much the dependent variable (the y-value) changes with change in the independent variable (the x-axis). We are interested in the "regression coefficient" which is the slope of the regression line. The discussion initially was for *linear* regression, in which the outcome is continuous.

Like all things in biostats, we must translate our one sample to the entire population by constructing a 95% confidence interval using the standard error of the regression coefficient.

The *coefficient of determination* is the proportion of the total variation that is due to the regression itself. That is, how much of the change in our dependent variable is due to change in the independent variable?

I then presented the other kinds of regressions, and I explored logistic regression in some detail, as it is extremely important in current research.

Finally I briefly presented Poisson regression.

And that brings us to the end of chapter B5. "Wait!" you say. "You said in your introduction to this chapter that you would explain how confounding is dealt with mathematically, but I don't see anything here that explains that!"

Um, yes, you are right. That will actually be explained in the next chapter. But in order to understand the stuff in the next chapter, you needed to gain a good understanding of this chapter first!

Biostats 7: Multivariable Regression

Multivariable regression in extension of the material presented in the previous chapter. Upon completion of this chapter, you will have a thorough understanding of mathematical models that deal with multiple confounders and prediction models.

Section B7.1 What is multivariable regression?

In the last chapter, I introduced single variable regression, which is the linear relationship between two factors:

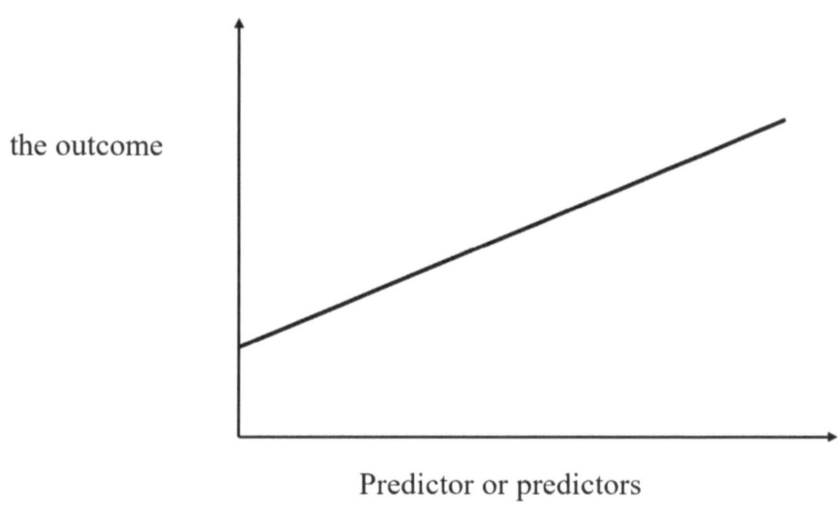

There is an outcome (also called the dependent variable) on the y axis, and the predictor (also called the independent variable) on the x axis. Note that I now put "predictor *or predictors*" on the x axis. And that is the difference: in simple (single variable) regression, there is one predictor, while in multivariable regression there are more than one. So I will start with an example.

Suppose we are examining a relationship between two factors. The independent variable is how many hours you spend studying biostatistics and epidemiology, and the dependent variable is how much fun you will have practicing medicine. Well, obviously there is a positive relationship between the two as shown:

$$Y = \beta_0 + \beta_1 x_1$$

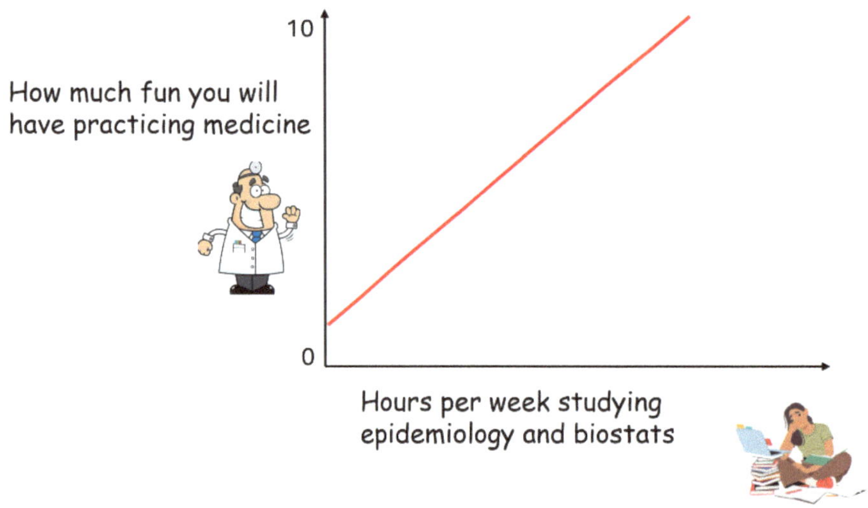

And the equation of the "best line" is $Y = \beta_0 + \beta_1 x_1$

1. Recall that β_0 is the __________________________ of the regression line, and β_1 is the _____________ of the regression line.

Now, if I plot all the data points, it is not a *perfectly linear* relationship:

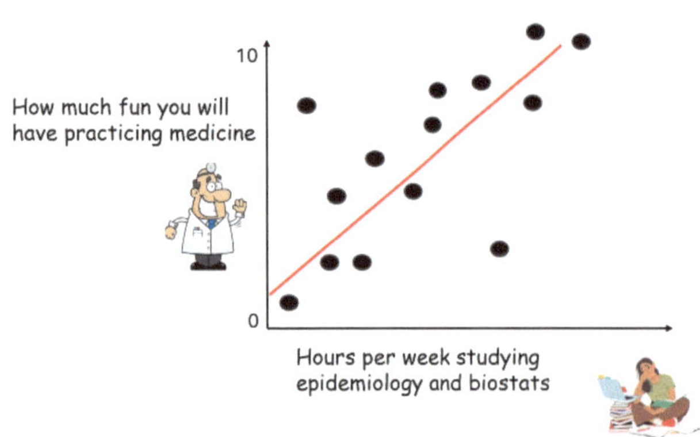

Why is that? Why are all the points not directly on the line? Well, because there are other factors that might be playing a role in how much fun you will have practicing medicine. For example, do you like the environment in which you work? Do you like your colleagues? Is your job intellectually stimulating? Do you have a good balance of professional and personal life, etc.? So there are many other factors that are also influencing how much fun you will have practicing medicine. And so we change our regression equation to a multivariable regression equation, which looks like this:

$$Y = \beta_0 + \beta_1 x_1 + \beta_x x_2 + \beta_x x_3 + \cdots$$

Multiple cofactors!

Y-intercept

Our y-intercept is still β_0 , but now we have x_1, x_2, x_3 etc, which are all the variables that are influencing the outcome y. We call these variables "cofactors." And all the βs are the slopes associated with each particular variable. That is, how much the outcome changes due to that particular variable.

The multivariable regression equation is a computer-generated equation that allows researchers to sort out the multifaceted nature of risk factors. We cannot easily draw and visualize by hand the relationship between the cofactors and the outcome as we could do with simple regression: multiple regression is way too complex!

2. A multivariable regression equation takes into account many different ____________________ that may be influencing the outcome. All the βs are the ______________ associated with that particular variable x. We cannot draw or visualize multivariable regression; it has to be generated by a _____________________________.

Why we need multivariable regression

To demonstrate why we need multivariable regression, I would like to present a study.

> Zhang, et al. Risk factors for deaths during the 2009 heat wave in Adelaide, Australia: a matched case-control study. *Int J Biometeorol* 2017 Jan;61(1):35-47.

In this study, researchers were researching the influence of several cofactors that might have contributed to deaths during a heat wave in Adelaide, Australia. There were quite a number of possible cofactors (independent variables) that they were considering. Here is the list:

	Cases (%)	Controls (%)	*P*
Demographic			
Non-European ethnic	7	1	<0.05
Married/De facto	14	65	<0.01
SEIFA ranking ≤3	19	12	>0.05
Main language speak at home/English	94	97	>0.05
Occupation/retired	70	74	>0.05
Education ≤ year 12	71	61	>0.05
Annual household income ≤70,000	75	69	>0.05
Living condition			
Institutional living	10	11	>0.05
North face building	56	83	<0.05
Living alone	68	27	<0.05
Having pet	30	48	<0.01
Air conditioning in house	49	89	<0.01
Air conditioning in bedroom	17	54	<0.01
Easy ventilation	51	80	<0.01
Support			
No relative or friend or carer visit	13	8	>0.05
No home delivery service	80	89	>0.05
Having private health insurance	19	62	<0.01
Having emergency button	13	32	<0.05
Having social activity more than once a week	40	90	<0.01
Health status			
Heart diseases	81	20	<0.01
Asthma	25	11	<0.05
Respiratory diseases	33	15	<0.05
High blood pressure	45	43	>0.05
Kidney diseases	33	5	<0.05
Diabetes	35	13	<0.05
Dementia	37	2	<0.05
Depression	68	13	<0.01
Confine to bed	13	1	<0.05
Neurological disease	6	5	>0.05
Cancer	27	23	>0.05
Taken more than two medicine	77	70	>0.05
Need assistance for daily activities ADL = 1	89	2	<0.01
Behaviour changes during heat wave			
Dress lighter than usual	84	95	>0.05
Stopping usual activities	59	63	>0.05
Use air conditioning	27	86	<0.01
Take extra bath	12	13	>0.05
Open windows	17	17	>0.05
Use of refreshment	53	83	<0.05

Wow! There are so many!

And you can see they did a case-control study, in which the cases were deaths, and the controls were people who lived in the same area, and experienced the same heat wave, but did not die. Let's consider one of the cofactors, diabetes, which I underlined. You can see that 35% of those who died had diabetes, while only 13% of those who did not die had diabetes, and so it certainly appears that diabetes is a strong risk factor for dying during the heat wave. A 2x2 table of the raw numbers would look like this:

	Cases	controls
Diabetes	26	22
No diabetes	56	142
totals	82	164

And the odds ratio is **2.9.** But the smart researchers would say, "Wait a minute…maybe there are confounders here. A lot of the diabetics probably also had heart disease, right? So maybe it is the heart disease that largely contributed to the deaths rather than the diabetes itself!" In other words, they would worry that heart disease is a confounder. So as presented in Epidemiology 4, a way that they could check for that would be to *stratify* the results by heart disease status:

	Cases	controls
Diabetes	26	22
No diabetes	56	142
totals	82	164

OR = 2.9

Heart disease

Diabetes	a	b
No diabetes	c	d

OR = 2.3

No heart disease

Diabetes	a	b
No diabetes	c	d

OR = 2.3

And now we see that the "adjusted" odds ratio is now 2.3. That is, diabetes, *when adjusted for heart disease status,* now shows an odds ratio of 2.3. Since the odds ratio went down (closer to the null) we say that indeed heart disease is a confounder, and a good amount of the apparent association between diabetes and deaths was actually due to the presence of heart disease. But the researchers might then say, "Hey wait a minute, what if more of the people with heart disease were confined to bed compared with people without heart disease? Could being confined to bed be acting as a confounder on heart disease?" And they would again stratify the results, now by "confined to bed" status:

	Cases	controls
Diabetes	26	22
No diabetes	56	142
totals	82	164

OR = 2.9

Heart disease

Diabetes	a	b
No diabetes	c	d

OR = 2.3

Confined

Diabetes	a	b
No diabetes	c	d

OR = 1.6

not confined

Diabetes	a	b
No diabetes	c	d

OR = 1.6

No heart disease

Diabetes	a	b
No diabetes	c	d

OR = 2.3

confined

Diabetes	a	b
No diabetes	c	d

OR = 2.1

not confined

Diabetes	a	b
No diabetes	c	d

OR = 2.1

And indeed "confined to bed" status is acting as a confounder to heart disease (which in turn is acting as a confounder to diabetes). But then the researchers might say, "Hey wait a minute, what if among those confined to bed, not having an air-conditioner may have played a roll…and once again, they stratify the results…and so on. You can see the problem. There were only 246 participants to start, and so once they stratify one time, or maybe two times, they start running out of people to fill the 2x2 cells.

What they really want to know is: is diabetes—*independent of all the other cofactors*—a risk factor for death during the heat wave? And so they would have to stratify the results many many times to account for all the other 45 or so cofactors listed! Mathematically we cannot do this, but the computer can, using multivariable regression. (Admittedly though, even the computer would have a tough time with so many cofactors, but it has no problem at all giving a regression equation for 4, 5, 6 or perhaps more cofactors). The multivariable regression gives us the regression coefficients (βs), which is how much each particular cofactor influences the outcome *independent of all the other outcomes.* That is, it gives us the value of each coefficient while *adjusting* for all the other variables in the equation.

3. Each β in multivariable regression is the regression coefficient for the valuable attached to it that is adjusted for all the other _______________________ in the equation.

Section B7.2: How multivariable regression helps clinicians and patients

Decision models

Decision models to help clinicians diagnose disease are often based on multivariable regressions. Here is an example. One of the critical decisions Emergency department clinicians are often called upon to make is determining if a patient complaining of chest pain are at risk of a heart attack or not. She often used decision models to help with this. An example would be:

$$Y = \beta_0 + \beta_1 x_1 + \beta_2 x_2 + \beta_3 x_3 + \beta_4 x_4 + \cdots$$

Odds of heart attack?

Does the pain radiate to left/arm or jaw?

Is diaphoresis present?

age

Is the pain pleuritic?

So the outcome, y, is the odds of a particular patient with chest pain having a heart attack. The x variables are cofactors as labeled. And the βs are the regression coefficients. The computer would tell us that the results would look something like this:

$$y = 0.7 + 1.4x_1 + 2.3x_2 + 1.1x_3 - 1.7x_4$$

The clinician would then be able to calculate the patient's odds of having a heart attack simply by filling in the equation. For example, if the patient with chest pain is 62 years old, and the pain does not radiate to the left arm or jaw, but the patient is diaphoretic (sweaty), and the pain is not pleuritic, then $x_1$would be coded as 0, x_2 would be coded as 1, x_3 would be coded as 62, and x_4 would be coded as 0. And then the odds would be calculated which would help the clinician decide whether or not to admit the patient and consult a cardiologist, etc.

By the way, the above model is fictitious, please do not use it when working in an emergency department! But here is a real example from the literature, a decision model to help the clinician decide the chance of surviving melanoma for at least 10 years:

> Schuchter, et al. A Prognostic Model for Predicting 10-Year Survival in Patients with Primary Melanoma. *Annals of Internal Medicine*: Volume 125, Number 5,1996.

Here is the list of cofactors they included in their decision model:

Lesion thickness
- <0.76 mm
- 0.76–1.69 mm
- 1.70–3.60 mm

Primary lesion on an extremity
Age at diagnosis ≤60 y
Female sex

And here is the multiple regression equation:

$$Y = -2.25 + 3.93x_1 + 2.25x_2 + 1.07x_3 + 1.47x_4 + 1.1x_5 + 0.71x_6$$

So the strongest cofactor—the one that gives the patient the highest chance of surviving ten year or more—is if the lesion thickness is < 0.76 mm. (x_1).

Example: the patient is a 65-year-old male, the lesion is 0.85 mm thick and is on his hand.

The equation would be:

$$Y = -2.25 + 3.93(0) + 2.25(1) + 1.07(0) + 1.47(1) + 1.1(0) + 0.71(0)$$

Section B7.3: Multivariable Logistic regression

Just like simple regressions that I discussed in chapter B5, multivariable regression comes in three main "flavors" (well, actually four, but the fourth will be discussed in a future chapter). The three types are:

Multiple linear regression
Multiple logistic regression
Multiple Poisson regression

As in simple regression, it is the outcome (the dependent variable) that determines which of the regressions we need to use. All of them can handle any kind of predictor (independent variable).

4. All the regressions can handle all kinds of ___________________________, but they differ in terms of what kind of ________________________ they have.

As I did in Biostats 5, I will present my "deep dive" into multivariable regression with attention to multivariable logistic regression.

The magic of multivariable regression

The most amazing and useful aspect of multivariable regression is that it allows researchers to identify confounding and effect measure modification in a quick and easy mathematical model (quick and easy for the computer, that is!)

Researchers can include several independent variables into their model, and the multivariable regression equation will give them the regression coefficients for each variable *independent of all the other variables.* What I mean by that is…well, let's look at our example. This is the fictitious study I presented in section B5.3 on the risk of being admitted to the hospital if you live in a warm state vs if you live in a cool state.

Here were the results:

State climate	Cases (hospital admission)	Controls (no admission)
Warm state	1253	1803
Cool state	899	1892

And this was the regression result:

$$\ln(odds\ of\ being\ admitted) = -0.74 + 0.\mathbf{38}x_1$$

and so the odds ratio is $e^{0.38} = \mathbf{1.46}$

But now the savvy researchers wonder if a person's weight might be playing into the results. That is, could weight be acting as a *confounder?* To answer this question, they run a new regression, and this time have two independent variables:

Our study on hospital admissions for CHF and climate, take 2:

Output: odds of being admitted for CHF

Inputs (independent variables):

x_1 warm state ? yes/no (categorical variable)

x_2 weight in kilograms (continuous variable)

Computer's multivariable logistic regression solution:

$$ln(odds\ of\ admission) = \beta_0 + \beta_1 x_1 + \beta_2 x_2$$

$$ln(odds\ of\ admission) = -1.1 + \mathbf{0.13}\boldsymbol{x_1} + 0.026x_2$$

So our regression coefficient for warm state, β_1, is now **0.13**. What does this mean? It means that this is our new regression coefficient for warm state *adjusted for weight.* In the first experiment, we found that β_1 was **0.38**. That was the *unadjusted* regression coefficient. And just like before, we can calculate our new odds ratio, which is now the *adjusted* odds ratio:

$$\ln(OR) = 0.13$$

$$OR = e^{0.13} = \mathbf{1.14}$$

Recall that we calculated the *unadjusted* odds ratio to be 1.43. When the adjusted odds ratio differs from the adjusted odds ratio, as the case here, by more than 10% (approximately), we say that the second variable (weight) is a *confounder*.

5. In multivariable regression, each regression coefficient gives us the odds ratio of its corresponding variable that is ______________________________ for all other variables.

6. Because our adjusted odds ratio is less than the unadjusted odds ratio, we know that our second variable, weight, is acting as a ______________________.

Translation: The odds ratio for being admitted to the hospital warm state vs cool state *adjusted for weight* is 1.14. And, "the odds of being admitted to the hospital if you live in a warm state, adjusted for weight, is 14% higher than the odds of being admitted to the hospital if you live in a cool state."

And now for more magic, we can do the same for weight:

$$ln(odds\ of\ admission) = -1.1 + 0.13x_1 + 0.026x_2$$

For weight: $OR = e^{0.026} = 1.026$

Recall that the unadjusted OR for weight was 1.035. So we can say that, just like weight was acting as a confounder for state climate, the reverse is also true: living in a warm vs cool state is acting as confounder for weight!

Translation: "For every one kilogram increase in weight, adjusted for state climate, there is a 2.6% increase in the odds of being admitted to the hospital."

7. In multivariable regression, each coefficient is the result adjusted for the other coefficients. Thus, β_1 is the regression coefficient of the variable x_1 that is adjusted for ________, and β_2 is the regression coefficient for ________ that is adjusted for __________.

If the results of our study were presented formally in a paper, it might look like this:

Table 1. Logistic Regression Results for Predictors of Hospital Admission Odds Ratios (95% CIs)

Predictor	Unadjusted	Adjusted
climate		
cool	reference	reference
warm	**1.46** (1.33, 1.60)	**1.14** (1.01, 1.29)
weight (kg)	**1.035** (1.030, 1.039)	**1.026** (1.020, 1.032)
Baseline odds		0.33

Please take a moment or two and examine the table to make sure you understand what everything is. The numbers presented are the exponentiated regression coefficients…so that means they are the odds ratios, followed by their 95% confidence intervals. The word "reference" is just that: living in a cool state is the "reference," so that the odds ratio of 1.46 means that there is a higher odds of being admitted in a warm state as compared to a cool state. And the "baseline odds" of 0.33 is the exponentiated y-intercept, which really has no direct meaning…it is the theoretical odds that would occur if all the x values were 0.

And so that is really the essence of why we need multivariable regression: we now have a mathematical method for accounting for several possible confounders.

Section B7.4: Effect measure modification in multivariable regression

Recall, or review if needed, my discussion on effect measure modification in section E4.4. Effect measure modification is a real biological interaction that is going on between two factors, (like cigarette smoking and asbestos exposure in the outcome of mesothelioma), so that when the results are stratified by the third factor (asbestos exposure) the outcome is very different.

Well it turns out that multivariable regression is a very useful and easy method for determining if interaction is present or not between any two variables. And that is an extremely important thing for researchers to determine.

I would like to present to you a fictitious simple example of the association between the independent variable of weight (in pounds), and systolic blood pressure.

Here are 10 people results:

Systolic BP	Weight (pounds)
110	100
100	130
110	150
170	160
112	180
120	190
180	200
132	220
190	220
220	240

If we graph the points, you would expect there to be positive trends between weight and systolic blood pressure:

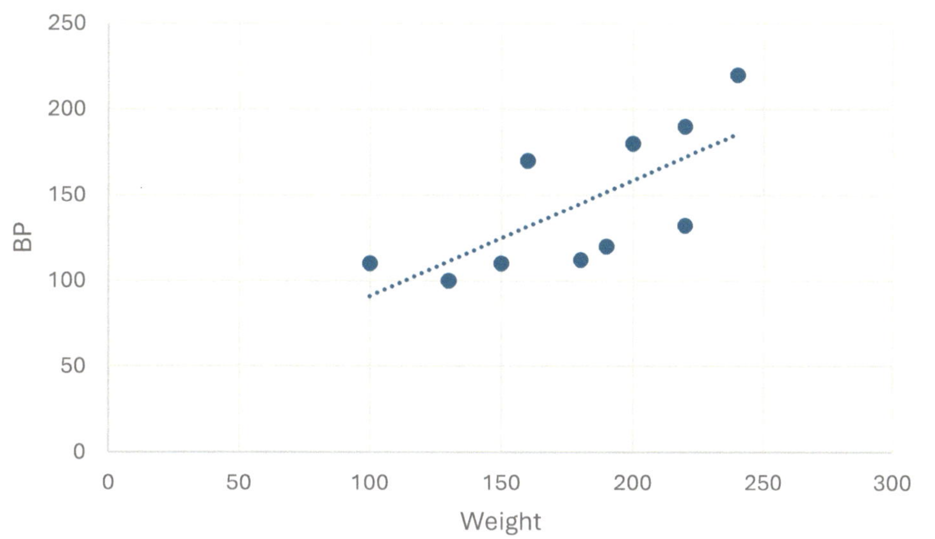

Indeed, if we run a simple regression, we get…

Oh,

8. Since the outcome is BP, the kind of regression we use is ____________________.

That's right. We use simple linear regression, and here is the output:

```
Coefficients:
            Estimate Std. Error t value Pr(>|t|)
(Intercept)   23.388     43.570   0.537   0.6060
weight         0.676      0.237   2.852   0.0214 *
```

So the regression coefficient is 0.68, and the y-intercept is 23.4

We can write our regression equation as follows:

$$y = 23.4 + 0.68(weight)$$

And since this is linear regression, the regression coefficient, 0.68, tells us that, on average, for every one pound increase in weight, systolic blood pressure increases by 0.68 mmHg. And someone who ways 200 pounds would be expected to have, on average, a systolic blood pressure of:

$$23.4 + 0.68(200) = 160\ mmHG$$

BUT, some of the people are men and some are women. If we now draw our graph so that the women are in blue and the men are in red, you see quite a difference:

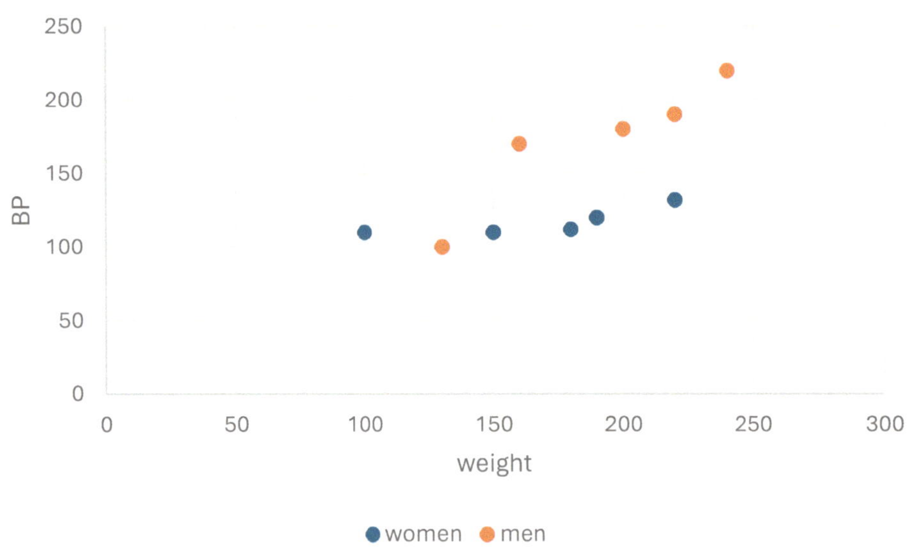

So, we now need to include gender into our regression and see what happens:

$$y = \beta_0 + \beta_1 x_1 + \beta_2 x_2$$

Where x_2 is gender: coded 1 if a man, and coded 0 if a woman.

And now we run the multivariable linear regression:

```
Coefficients:
            Estimate Std. Error t value Pr(>|t|)
(Intercept)  26.1130    31.0628   0.841   0.4283
weight        0.5398     0.1751   3.083   0.0177 *
gender       43.3243    14.6436   2.959   0.0211 *
```

Our new regression equation is:

$$syst\ bp = 26.11 + 0.54(weight) + 43.32(gender)$$

So now, a man who weighs 200 pounds would be expected to have, on average, a bp of:

$$26.11 + 0.54(200) + 43.32 = 177.4$$

While a woman who weighs 200 pounds would be expected to have, on average, a bp of:

$$26.11 + 0.54(200) + 43.32(0) = 134.1$$

And…what about confounding? Well, the *unadjusted* regression coefficient for weight was **0.68**; the adjusted regression coefficient is now 0.**54**

It appears, then, then gender is acting as confounder here!

9. Since the regression coefficient changed by more than 10% when adding a second variable, we say that the second variable acted as a ___________________________.

BUT let's look again at our graph, and this time add in our regression lines;

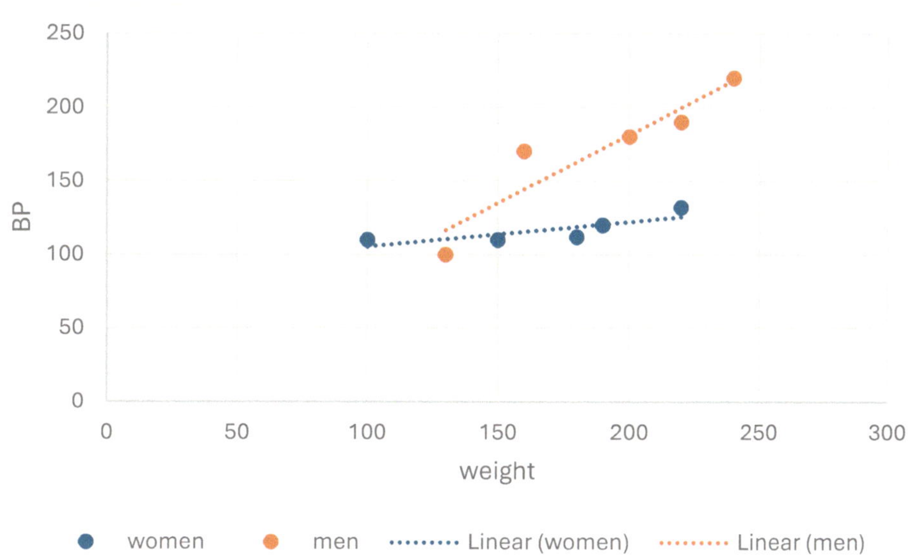

We now notice that the regression lines are not nearly parallel. This tips us off that what appeared to be confounding between the two variables is actually something even more important: this is *effect measure modification*, which is also known as an *interaction* between weight and gender. Being a man is influencing bp a lot more that being a woman does.

We now must run our regression again, and this time we add in *interaction* term, which is the *product* of weight and gender as such:

$$y = \beta_0 + \beta_1 x_1 + \beta_2 x_2 + \beta_3 (x_1 * x_2)$$

We run our regression again:

```
Coefficients:
              Estimate Std. Error t value Pr(>|t|)
(Intercept)    88.6377    26.4037   3.357   0.0153 *
weight          0.1676     0.1527   1.097   0.3145
gender        -92.3877    40.0943  -2.304   0.0607 .
weight:gender   0.7574     0.2179   3.476   0.0132 *
```

We see that our regression coefficient for the interaction, β_3 is 0.76, but more importantly, when we look all the way over to the right, we see the p-value (labeled as "pr") is 0.013, which is less than 0.05, so is statistically significant. And when we see a statistically significant interaction coefficient, we indeed conclude that there is an interaction occurring, and we have to deal with this!

So, what can we say now?

A man who weighs 200 pounds would be expected, on average, to have a bp of

$$88.7 + 0.17(200) - 92.4(1) + 0.76(200 * 1) = 152mmHg$$

And a woman who weighs 200 pounds would be expected, on average, to have a bp of

$$88.7 + 0.17(200) - 92.4(0) + 0.76(200 * 0) = 92.1mmHg???$$

So this doesn't really make any sense. No one had a bp of less than 100 mmHg, so what gives?

Here's the deal: when a significant interaction is present, *we can no longer make any predictions based on our regression.* We have to go back to square one and accept the fact that all our regression coefficients are meaningless, and we must start all over by perhaps calculating the outcomes for men and women separately. That is why the presence of interaction is such a big deal, and it is of paramount importance that researchers look for any possible interactions occurring!

Let's extend this argument a bit. I would like to fudge the data a little by changing one of the points:

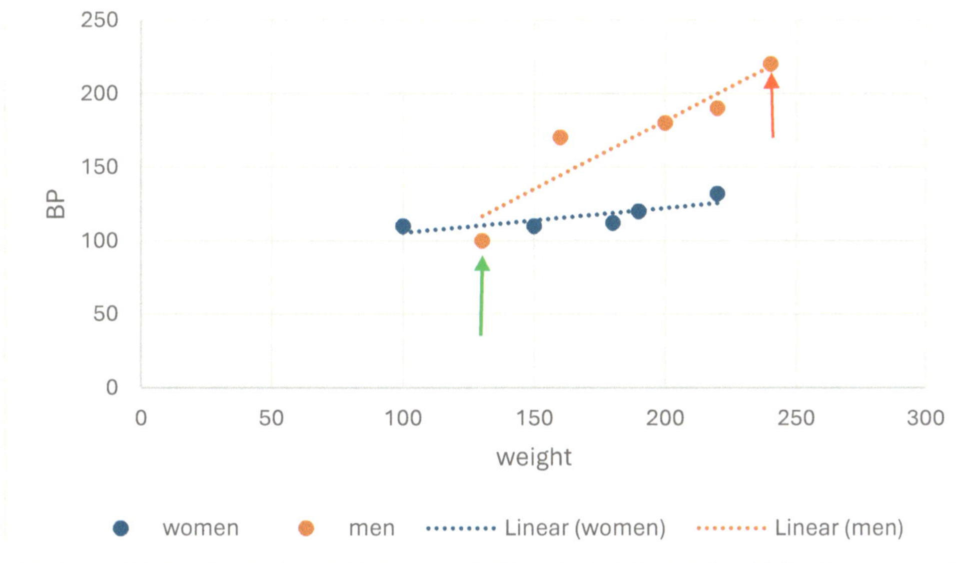

The green-arrowed point is a man who weighs 130 and has a bp of 100. Let's change his bp to 170, and the red arrow is a man who weighs 240 and has a bp of 220. Let's change his bp to 190. Now we see that the slopes are very similar:

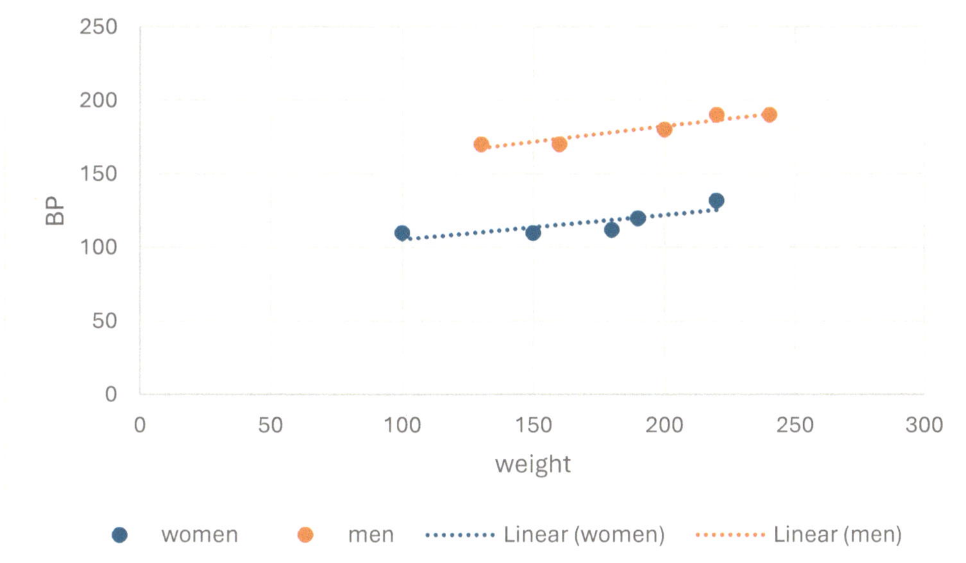

Now let's run the multivariable regression with this data, first without the interaction term:

```
Coefficients:
            Estimate Std. Error t value Pr(>|t|)    
(Intercept) 84.93366    6.87422  12.355 5.23e-06 ***
weight       0.18968    0.03874   4.896  0.00176 ** 
gender      59.02703    3.24064  18.215 3.72e-07 ***
```

Now we run it with the interaction term. What do we expect will happen?

10. Since the slopes for men and women looks very much the same, we do not expect there to be significant __________________________ present between weight and gender.

```
Coefficients:
              Estimate Std. Error t value Pr(>|t|)    
(Intercept)   88.63768    9.89755   8.956 0.000108 ***
weight         0.16763    0.05726   2.928 0.026367 *  
gender        50.98732   15.02953   3.392 0.014631 *  
weight:gender  0.04487    0.08168   0.549 0.602628    
```

Now we look all the way across at our p-value for the interaction term: it is 0.60, not at all significant. So now we have proven mathematically that there is no significant interaction occurring between weight and gender, and so we *scrap this model entirely,* and accept our previous model (the one without the interaction) as our preferred model!

Preferred regression model:

$$Systol\ bp = 84.9 + 0.19(weight) + 59.0(gender)$$

And we can proceed to make our predictions as we did before!

And that really sums up what I wanted to say about effect measure modification in multivariable regression. Remember that multivariable regression is a very useful to detect interactions between any variables!

Section B7.5: Assumptions of Multivariable regression

Nothing in biostats is perfect, and although "magic," multivariable regression is no exception. Researchers must be careful about a few things before "accepting" their multivariable regression.

1. There must be a **linear relationship** between continuous predictors and outcomes. This makes sense; remember that the regression coefficient is the slope of a line; we cannot have a slope of curved line! (But unfortunately, our computer will still spit out results even if it's not a straight line!). For example, in a situation like below, we cannot use regression!

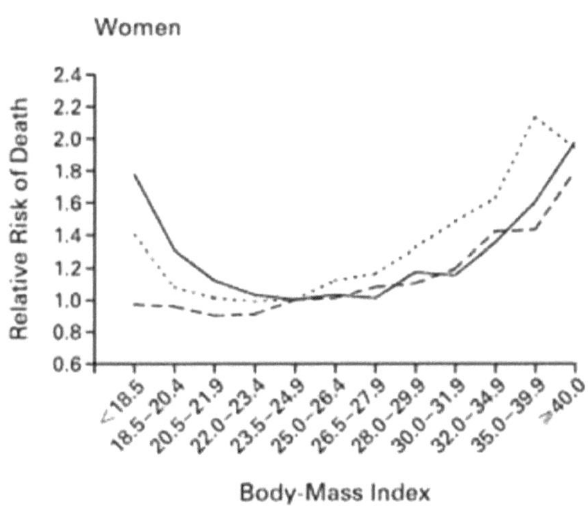

   The best way to test for linearity is to perform a scatter plot, and visually inspect the relationship between the *adjusted* variable and the outcome.

2. **Variables must not be "collinear."** Often times variables might be measuring basically the same thing. If some of them are highly correlated, it creates a problem in the analysis, as there are two (or more) factors basically measuring the same thing. This can affect the precision of the coefficients rather severely, and can make it difficult to reject the null hypothesis (because standard errors will be higher than they should be, and confidence intervals wider than they should be).

   We can check for collinearity by performing a "correlation matrix" of all the factors by calculating correlation coefficients (r) between all the factors. Here is an example of a correlation matrix for my example of cigarette smokers vs nonsmokers:

```
          group        time         died        college     stress
group    1.00000000 -0.36952722  0.42008403  0.04003204  0.2400000
time    -0.36952722  1.00000000 -0.35749028 -0.06764395 -0.1804765
died     0.42008403 -0.35749028  1.00000000  0.09929932  0.5001000
college  0.04003204 -0.06764395  0.09929932  1.00000000  0.2001602
stress   0.24000000 -0.18047651  0.50010003  0.20016019  1.0000000
```

If there is a significant collinearity between any two variables, the correlation coefficient will be 0.8 or higher. My example passes the test; all the variables are much less than 0.8. And if you do see high correlation, then the decision must be made to eliminate one of the factors from the model. A common example we see in epidemiologic research that can be problematic is when we are using many measures of socio-economic indicators as cofactors. We can imagine, for example, that if we are measuring say income, and education level, we are often measuring the same thing!

These are the two most important things to worry about. There are a few others that I will just mention, but not expect you to know in detail:

3. **Each observation in the dataset must be independent** of one another.
4. **The residuals in the model must have constant variance.** (This is called "homoscedasticity" in case you ever see the term!
5. **All the residuals in the model must be approximately normally distributed**

Summary of Biostats 7

Multivariable regression is an extremely powerful tool to aid clinicians, patients and researchers. It is a computer-generated mathematical equation that enables us to predict an output given a set of independent variables.

Logistic and Poisson regression both use the logarithmic scale; the exponentiated regression coefficient is equal to the measure of association (odds ratio or incidence rate ratio).

Multivariable regression can assess for confounding by giving us regression coefficients for each variable *independent* of all the other variables.

Multivariable regression also can check for effect measure modification (interaction) between variables.

Multivariable regression is not perfect and must be checked for several assumptions before accepting it as a valid model.

Biostats 8: Survival Analysis

Section B8.1: Introduction and why we need it

Survival analysis has become one of the most utilized tools in modern epidemiologic research. It is very important to understand it. It is used when the outcome is binary (yes/no…did an event occur?), and when we know the time to event for every participant in the study. It is therefore similar in some respects to Poisson regression that I discussed in Biostats 6, because in Poisson regression, time is also an element, as the effect measure is the incidence rate and the measure of association between two factors is the incidence rate ratio. But in Poisson regression, we only know the time for a *group* of people, rather than the specific times for each individual person. (If 10 people followed for 5 years had an event, then the incidence rate ("person-time incidence rate") is 10 cases/50 p-y). But in survival analysis, we know the time to event for each individual person, and this enables us to perform more precise calculations. To show why this is important, I would like to present a very simplified longitudinal study.

Let's say we have a group of 20 people whom we will follow for 10 years and see if they have an outcome (an "event"):

PPPPP
PPPPP
PPPPP
PPPPP

time 0 yr 10 yr

At the end of the ten-year period, we record 4 events (the events are in red)

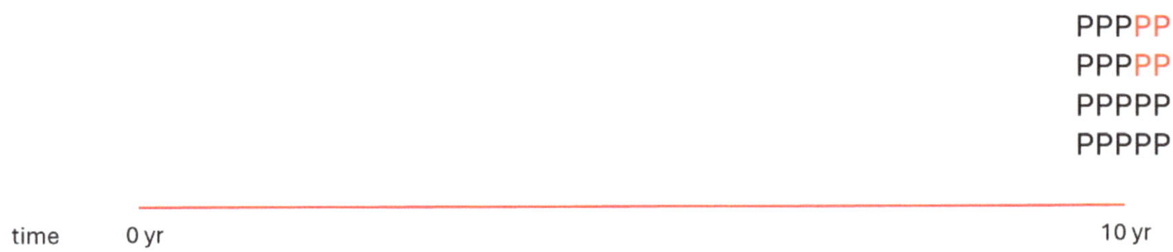

$$I_c = risk = \frac{4}{20} = 0.2$$

We calculate the cumulative incidence as above to equal 0.2. We interpret this cumulative incidence as "the risk of an event for each person followed for 10 years is 0.2." Or, we can think of it as "there is expected to be 2 events for every 10 people followed for 10 years."

But in the real world of epidemiologic research, when we do a longitudinal study like this, we cannot recruit all the people at the start of our study. Instead, many people may enter the study a few years into the study, or at certain points as shown here:

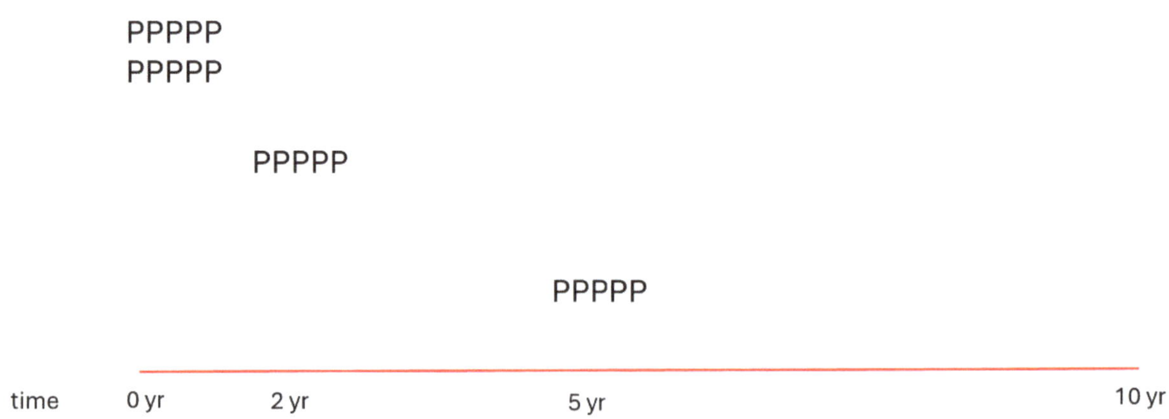

So now, 10 people entered the study at the beginning of the observation period, another 5 people joined at the 2 year point, and another 5 joined at the 5 year point. So when this happens, we can get more precise by using person-time incidence rates as shown below:

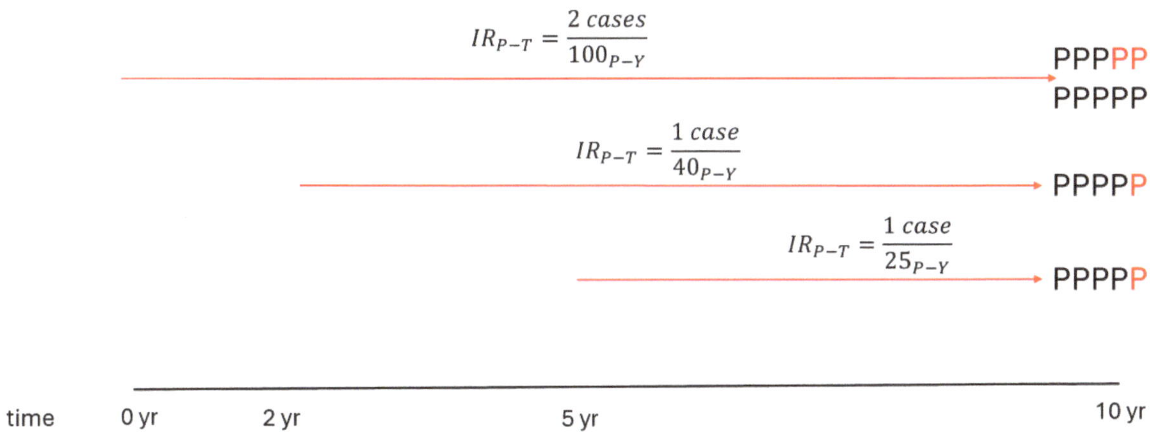

$$IR_{P-T} = \frac{4\ cases}{165_{P-Y}} = \frac{0.024\ cases}{P-Y} = \frac{0.24\ cases}{10_{P-Y}} \qquad I_c = risk = \frac{4}{20} = 0.2$$

The top red line are our participants who started the study at the beginning. There were two cases in that group, so the incidence *rate* is 2 cases per 100 person-years. (Make sure you understand the denominator: since there were 10 people followed for 10 years, it is 100 person-years). The middle red line are the participants who joined the trial at the 2-year point. There was one case in this group. Since 5 people were followed for 8 years, the denominator is 40 person-years, and the incidence rate of this group was 1 case per 40 person-years. The bottom red line are the participants who joined at the 5-year point, and there was 1 case, so the incidence rate of this group was 1 case per 25 person-years.

Then we add the three different rates, and get 4 cases per 265 person-years, which equals 0.24 cases per 10 person-years. (This is interpreted as 0.24 cases for each person followed for 10 years). So, we now have more precise information than our initial cumulative incidence of 0.2. And the more precise information was because we used person-time incidence rates.

But here is the other problem that often occurs in epidemiologic research: people drop out of the study, and we do not know if they had an event or not. This is a common problem, and can lead to significantly inaccurate data as shown below:

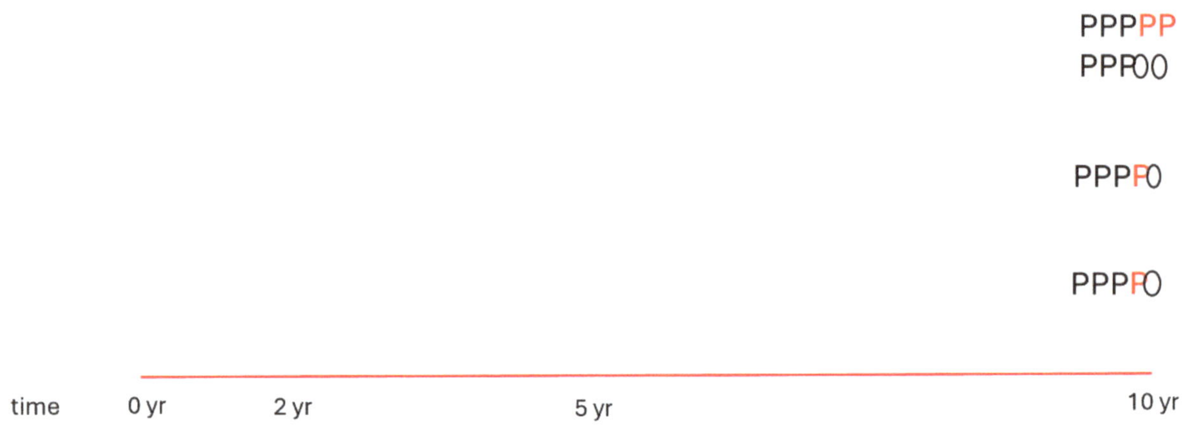

The ovals represent people who dropped out of the study: 2 from the first group who started at the beginning of the trial, 1 from the second group which started at the 2-year point, and one from the third group which started at the 5-year point. We lost contact with these people, so we do not know if they had an event or not. What do we do with these people? Do we assume they had an event? Do we assume they did not have an event?

Well, we can try assuming that they did not have an event:

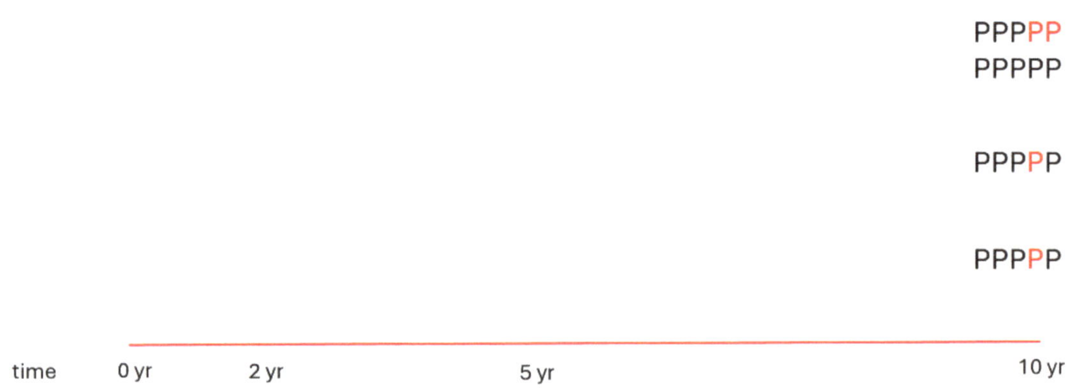

$$IR_{P-T} = \frac{4\ cases}{165_{P-Y}} = 0.024 = 0.24\ cases/10_{P-Y}$$

Our results are as they were before.

Or we can assume that they did have events:

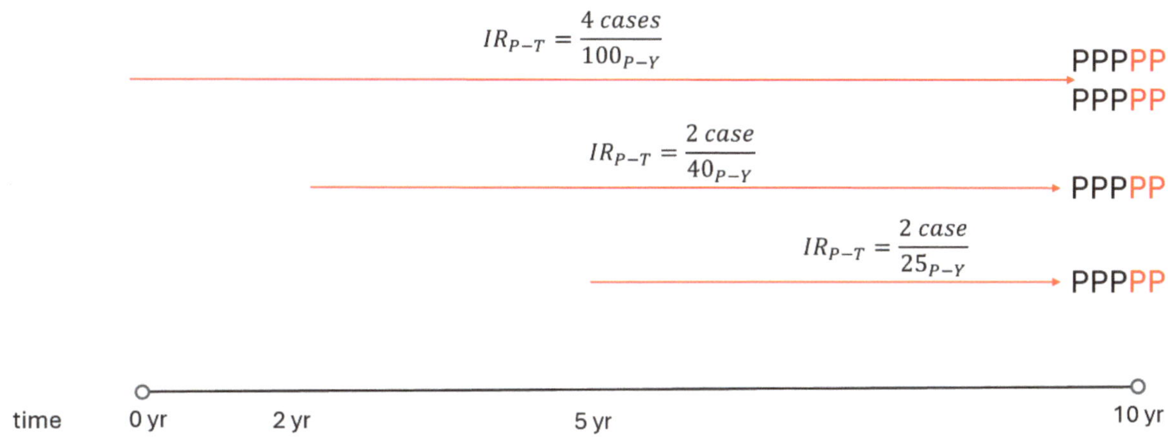

$$IR_{P-T} = \frac{8\ cases}{165_{P-Y}} = 0.048 = 0.48\ cases/10_{P-Y}$$

We see a very different result of 0.48 cases per 10 person-years. So we have no way of knowing if our result is 0.24, or 0.48, or somewhere in between! Luckily, we can solve both problems quite well with *survival analysis*.

Survival analysis incorporates three concepts which I will discuss in some detail. The three concepts are:

Kaplan-Meier Survival Function

Hazard Ratios

Cox Proportional Hazard Regression

Section B8.2: Kaplan-Meier Survival Function

Kaplan and Meier invented their survival function back in the 1950s to deal with two problems inherent in measuring survival times: one is that survival times do not follow a normal distribution, and two is the problem of people dropping out of the study (so-called "censoring"). Their survival function is a graph that looks like this:

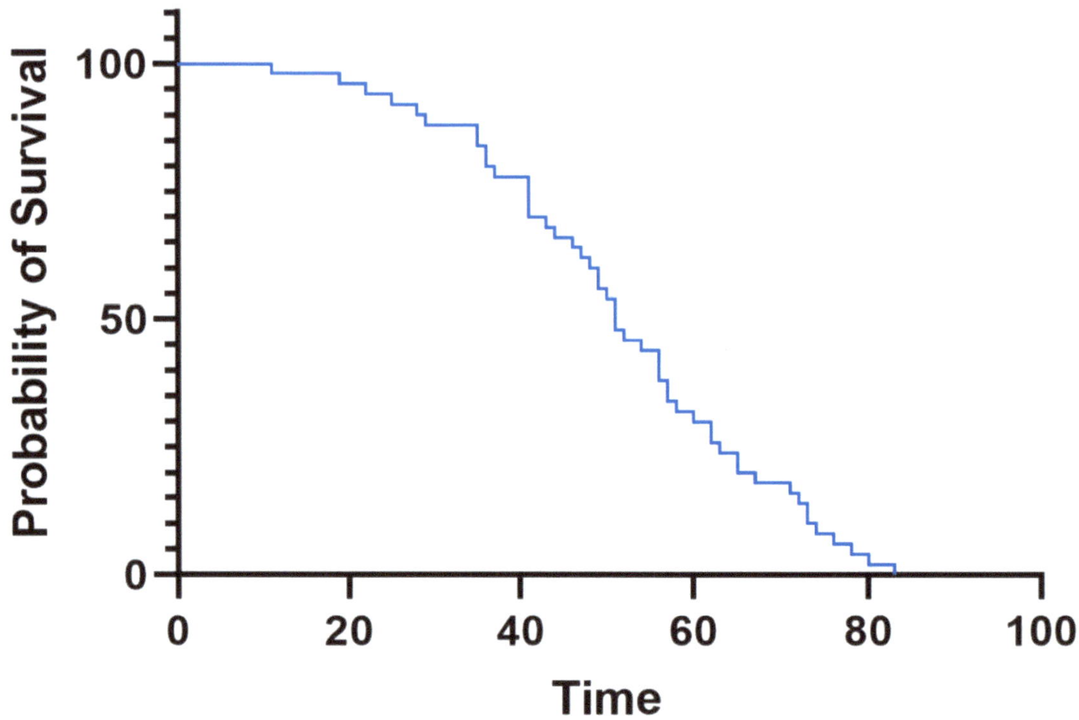

On the x-axis is time, and on the y-axis is probability of survival. And I would like to point out that the word "survival" is not necessarily survival in the strict sense, i.e. staying alive, but rather being *free of an event.* And that event can be anything you can imagine: a disease occurring, a hospital admission, a relapse, a side effect of a drug, etc. (But of course, it can also mean "survival" in the strict sense!)

1. In Kaplan-Meier survival function, we plot probability of survival on the ___- axis, and time on the ___-axis.

In the language of logic, we say that $S(t) = P(T > t)$. That is, the survival function at time t is the probability of surviving beyond time t.

So if I draw a line up from t = 40, and then across to the y-axis, I see that the probability of surviving beyond time of 40 is about 77%.

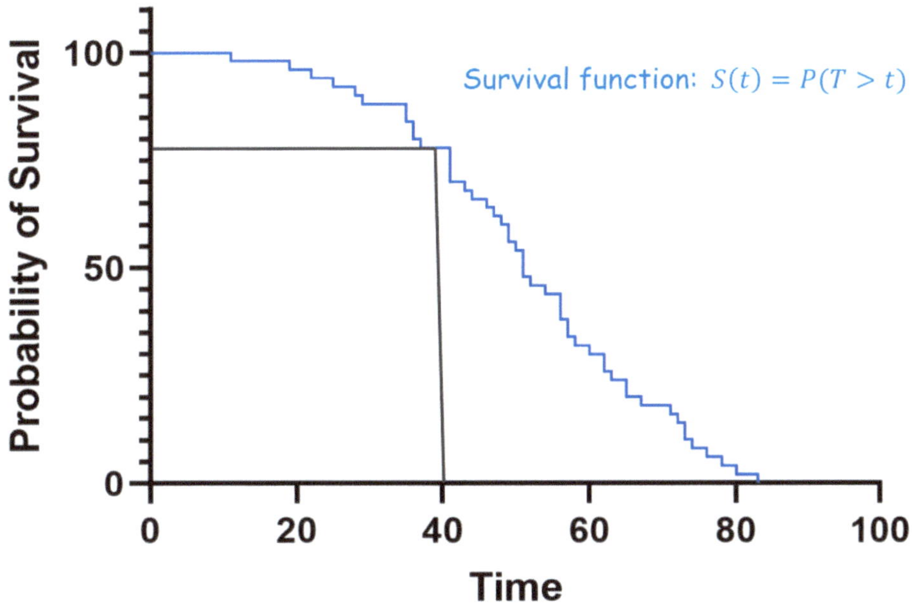

Likewise, the probability of surviving beyond time 60 is about 30%:

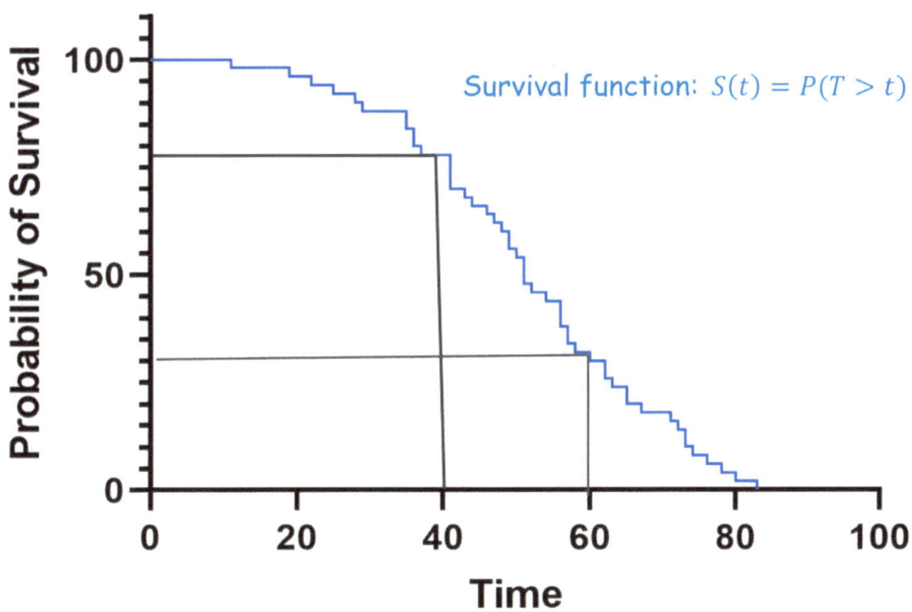

We say $S(60) = 30\%$

We define a "median survival time" as the time at which half the population is still alive:

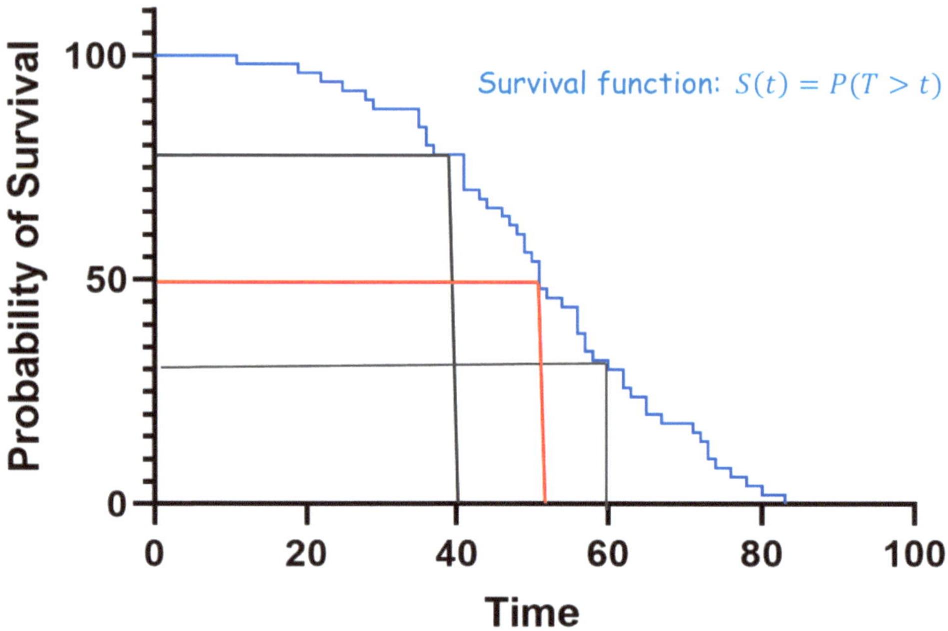

The "median survival time" here is approximately 52.

2. At the median survival time, a person has a ____ % chance of ______________________.

Please also know that in the medical literature we often see an "upside-down" K-M curve, like this:

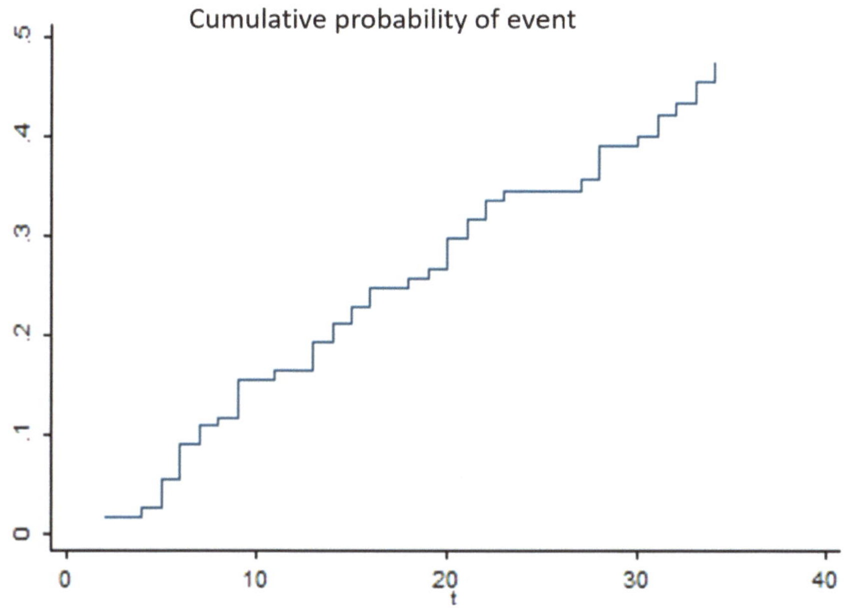

So now the y-axis is the probability of an event occurring, rather than the probability of being event free.

Dissecting the Kaplan-Meier curve

Here is a K-M curve that the computer generated when I fed it some fictitious data about 50 fictitious smokers followed for 20 years, and recording when they fictitiously die:

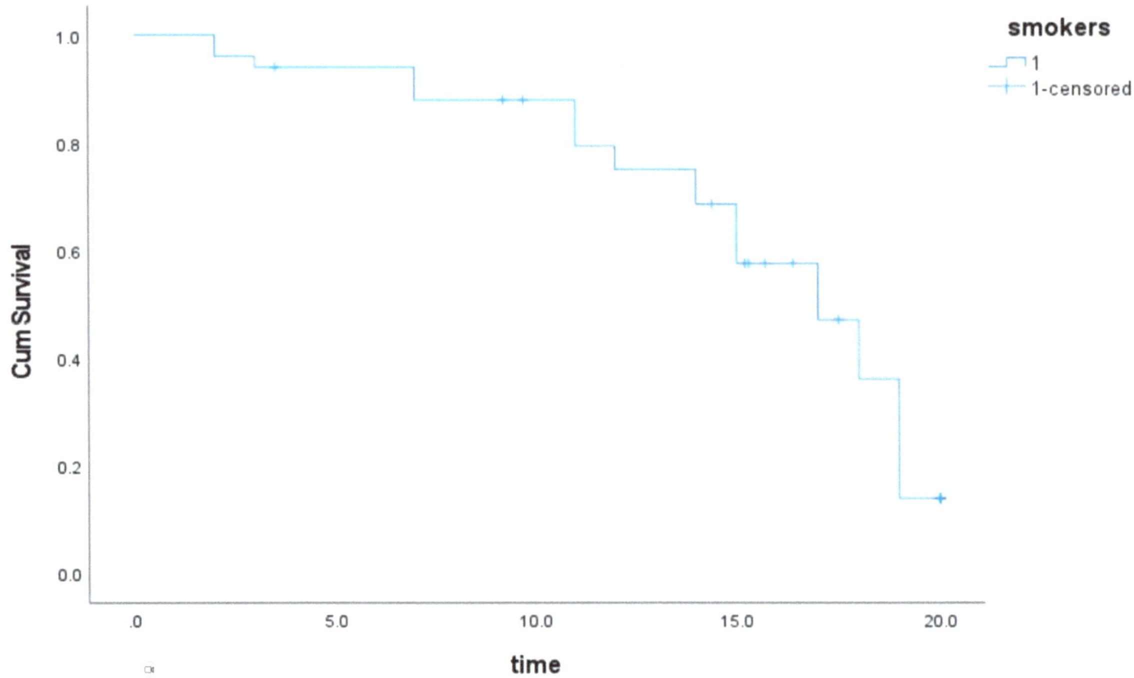

Each of the vertical lines represents times at which a person or persons died. Each of the littles notches in the horizontal lines represents when a person withdraws from the study and is lost to follow-up. In the following figure, the vertical lines (deaths) are pointed out by the purple arrows, and the notches representing the "censored" people are pointed out by the yellow arrows:

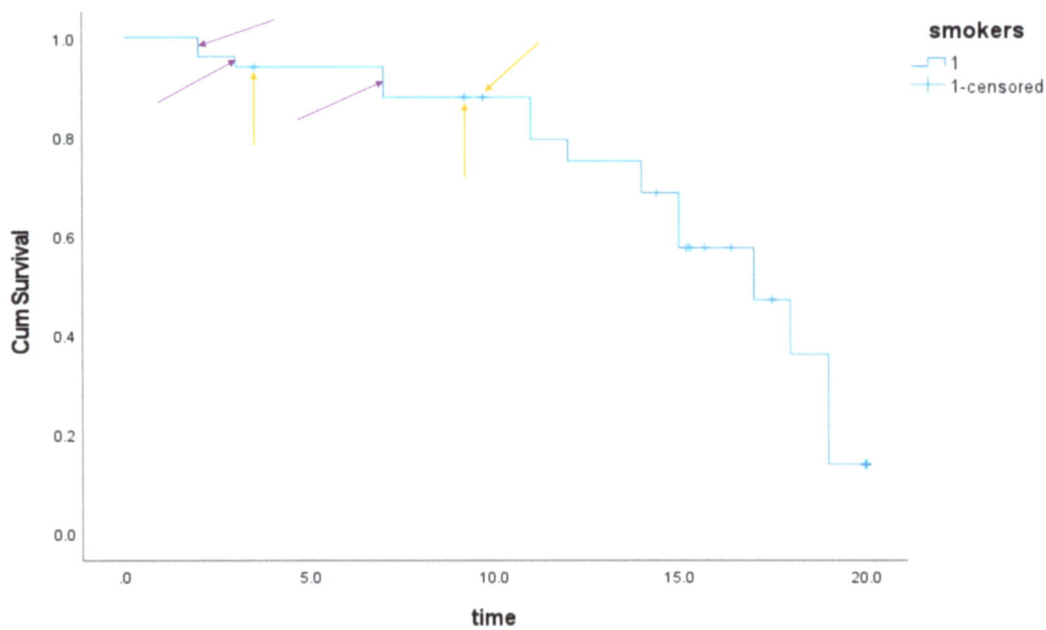

Censoring

This concept of "censoring" needs a bit more discussion. When a participant drops out of a study, and we lose contact with her, we only have partial information about that participant. We know she was event-free up to a certain point, but we don't know if and when she went on to have an event. And so we say that participant is "censored." (Specifically, biostatisticians call this "right censoring," as opposed to "left censoring." "Left censoring" is not a problem in most longitudinal studies and refers to the fact that we may not know how long *before* the study started that a participant may have had an event…in epidemiologic studies we are very careful to make sure that participants did not suffer an event before the trial started!)

Take a look at the figure below and follow with me what happens to each of these six participants in a twenty-year longitudinal study.

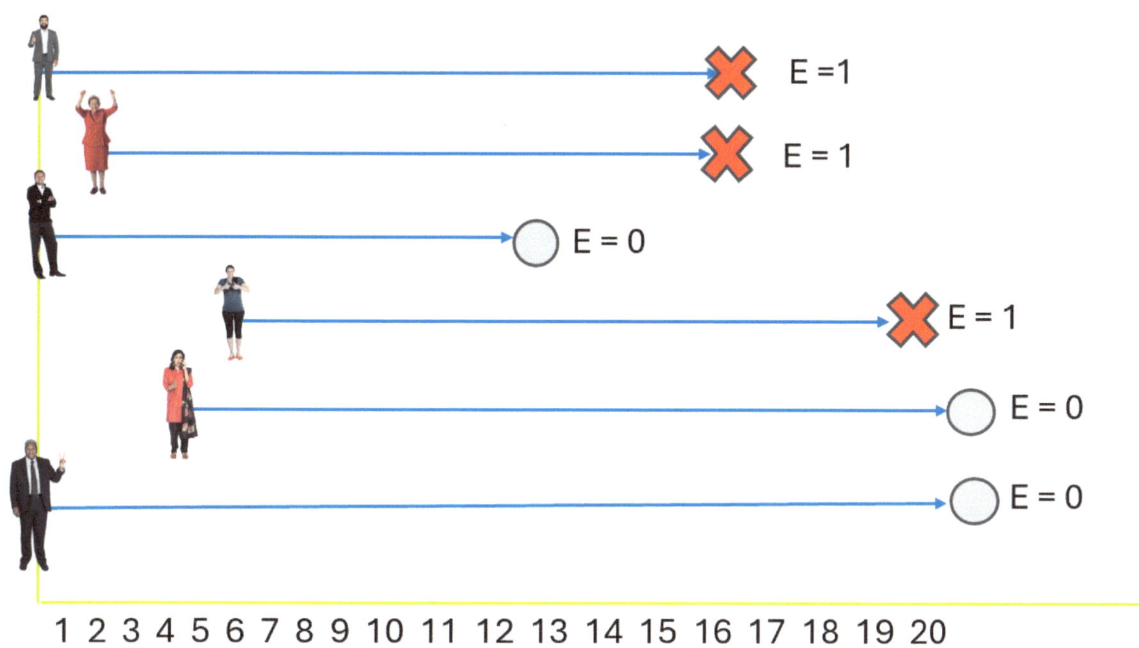

The person at the very top entered the trial at the beginning, and then at year 16 of the trial had an event (red X). The "E = 1" means that when there is an event, we code it as a "1" in the computer. The next person (in the red dress) entered the study at year 2, and then at year 16 also had an event. The next person down entered the study at the beginning, and then at year 12 dropped out and we lost contact. He had no event up to year 12, that is all we know, so he is "censored." The computer codes this as a "0." The next person down entered the trial in year 6, and then in year 19 had an event. The next person down entered the study in year 4, and went all the way to the end of the trial period without an event. She is coded as a "0". And this is an important point: although she did not withdraw, and we never lost contact with her, she is still officially considered "censored." Why? Well, strictly speaking, we don't know *when* she'll have an event, because our study ended! Strictly speaking, we therefore only know partial information about her!

The main point is that in longitudinal studies in which we know the time to event for each participant, and we are using survival analysis, there are only two possible outcomes: either an event occurred, or the participant is censored. That is all!

OK, back to our simulation: the last person at the bottom started at the beginning of the trial and went all the way to the end without an event. How do we classify this participant? He also censored!

3. In survival analysis, only one of two things can happen: either a participant has an event or the participant is ________________ .

So then the method of K-M survival dictates that we assume all participants started at day 1 when we calculate their time to event or time to censoring:

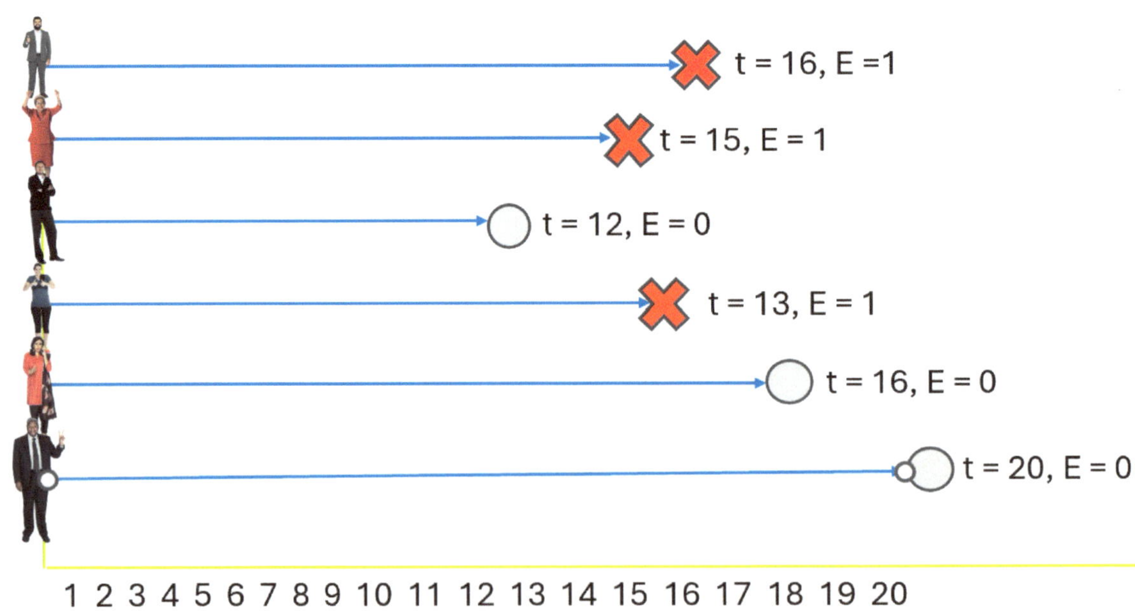

So we would code each person into the computer, and code a "1" if they had an event, or a "0" if they were censored, and then code each of their times.

And that is how we deal with censored subjects: we code the times that we lost contact from them…at least up till this point they had no event. And although that is only partial information, it is not bad!

Here is a portion of my data (the cigarette smokers followed for 20 years, and how I coded them into the computer:

1	group	time	died
2	1	2	1
3	1	2	1
4	1	3	1
5	1	3.5	0
6	1	7	1
7	1	7	1
8	1	7	1
9	1	9.2	0
10	1	9.7	0
11	1	11	1
12	1	11	1
13	1	11	1
14	1	11	1
15	1	12	1
16	1	12	1
17	1	14	1
18	1	14	1
19	1	14	1
20	1	15	1
21	1	15	1
22	1	15	1
23	1	15	1
24	1	15	1
25	1	14.4	0
26	1	15.2	0
27	1	15.3	0
28	1	15.7	0
29	1	16.4	0
30	1	17	1
31	1	17	1
32	1	17	1
33	1	17	1

(The third column "died:" coded as 1 if they died, and a 0 if they were censored)

And the computer then spits out the K-M curve:

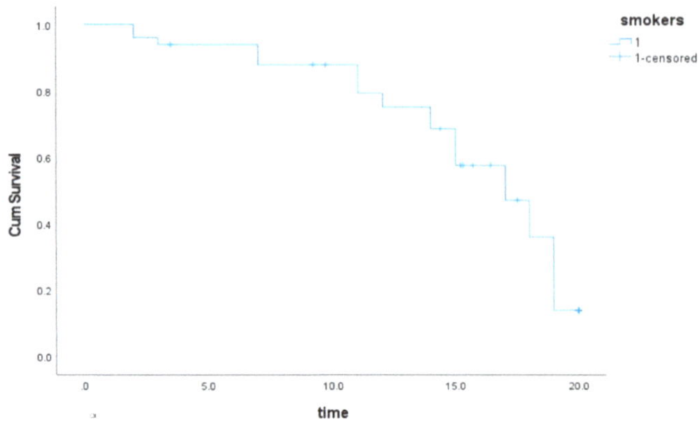

So now it's time to get to the nitty gritty and show you exactly how a K-M curve is constructed. I will zoom in on the first part of the curve:

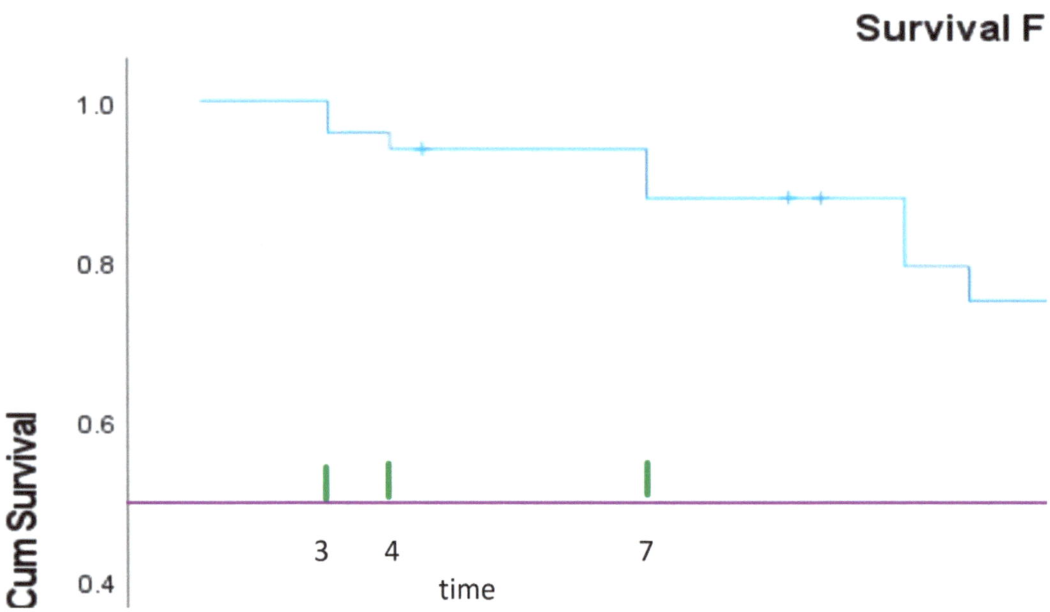

And now I will label some points that we can go through:

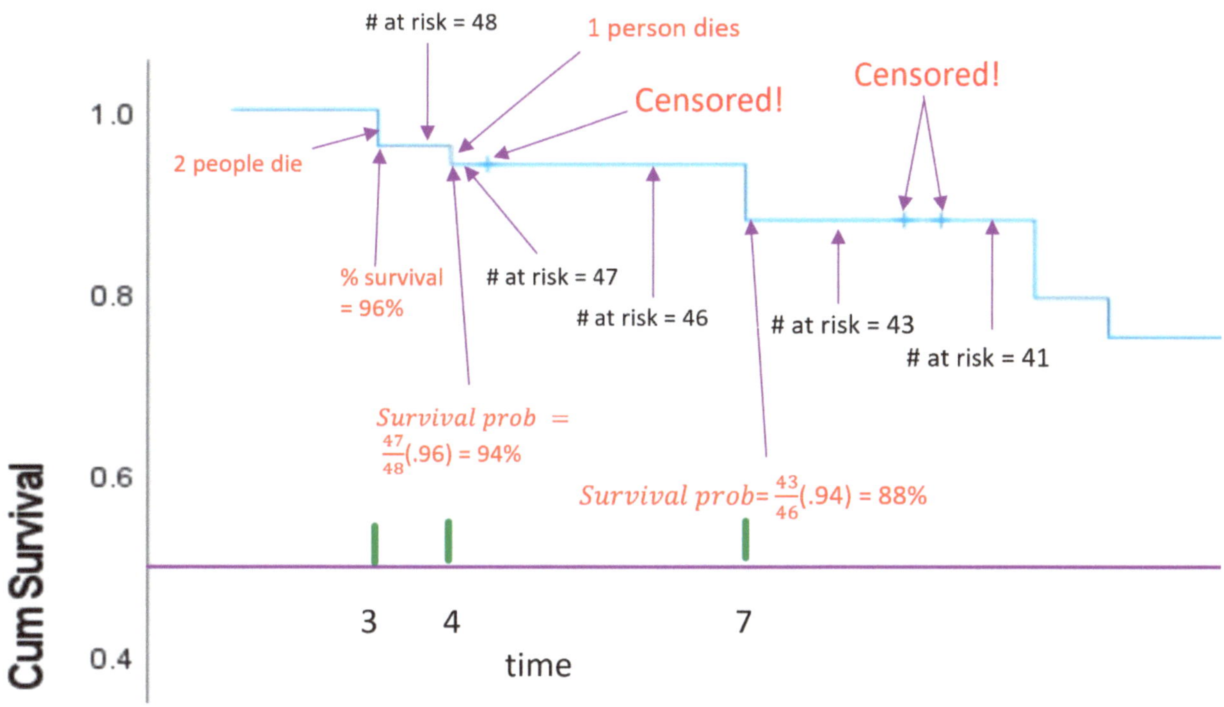

So follow with me as we start from the left. Initially, all of the 50 people are alive. Thus the probability of survival at time = 0 is 100% (1.0). Then at time = 3, two people die, and so you see the vertical line down. So, from time = 3, 48/50 people have survived, so the survival probability is 96%. Then, since 2 have died, the number at risk is down to 48. Then at time = 4, one person dies. So the probability of survival is 47/48, which is 98%. But…98% of what? Since we are talking about cumulative survival, it's 98% of the 96% that was remaining. So, it's .98(96%) = 94%. And now, since one person died, the number at risk is down to 47. And then soon thereafter (like at time = 4.3), one person drops out and is "censored." And because of that, as we approach t = 7, the number at risk goes down by one to 46. Then at t = 7, three more people die, and so the cumulative survival probability is now 43/46, or 93.5%. But…93.5% of what? Of the 94% that we started with at this time. So, it's actually 43/46(94%) = 88%. Indeed, if we drew a horizontal line from this point back to the y-axis, we would be at 0.88:

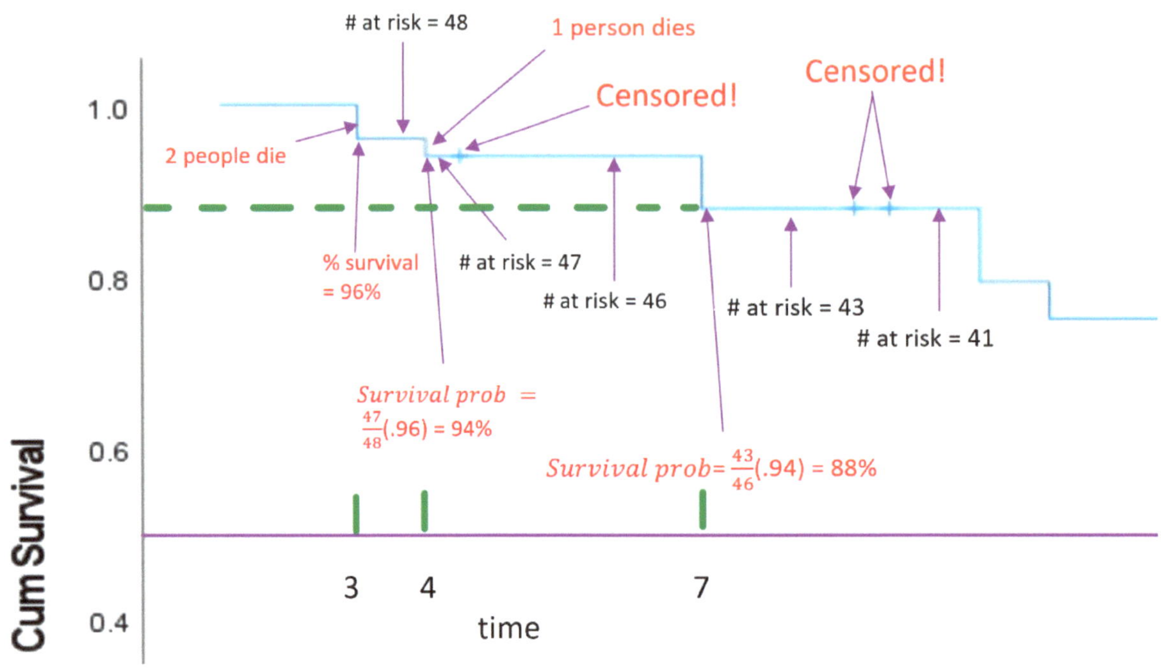

Continuing on, the # remaining at risk after t = 7 is 43. Then we see two more are censored, and so the number at risk is down to 41.

And that is how it's constructed!

Comparing two groups

Of course, we are usually interested in comparing two groups. To demonstrate, I created a second group in my fictitious longitudinal study, a group of nonsmokers, and added their data. Here is the output:

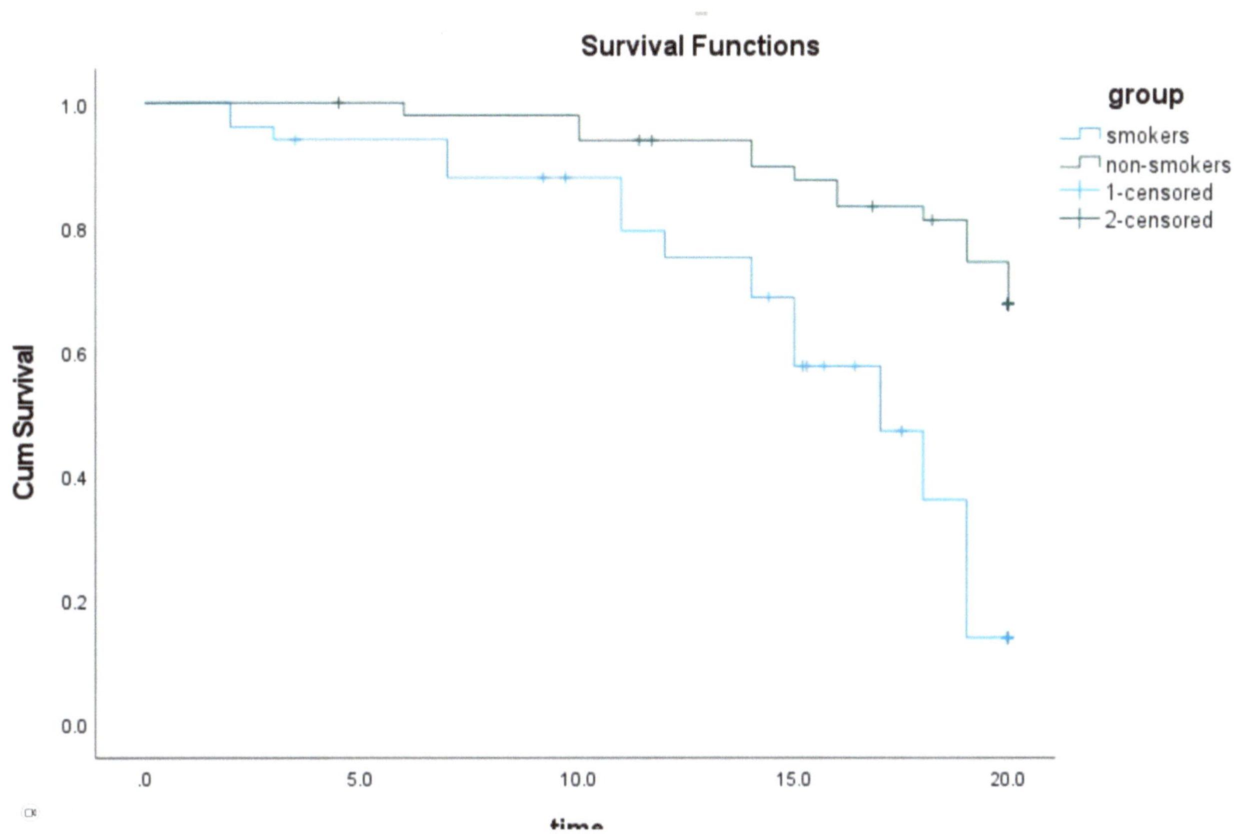

The new group, in green, is on top. As is typical of K-M curves, the group on top does better: they have a better survival. This is demonstrated by looking at time = 15 years:

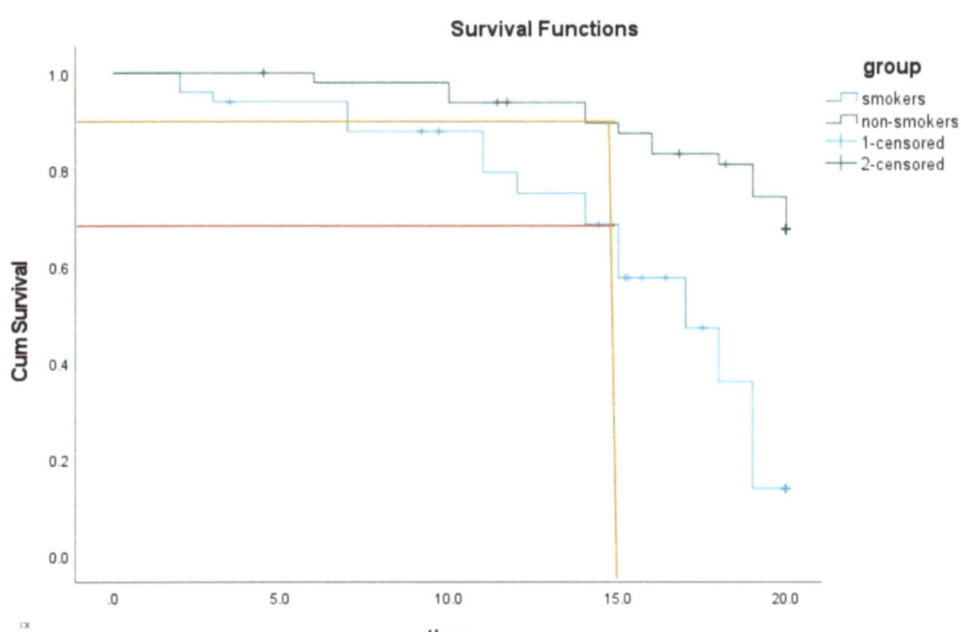

The survival probability for the smokers is about 68%, while the survival probability for the nonsmokers is about 90%.

But if our data are presented as upside-down KM curve, we see:

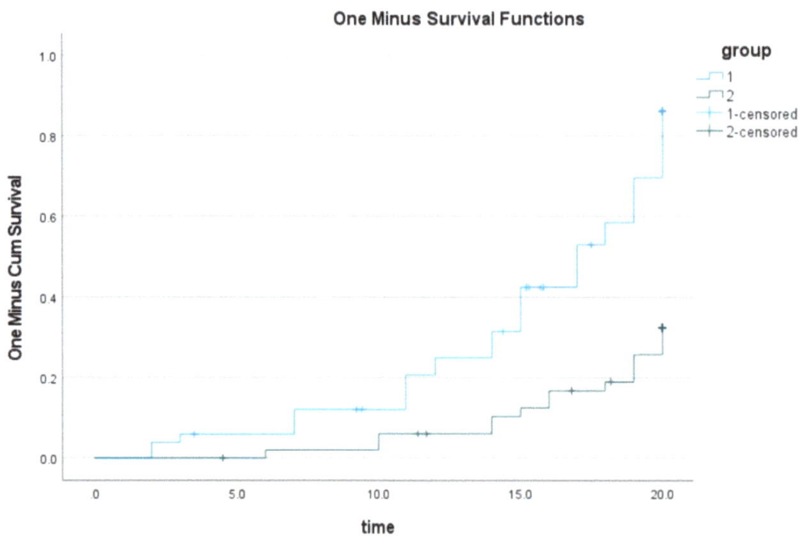

Now the curve on the bottom does better…they have a lower probability of an event occurring.

4. In K-M survival, the group on top does ______________________, because they have a higher probability of being event-free. But if the data is presented as an upside-down K-M curve, then the group on the top does ______________, because they have a higher probability of having an ________________.

In my example, it seems pretty clear just by looking at the graphs that one group is surviving significantly better than the other. But sometimes it is not so clear just by looking:

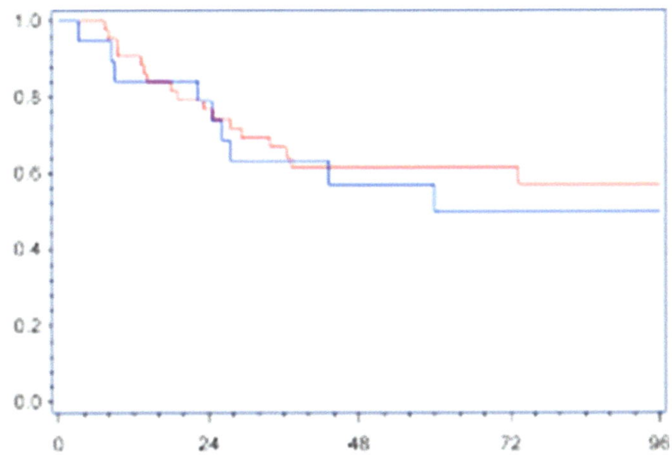

Is there a significant difference in survival between these two groups? We do not know; we need a mathematical tool to tell us how different they are.

The log-rank test

The Log-Rank test is used to compare the survival curves of two or more independent groups. The log- rank test is very similar to a test I have already talked about, in Section B3.5, the Chi-square test. Recall the formula for chi-square:

$$\chi^2 = \Sigma \frac{(Observed - Expected)^2}{Expected}$$

With slight difference when comparing two curves:

$$\chi^2 = \Sigma \frac{(\sum Observed - \sum Expected)^2}{\sum Expected}$$

So now we have two different curves. One for the group that received the treatment in question, and one for the group who did not receive the treatment. We do the same here as we did in Chapter 3. You have to take each time block, and calculate an "expected" occurrence, and you do this for each curve. I won't go through it step-by-step because I already did it in Chapter 3, but just a couple of points here: The "expected" frequency is calculate by:

$E = N_x \left(\frac{O_x}{N_t}\right)$ The subscript x refers to each particular curve, while the subscript t refers to total number. N is the "number at risk" as we discussed.

It's actually a bit simpler than the chi-square described in chapter 3, when we had to go through each cell, one-by-one, and calculate the differences between the observed and expected. Here we just sum up all the observed, and sum up all the expected, and plug them in the equation. We add the results for each curve. For example, if there are three curves, then:

$$\chi^2 = \frac{(\sum Observed - \sum Expected)^2}{\sum Expected} \text{ for curve 1 plus } \frac{(\sum Observed - \sum Expected)^2}{\sum Expected} \text{ for curve 2 plus } \frac{(\sum Observed - \sum Expected)^2}{\sum Expected} \text{ for curve 3.)}$$

We end up with a chi-square value, and the null hypothesis is that the curves are identical, and there is no difference in survival times. The larger the chi-square, the more likely it is that we can reject the null hypothesis.

5. The ________________ test is used to tell us if indeed the independent groups have statistically different survivals.

Here are the computer results for my two groups:

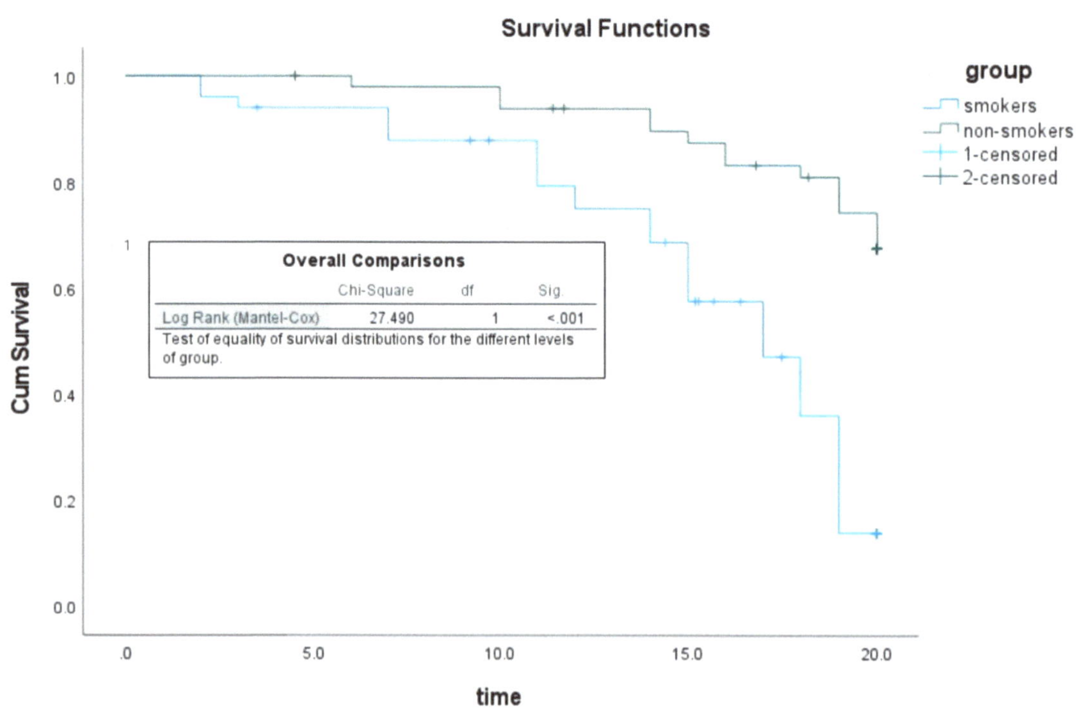

Note that the chi-square value is quite high, and the p-value is < 0.001, indicating that there is indeed a statistically significant difference in survival between the two groups.

And here is an example from the literature:

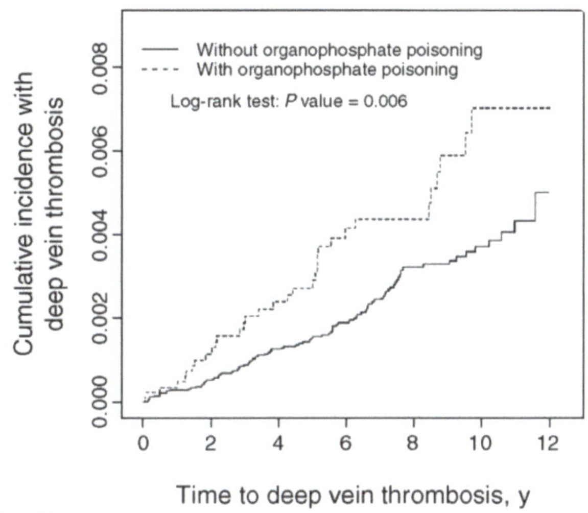

Organophospate poisoning, No.						
At risk	9223	7054	5788	4483	3110	1496
DVT events	0	9	8	9	1	6
Non-organophospate poisoning, No.						
At risk	36,892	33,444	28,152	22,064	15,317	7476
DVT events	0	19	23	16	25	5

FIGURE 1

Cummulative incidence of deep vein thrombosis in patients with organophosphate poisoning and comparison patients.

Lim et al.Increased Risk of Deep Vein Thrombosis and Pulmonary Thromboembolism in Patients With Organophosphate Intoxication. *Medicine* (Baltimore). 2015 Jan; 94(1): e341.
Published online 2015 Jan 9.

Note that the long-rank test shows a p-value of 0.006, indicating that there is a significant difference between the two groups.

6. Because this is an upside-down K-M curve, the group without organophosphate poisoning does ____________________ than the group with poisoning, in terms of being free from event occurring.

However, from the same paper,

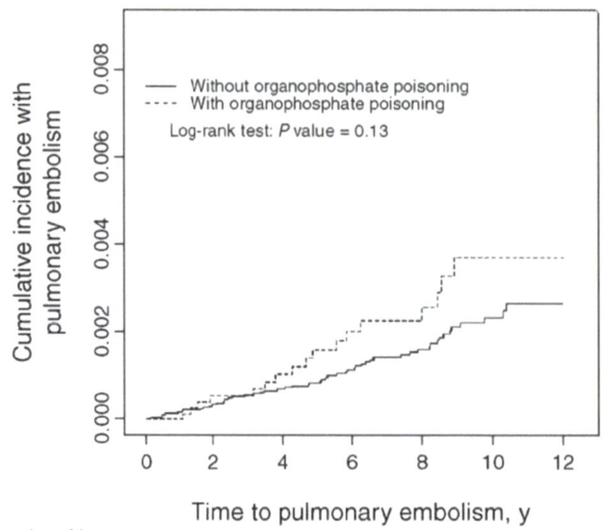

Organophospate poisoning, No.						
At risk	9223	7057	5793	4490	3111	1498
PE events	0	4	3	5	2	3
Non-organophospate poisoning, No.						
At risk	36,892	33,450	28,165	22,078	15,340	7485
PE events	0	12	11	11	9	9

FIGURE 2

Cummulative incidence of pulmonary thromboembolismin in patients with organophosphate poisoning and comparison patients.

Point here being that even though these curves *look* different, the log-rank test tells us that they are not statistically different.

And that is how Kaplan-Meier survival function works; it is time to move on to topic #2

Section B8.3: The Hazard Ratio

Whenever a paper uses survival analyses and KM curves, the measure of association between groups is the *hazard ratio.* The hazard ratio between two groups is the ratio of hazards between the groups. I should point out at the outset that the concept of hazards and hazard ratios is an esoteric one. It was invented by the renowned British statistician Sir David Cox (more on him later!) in the late 1960s in conjunction with Kaplan and Meier, and the three concepts presented in this chapter: K-M survival, hazard ratios and Cox Proportional Hazards are all intertwined in a complex way so that even many biostatisticians do not fully grasp it. My goal then, is to present it in a pragmatic way so that you will have a solid general understanding of what it means when you read the literature.

The best way to understand the hazard ratio may be to compare it to what we already know. It is often compared to, or confused with, the **relative risk**, which you should know well at this point. Let's look again at my fictitious longitudinal study that compared cigarette smokers vs nonsmokers.

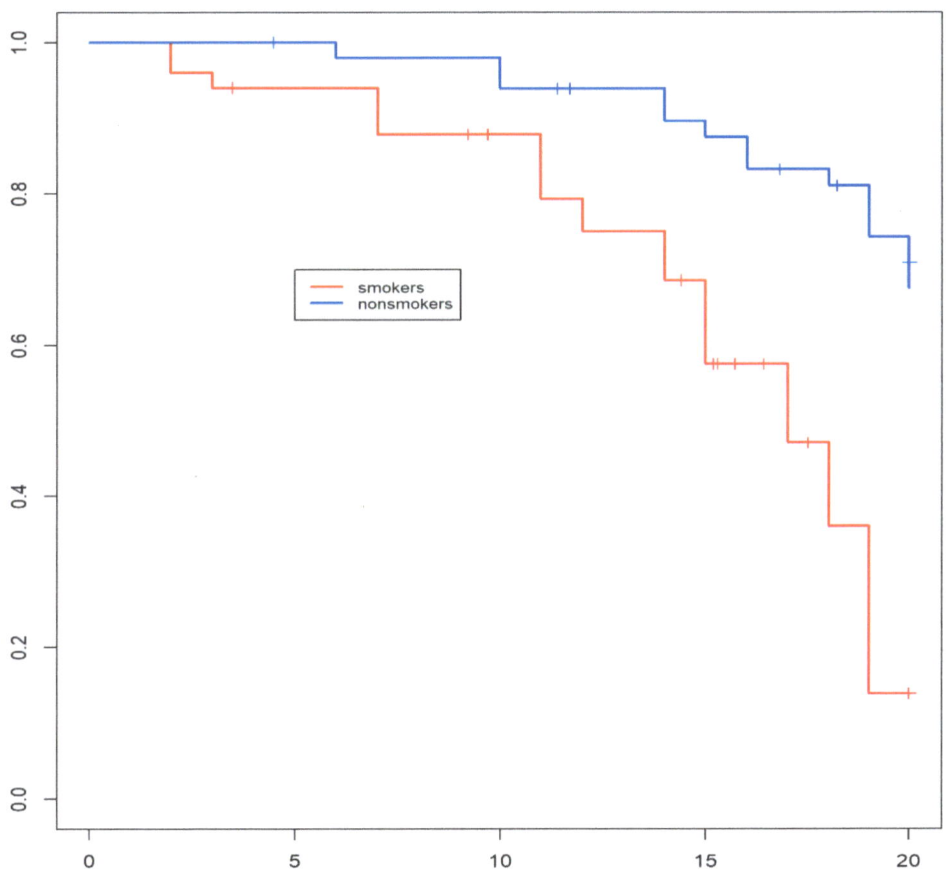

To remind you, there were 50 people in each group, and simply followed for the event of death over a 20-year period. If you were to look at the spreadsheet that I fed into the computer, you would see that in the smoking group there were 36 events over the 20-year period, while in the nonsmoking group there were 15 events. So if we were to ignore the factor of time and just calculate the RR (relative risk)…well, the risk (cumulative incidence) of an event in the smoking group is 36/50, and the risk (cumulative incidence) of an event in the nonsmoking group is 15/50. And so:

$$RR = \frac{36/_{50}}{15/_{50}} = 2.4$$

7. The relative risk does not take into account ________________ and is simply the ___________ (also called the "cumulative incidence") of one group as compared to the _____________ of the other group.

To interpret this relative risk we would say the risk that a smoker has of dying over a 20-year period is 2.4 times the risk that a nonsmoker has of dying.

But we know the time to event for each individual person in the trial. Therefore, we can calculate more precise information. The computer calculates the **hazard ratio**, and it comes out to **4.897.** (You cannot calculate this by hand like you can with the RR, the computer needs to calculate with HR).

The hazard ratio of **4.9** is translated as: a*t a given instant in time*, a smoker is 4.9 times as likely to die as is a nonsmoker.

Why is there such a big difference between the relative risk and the hazard ratio? It is because the hazard ratio takes into account the time factor. A characteristic of survival analysis is that the risk tends to increase as time goes on; there is often a As in most survival studies, the risk of dying goes way up as time goes on, and the hazard ratio is a computer-generated average of all these risks. It takes the small risks toward the beginning and the high risks toward the end and gives us an average. So perhaps the translation is better stated: *On average,* at a given instant in time, a smoker is 4.9 times as likely to die as a nonsmoker.

A hazard ratio is a ratio of hazards, and a *hazard* is the risk at a given point in time. Let's zoom in on the upper left section of the K-M curves:

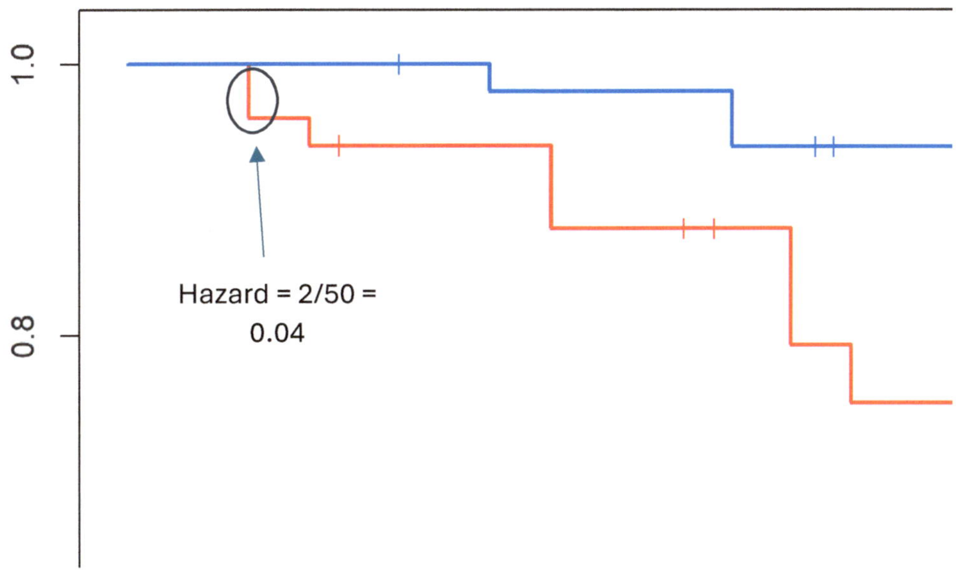

I have circled the first vertical drop of the smokers group. At this particular instant in time (t = 2), 2 people out of 50 died. Therefore, the instantaneous risk, or the hazard at t = 3 is 2/50 = 0.04,

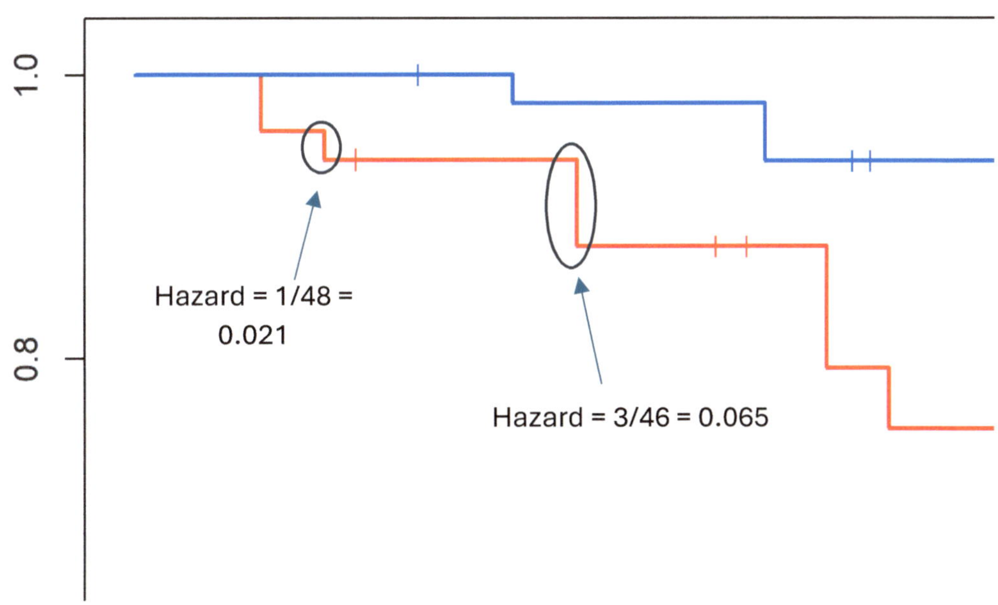

At the second vertical drop, one person died, but only 48 people were at risk, so the instantaneous risk (the hazard) at tie t = 4 is 1/40 = **0.021**.

At the third vertical drop at t = 7, 3 people died and there were 46 at risk (one was censored a bit after time 4), so the instantaneous risk at time = 7 is 3/46 = **0.065,** and at the 4th vertical drop (no circle), 4 people died and 41 were at risk, so the hazard at this time is 4/41 = **0.098.**

So, unlike cumulative risk, which is one "lump sum" calculated at the end of the trial, the hazard is different at every point measured, and in general increase as the survival study progresses. (And that makes sense if you think about it: if you were lucky enough to survive till the age of 90, you can imagine that your risk of dying at any moment is WAY higher than that risk was when you were 30!)

If I were to plot all the hazards from the smokers group onto the graph, it would look like this:

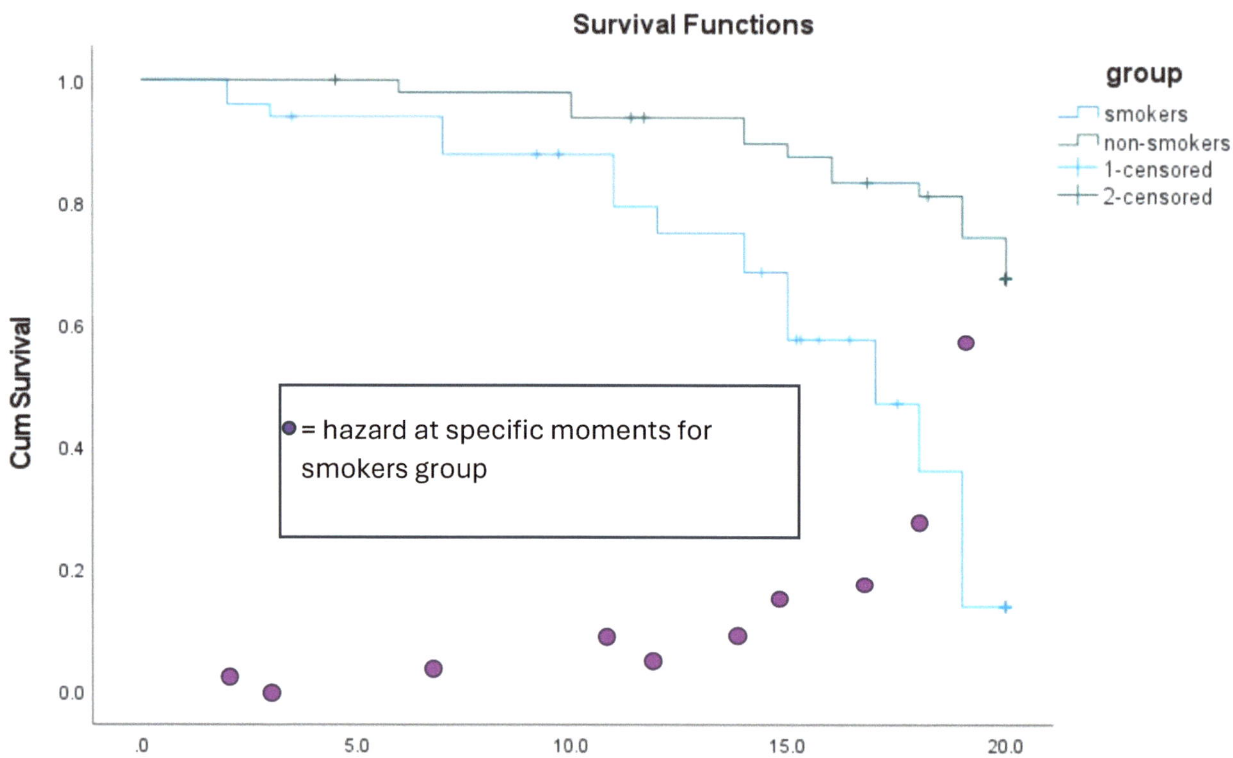

You can see how the hazards increase, especially toward the end of the study! And what about the hazard *ratio* between the two groups? Well, it also changes *a little* as time goes on, but not nearly as much as the individual hazards are changing, and that is because the hazards of *both* groups are increasing with time. Let's focus in on another area of the K-M plots, where events in both groups are happening simultaneously:

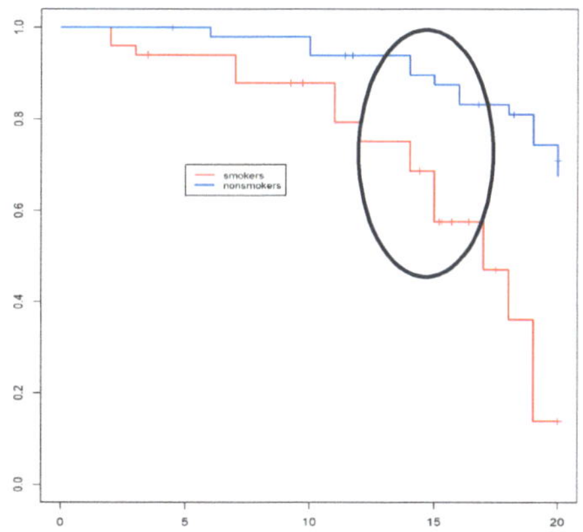

Here is the zoom in:

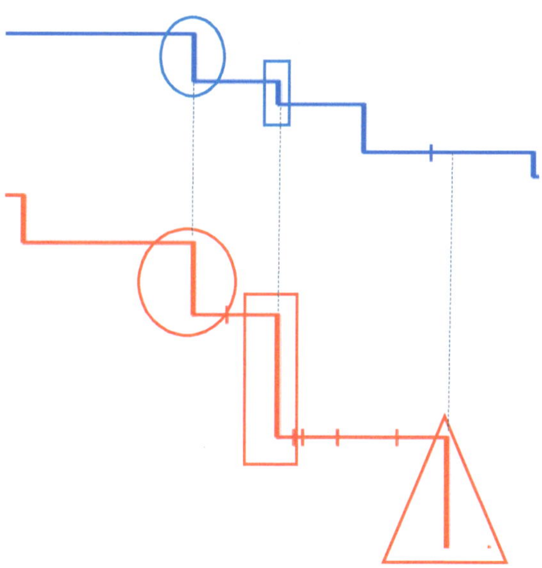

At the red circle in the smokers group, the hazard is 3/35 = 0.086, while the simultaneous hazard in the blue smokers (nonsmokers) is 2/45 = 0.044. So the hazard *ratio* at that moment in time is 0.086/0.044 = 1.95.

At the red rectangle, the hazard is 5/34 = 0.15, while the simultaneous hazard in the blue rectangle is 1/43 = 0.023. And so the hazard ratio at this moment in time is 0.15/0.023 = 6.5.

That is a big difference in hazard ratios! (That is unusual and is occurring here because there are relatively few participants in our study. In larger studies, the survival curves are a lot "smoother," and not so much variation in the hazard ratios are seen).

And here's where it gets weirder: at the red triangle, the hazard is 4/25 = 0.16. But in the blue nonsmokers group there were *no* events at that particular moment in time so the hazard is 0. And so the hazard ratio at this moment is 0.16/0 = undefined??

And so this demonstration of how the hazard ratio changes from moment to moment, and how at times it's even undefined is just to demonstrate to you that the hazard ratio—the great measure of association that is used in survival analysis—cannot be calculated by hand precisely. The computer does some sort of "weighted average" of all the hazards and gives us a hazard ratio that is the "best estimate."

For those of you who really want to know what is going on mathematically, it is something like this: the computer calculates the hazard at ever point in time, and then calculates a "cumulative hazard," which is the sum of all hazards, and then the hazard function is the derivative of the cumulative function curve. So there you go.

But here's the key point: The hazards can change wildly over the course of the survival analysis time period, but the hazard *ratio* between the groups stays *pretty much* the same (on average…despite the little differences from point to point, and occasional outlier big differences as I demonstrated!).

I would like to show you one more example of this relationship between K-M curves and hazards. Here is a very simple example of a two-group K-M plot:

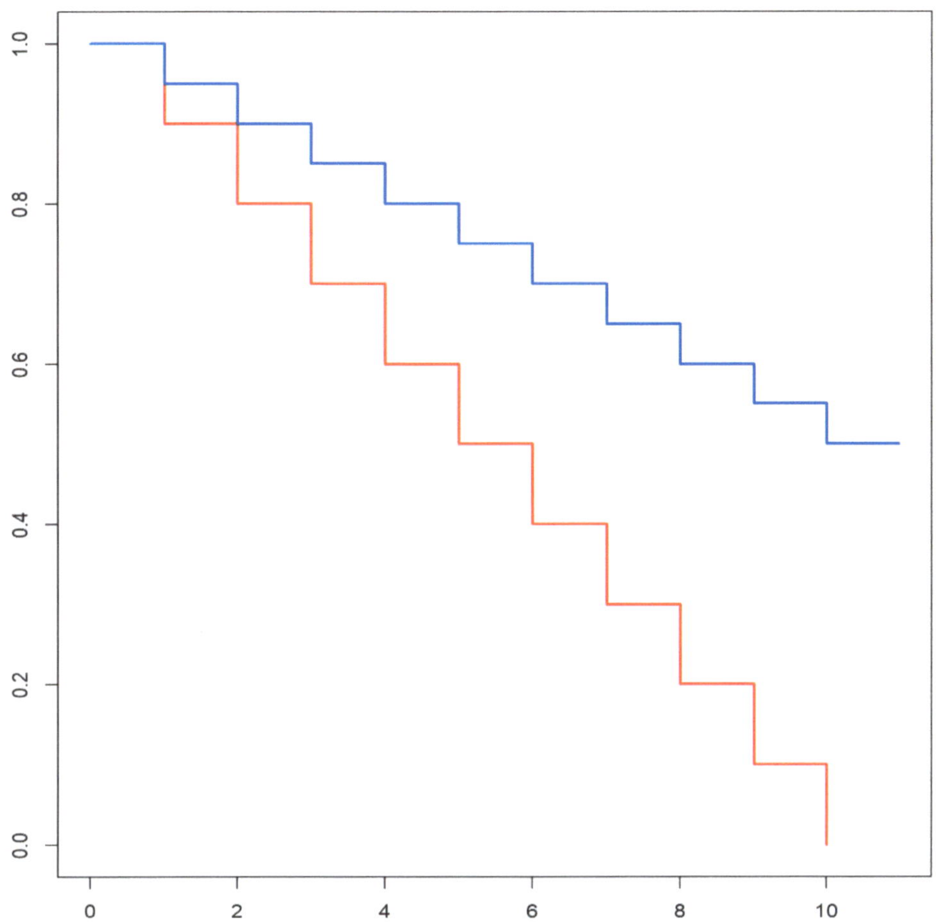

Two groups here: the group in red has 10 deaths every year, and the group in blue has 5 deaths every year. Nice and simple. If 10 people die/year in one group, and 5 people die per year in the other group, then the survival function (the y-values) go down in equal stepwise fashion, as shown by the spreadsheets:

The red group:

time	n.risk	n.event	survival	std.err	lower 95% CI	upper 95% CI
1	100	10	0.9	0.0300	0.8431	0.961
2	90	10	0.8	0.0400	0.7253	0.882
3	80	10	0.7	0.0458	0.6157	0.796
4	70	10	0.6	0.0490	0.5113	0.704
5	60	10	0.5	0.0500	0.4110	0.608
6	50	10	0.4	0.0490	0.3146	0.509
7	40	10	0.3	0.0458	0.2224	0.405
8	30	10	0.2	0.0400	0.1351	0.296
9	20	10	0.1	0.0300	0.0555	0.180
10	10	10	0.0	NaN	NA	NA

The blue group:

time	n.risk	n.event	survival	std.err	lower 95% CI	upper 95% CI
1	100	5	0.95	0.0218	0.908	0.994
2	95	5	0.90	0.0300	0.843	0.961
3	90	5	0.85	0.0357	0.783	0.923
4	85	5	0.80	0.0400	0.725	0.882
5	80	5	0.75	0.0433	0.670	0.840
6	75	5	0.70	0.0458	0.616	0.796
7	70	5	0.65	0.0477	0.563	0.751
8	65	5	0.60	0.0490	0.511	0.704
9	60	5	0.55	0.0497	0.461	0.657
10	55	5	0.50	0.0500	0.411	0.608

But what about the hazards? Remember, the hazard is the *instantaneous* risk, which increases as time goes on. At time 6, for example, the hazard in the red group is 10/50 = 0.2, while the hazard at time 7 in this group is 10/40 = 0.25, and so on. I can graph the hazards at each time with red dots:

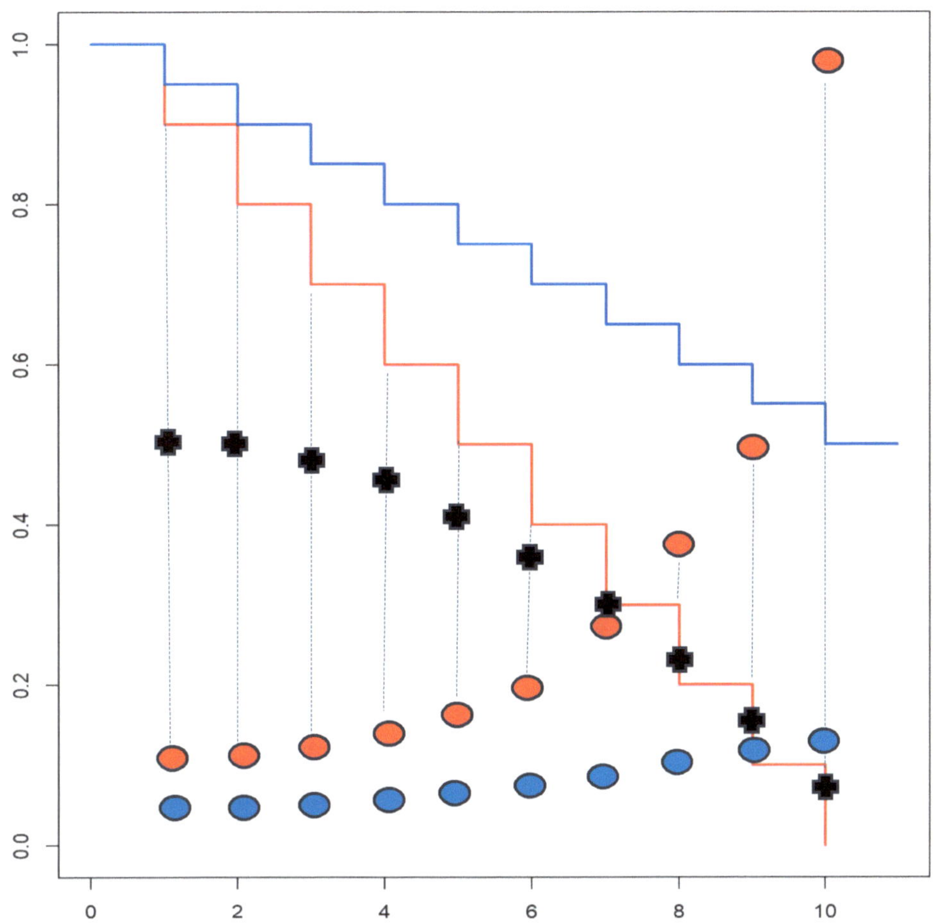

figure 7.1

Does it make sense to you that the hazard function curves dramatically upward? If you think about it, since 10 people die each year and you made it to say time 9…well, there are only 20 people left, so your risk is 50%. And if you were lucky enough to make it to time 10, well there are only 10 people left, so your hazard becomes 100%!

The blue group of course does much better because only 5 of these people die each year, and their hazards are plotted with blue dots.

And finally, the black crosses are the hazard ratios (blue/red). It slowly diminishes over time (if I had chosen to graph the hazard ratio as red/blue, I could not fit it in this graph, as it increases from 2 to over 11 as time goes on.

So I hope you have a general sense of hazards and hazard ratios and how they relate to the K-M survival function.

Key points:

The K-M survival function gives us the probability of surviving (or being free from an event) from a certain point onward.

The hazard is the *instantaneous risk* of having an event at a certain point, given that you have survived up till that point

The hazard function and the hazard ratio cannot be calculated by hand; they are calculated by the computer.

In the world of modern epidemiologic research, we usually obtain our hazard ratio via the Cox Proportional Hazards model, which will be covered in the next section!

One final point:

If you are really having trouble with the concept of hazards and hazard ratios, do not fret. If all else fails, know that the hazard ratio is very similar to the *incidence rate ratio*, if the incidence rate is calculated for every person individually. For example, in the red group above, we would say that there were 10 events at year 1 (out of 100 at risk). That translates to an incidence rate of 10 cases/100 person-years. At year 2, there were 10 cases per 90 people at risk, so that would be an incidence rate of 10 cases/90 person-years, and so on. Then, if you make all the denominators the same and add them up, you come up with a total incidence rate. Do the same for the blue group, and the ratio of the two is the incidence rate ratio. This will be almost identical to the hazard rate that the computer will spit out. So, in a way, you can calculate the hazard ratio by hand if you want to…as long as there are no possible confounder or interactions present. (And since that is very rarely the case, we are "stuck" having to rely on the computer to calculate our hazard ratio for us using Cox Proportional Hazards model!)

8. The hazard ratio is very much like the ____________________ ___________ ratio when calculated for each individual participant.

Section B8.4: Cox Proportional Hazards

Cox Proportional Hazards model is a type of regression that was invented by the one and only Sir David Cox, the British biostatistician who is generally considered the hero of the biostatistics world (if you can grasp such a concept!) I mean, he was knighted by Queen Elizabeth II, and worked on biostats well into his 90s until he died in 2015. His model is a tool to handle the mathematics of survival analysis with several cofactors (independent variables).

Recall that, similar to all the other types of regressions I discussed in Biostats 5 and 6, when there are multiple cofactors present, we may be interested in the effect of each cofactor *independent of all the others.* And we want to know if certain cofactors are acting as confounders to the factor of interest. And we would also need to check to see if any possible interactions (effect measure modification) is present.

First point: Similar to logistic regression and Poisson regression, the outcome here is binary. (That is obvious since we are talking about survival analysis, in which the outcome is: did an event occur? Yes/no).

9. The only kind of regression that deals with a continuous outcome is ____________________ regression.

So recall in linear regression we have:

$$continuous\ dependent\ variable = \beta_0 + \beta_1 x_1 + \beta_2 x_2 + \cdots$$

And in logistic regression, we have:

$$ln(odds\ of\ event) = \beta_0 + \beta_1 x_1 + \beta_2 x_2 + \cdots$$

And in Poisson regression we have:

$$ln(incidence) = \beta_0 + \beta_1 x_1 + \beta_2 x_2 + \cdots$$

Similarly, in Cox regression we have:

$$\ln(hazard) = \ln(h_0(t)) + \beta_1 x_1 + \beta_2 x_2 + \cdots$$

Since hazard is a proportion, we must deal in logarithms, just like logistic and Poisson. So the left side is the *ln* of the hazard. The right side is a bit different from the other two because of the first term that is circled. In the other three types of regression, the β_0 is our "intercept term," meaning it is the value of the output when all the covariables (x_1 , x_2, etc.) are all zero. It is the "baseline" value, and it is "fixed" (it does not change with time). In Cox, the first term is *sort of* like an intercept term in that it is also the baseline value when all other cofactors are set to zero, but notice that it is a function *with respect to time,* meaning that it *does* change over time. It is not "fixed" like the intercept term in logistic and Poisson. And this is consistent what we now know about hazards: they change over time!

(And just like the other multivariable regressions, the cofactors can be any type of variable: continuous, categorical, or binary).

10. Cox regression is similar to the other regression types that deal with binary outcomes: logistic and Poisson, except that in Cox, the intercept term is time - ___________________________.

Cox regression has the same "magic" as logistic and Poisson, and following along the argument that I presented in Section B5.3:

For a simple Cox regression (only one cofactor) we have:

$$ln(hazard) = \ln(h_0(t)) + \beta_1 x_1$$

When we compare two groups, we have:

$$\text{group a: } x_1 = 1; \; ln(hazard_a) = \ln(h_0(\text{t})) + \beta_1$$
$$\text{group b: } x_1 = 0; \; ln(hazard_b) = \ln(h_0(t))$$

And so,

$$ln(hazard_a) - ln(hazard_b) = \boldsymbol{\beta_1}$$

$$\beta_1 = ln\left(\frac{hazard_a}{hazard_b}\right) = ln(HR)\,!$$

So just like in logistic and Poisson, the regression coefficient, β_1, is the ln of the measure of association (in this case the hazard ratio).

Let's revisit my fictitious longitudinal study comparing a group of smokers with a group of nonsmokers.

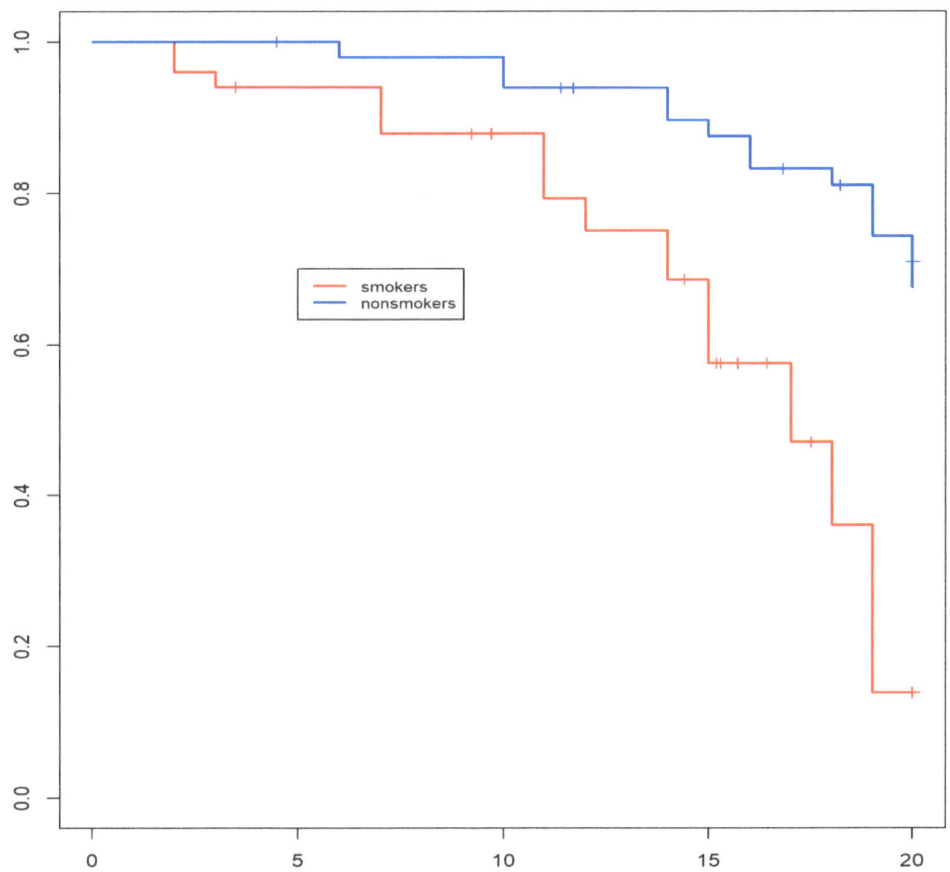

We now ask our computer to do a Cox hazards regression. We get the following results:

```
               coef exp(coef) se(coef)     z Pr(>|z|)
cigs$group1 1.5887    4.8974   0.3187 4.984 6.22e-07 ***
```

"cigs$group" is just "groups"

"coef" is our β , which is our regression coefficient: the thing we care about!

"exp(coef)" is just e^{β}

"se(coef)" is the standard error of the coefficient. (Just like all regressions, the computer calculates the standard error along with the coefficient).

"z" is the z-score. You remember, how many standard errors away from the null is our coefficient. (You know that this is just 1.5887/.3187…how many standard errors away from the null (which is 0) is 1.5887?)

"Pr" is the p-value.

So in my example, the regression coefficient, after exponentiating, is **4.8974**. What does that mean? It means the hazard ratio is **4.8974**. (The way I coded it, the hazard ratio is smokers/nonsmokers, but you could simply take the reciprocal of 4.8974, and find that the hazard ratio for smokers/nonsmokers is **0.2042**.

Translation: the instantaneous risk of dying if you're a cigarette smoker is almost 5 times the instantaneous risk of dying if you're a nonsmoker.

And we see the p-value is very high, meaning the hazard ratio is statistically significant.

Multivariable Cox Regression

In my experiment, I would then wonder about possible confounding. I would consider adding cofactors. How about stress level? Could that be contributing to the difference in survival? So, first, let's think about it: Is stress level a risk factor for the outcome? Yes. Is it associated with the exposure? Yes, in general, cigarette smokers may be more stressed than nonsmokers. So stress level does meet the definition of a possible confounder. So, in addition to coding each person's time of death along with their group (smoker vs nonsmoker), I also code whether or not they have a high level of stress (coded as 1 if they have a high level of stress, and 0 if they do not).

So we run a *multivariable* Cox regression, and here are the results:

```
                coef exp(coef) se(coef)      z Pr(>|z|)
cigs$group1  1.3121    3.7140   0.3297 3.980 6.89e-05 ***
cigs$stress1 1.2047    3.3357   0.3367 3.578 0.000346 ***
```

Our regression coefficient is now 1.31, and exponentiated, the hazard ratio now is **3.71.**

Translation: The instantaneous risk of death at a given point in time for cigarette smokers, *adjusted for stress level* is 3.71 times the risk for nonsmokers. Recall that before we added stress into the regression the hazard ratio was 4.90. So since adding stress caused the hazard ratio to decrease significantly, we can say that indeed stress acted as a confounder, and we must adjust for it.

Note that we can also use this regression to say: The instantaneous risk of death at a given point in time for people with high stress, *adjusted for cigarette smoking* is 3.34 times the risk for people without high stress.

11. In all types of multivariable regression, each regression coefficient gives us the measure of association ____________________ of all the other variables in the regression.

The regression equation for this model would look like:

$$ln(hazard) = ln(h_0(t)) + \beta_1 x_1 + \beta_2 x_2$$

Where x_1 is the group (coded as 1 if smoker and as 0 if nonsmoker), and x_2 is stress (coded as 1 if high stress and 0 if no stress).

And our results:

$$ln(hazard\ of\ dying) = ln(h_0(t)) + 1.31x_1 + 1.20x_2$$

Notice that the "intercept" term, $ln(h_0(t))$ has no coefficient; we do not know what it is, and that is because, unlike all other types of regression, in Cox regression the "intercept" term is a function of time. Since it is always changing with time, Cox regression cannot find a value for this. So, unlike other types of regression, we cannot use our regression equation to calculate an output. That is, we cannot say what the "hazard" would be given certain values for x_1 and x_2. And that is the one disadvantage inherent in Cox regression: since there is no intercept term, we cannot use it for predictions. We can only use it to calculate hazard *ratios* between groups.

12. Cox regression, unlike all other types of regression, cannot be used to predict the outcome for ____________ of the groups because it cannot give us an intercept term. It can only be used to calculate the hazard ________________ between the groups.

Notice that the two cofactors I have chosen are group status, (smoker vs nonsmoker), and stress status (high level or not) are both *binary* variables. But just like all other types of regression, Cox regression can also handle *continuous variables.* I could have, for example, chosen weight as another cofactor instead of stress. If I did, the regression equation might have looked like this:

$$\ln(hazard\ of\ dying) = \ln(h_0(t)) + 1.26x_1 + 0.08x_2$$

Where x_1 is group status, and x_2 is weight in kilograms. If I did this (I cannot do this in reality, because I don't have data for weight of each participant, so these results are made up!), then the hazard ratio for weight is $e^{0.08} = 1.08$. The translation for that would be: for every 1 kilogram increase in weight, the hazard ratio increases by 8%.

Now, let's say I'm thinking about education level as a possible confounder. (I have included coding for education level, so we can really do this!).

We can run a regression now with all three cofactors: group (smoker/nonsmoker), stress (high or not high) and education level (college or no college).

We get the following results:

```
                    coef exp(coef) se(coef)     z Pr(>|z|)
cigs$group      1.31360   3.71955  0.33024 3.978 6.96e-05 ***
cigs$stress1    1.20190   3.32643  0.33888 3.547  0.00039 ***
cigs$college1   0.02032   1.02053  0.28522 0.071  0.94320
```

The coefficient for college is 0.02, but the p value is non-significant. This means that college education *did not* affect our results significantly, and we therefore *eliminate it* from our model, and our accepted hazard ratios are as before:

Hazard ratio for group status, adjusted for stress: 3.714

Hazard ratio for stress level, adjusted for group status: 3.34.

13. If the regression coefficient for a cofactor is not statistically significant, we ____________ the model completely.

Interaction

In section B6.4, I discussed how multivariable regression handles interaction. Cox regression is no different. So I might wonder, in my example, if there is an interaction between stress and smoking…perhaps it is more than just confounding, perhaps there is some biological "thing" happening, so that for some reason only smokers suffer the effects of stress and die, while nonsmokers just don't (for whatever reason). So we need to run another regression, and this time add an interaction term:

$$\ln(hazard) = \ln(h_0(t)) + \beta_1 x_1 + \beta_2 x_2 + \beta_3 (x_1 * x_2)$$

And here are the results:

```
                               coef exp(coef) se(coef)      z Pr(>|z|)
cigs$group                   2.0894    8.0804   0.6045  3.457 0.000547 ***
cigs$stress1                 1.9201    6.8216   0.5849  3.283 0.001029 **
cigs$group:cigs$stress1     -1.1172    0.3272   0.7001 -1.596 0.110580
```

The coefficient for the interaction term is -1.1172, but the p-value is 0.11, indicating that no significant interaction is occurring between the variables. We don't have to worry about it, and eliminate this model.

Proportional Hazards

As you know, nothing in biostats is perfect, and Cox regression is certainly no exception. The reason it's called "Cox proportional hazards regression" is because of the main assumption that the hazards between groups have to be proportional over time. And the authors of any study that use Cox regression understand this and must check to make sure the proportionality requirement is met.

The quickest and easiest way to test the proportionality assumption is simply to examine the K-M curves. If they cross, then it is an obvious violation:

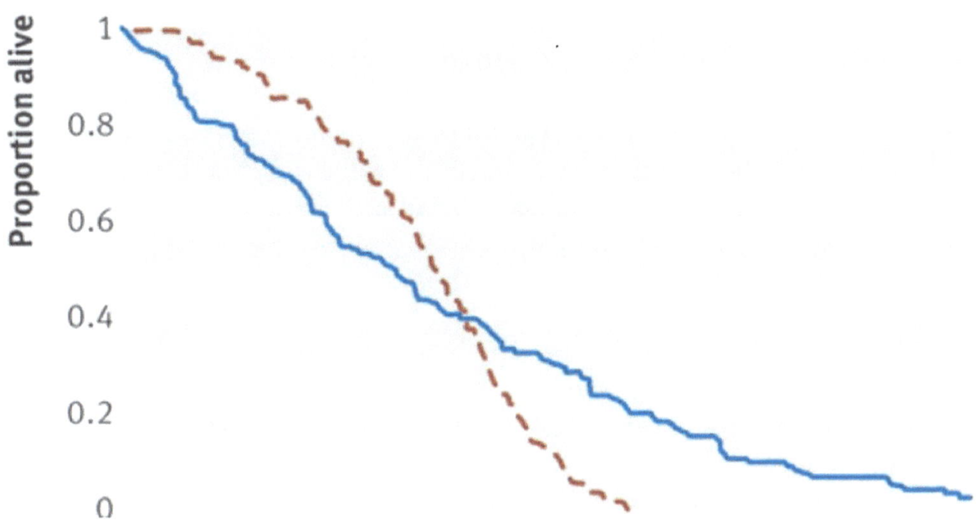

And we cannot use Cox regression!

Also, something like this is a problem:

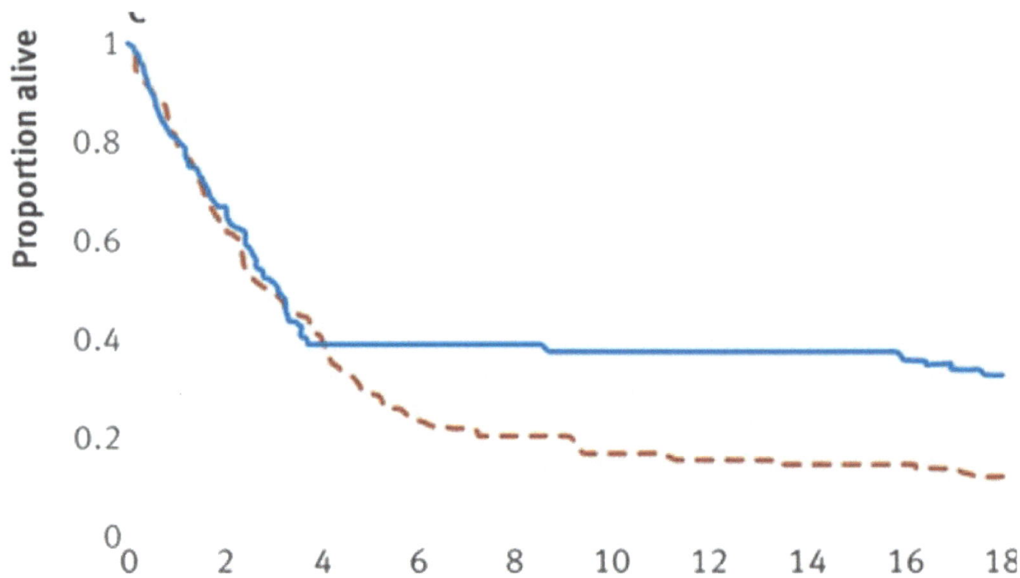

Although a bit more subtle, the proportionality assumption is also violated here. You can see that between time = 0 and time = 4, the people were dying at the same rate, and then a sudden change at time = 4 when the people in the blue group stopped dying, while the people in the red group continued to die. The hazard ratios cannot be proportional for the length of the study. (This is actually called "delayed treatment effect.")

If visually inspecting the K-M curves does not lead to an obvious decision concerning proportionality, a better way to visualize whether or not the proportionality assumption is violated is by plotting the "log-log" curve of the survival function. (The *ln* of survival on the y-axis, and the *ln* of time on the x-axis). And that is because proportionality is on the logarithmic scale. So, for example, remember the very simple K-M example I gave earlier, and I calculated the individual hazards and then the hazard ratios? (figure 7.1).

Here is the K-M curve again:

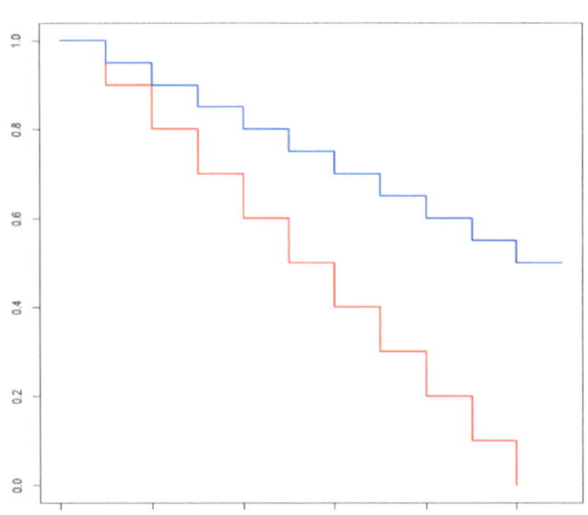

Now I will plot the “log-log”plot, which is the ln of the survival on the y-axix, and *ln* of time on the x-axis:

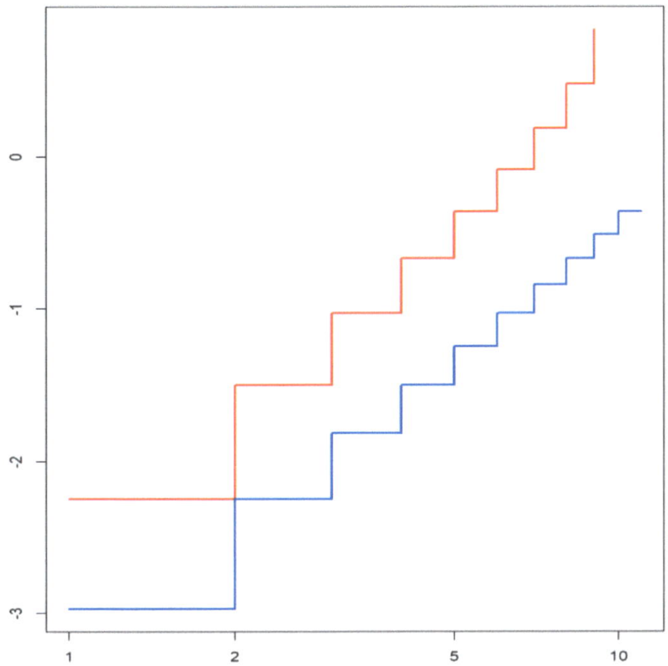

The log-log plot shows parallel lines…the proportionality assumption is satisfied! (And the reason I pointed this out is, if you look at the hazard ratios in figure 7.1, you see that the hazard ratios do change over time, but they are proportional!)

Now my example of cigarette smokers vs nonsmokers: Here is the log-log plot:

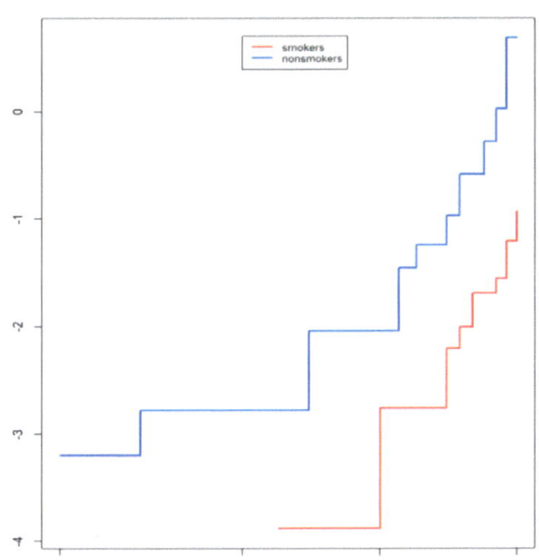

The lines are basically parallel…the proportionality assumption is satisfied!

There are other tests to check for proportionality, including "Schoenfeld residuals plotting" and "goodness of fit" testing. The details of these topics are out of our scope in this book. (That is, I do not know the details of these tests!)

Summary Biostats 8

I began with a discussion on survival analysis and why we need it: how it deals with the problem of censoring, and how it gives us more accurate information when participants join the trial late.

Then I discussed Kaplan-Meir survival function in detail. The survival function is the probability of surviving beyond a particular time. It is also called "cumulative survival." I then "dissected" a curve. Before the "dissection," I explained the concept of **censoring** in detail. Censoring (also called "right censoring") is when we only know partial information about a participant because they drop out and we lose contact.

Two groups of K-M curves are compared with the "log-rank" test, to see if they are different from each other, statistically speaking.

Survival analysis uses the **hazard function,** which is the instantaneous risk of having an event (assuming survival up to that point), and when comparing two groups, we use the **hazard ratio.**

Cox regression is used to evaluate the data in survival analysis. The exponentiated regression coefficients obtained are the hazard ratios for each cofactor, adjusted for all the other variables.

I discussed confounding and interactions with Cox regression, and ended the chapter with the proportional hazards assumption, and how to check for it.

And that's about it for this rather long and rather difficult chapter! Hope you hung in there!

Biostats 9: Meta-analysis

The meta-analysis is a very powerful tool in the world of epidemiologic research. Very often when individual studies are done to explore a particular hypothesis, they yield conflicting results. For example, a recent topic of interested in internal medicine is the association between statin drugs (simvastatin, atorvastatin, lovastatin, et al) and the development of type II diabetes. (When the studies were done to test the association between statin drugs and possible decreased risk of cardiovascular diseases, researchers also commented on side effects, and one possible side-effect seemed to be an increased risk of developing type II diabetes). But the problem is that only some of the studies showed the association and others did not. For example, the JUPITER[1] trial showed an association, with an odds ratio of **1.26 (95% CI from 1.04 to 1.51**) (meaning those who took statins had a 26% higher odds of developing type II diabetes compared to those who did not take statins). But the ASCOT-LLA[2] trial did not show a significant association (odd ratio = **1.14 (95% CI from 0.89 to 1.46).**

Note: If you are not entirely sure as to why the ASCOT-LLA results are *not* significant, please review Section B1.6!

So what is a clinician to do when some of the studies show an association and others do not? What do we tell our patients? The strategy that is often used in epidemiology is to *combine* all the studies together. We then have the luxury of many more trial participants, and, as you recall, the more participants the better. As we increase the number of participants, we improve our precision as the standard errors and confidence intervals become smaller. Say, for example, that each study only has 100 or so participants. That is a relatively small number, so we know that it would be difficult to show statistically significant results. But if we have 10 of these studies, and combine them, now we have 1000 participants to analyze, and have a much better chance of proving our hypothesis!

Section B9.1: Meta-analysis basics

And here is an example of a meta-analysis that was done in 2010[3] to examine this possible association further. They identified 13 studies that fit their criteria. Here are the results:

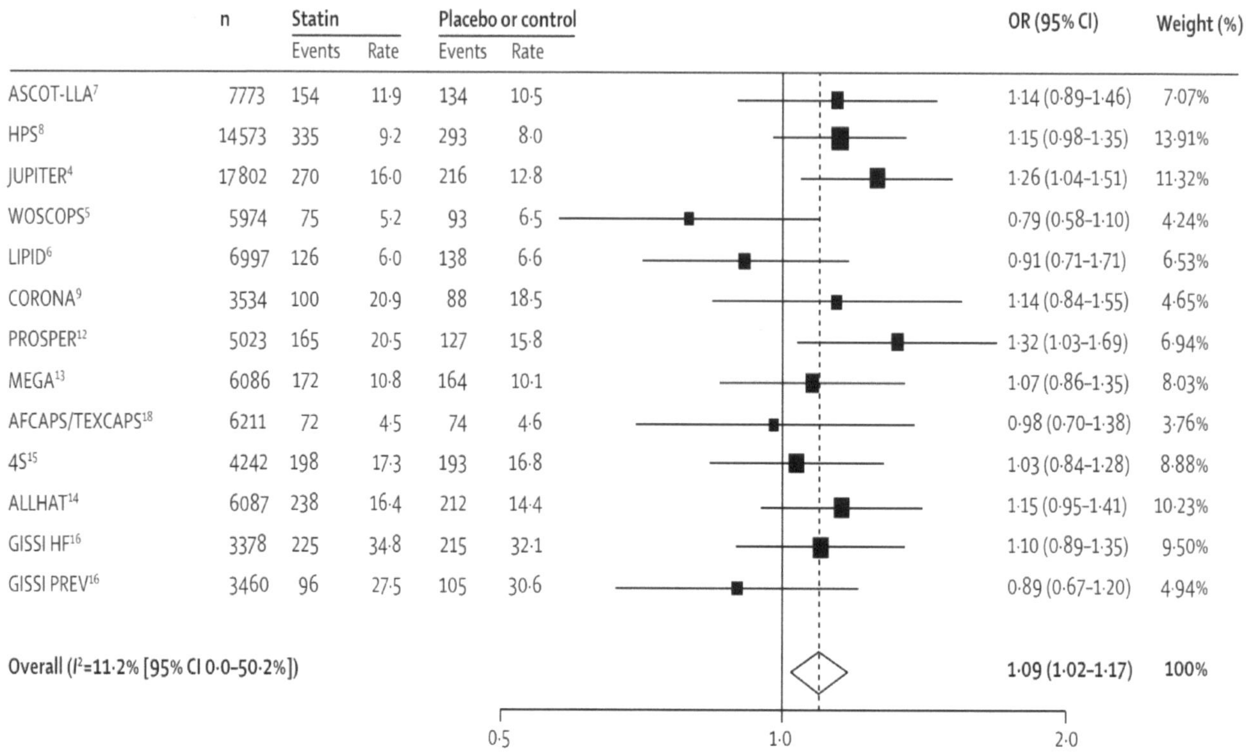

Figure B9.1

Typical for many meta-analyses, the results are displayed as a "forest plot" shown above. (By the way, the forest plot is sometimes known as a "blobbogram," which I just love).

I will zoom in on the top part, so I can dissect it:

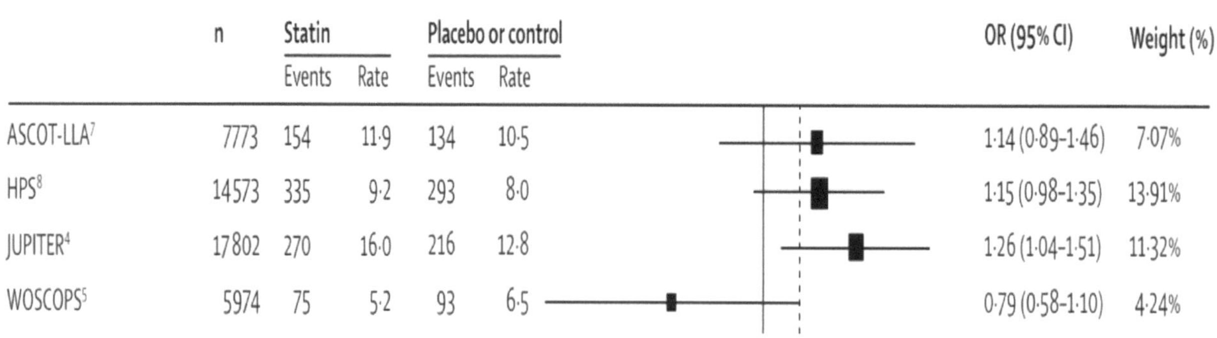

Figure B9.2

On the left side are the numbers for each individual study, and then on the right side we see the blocks and horizontal lines. The blocks represent the measure of association, and the horizontal lines are the 95% confidence intervals, so that each study's results are easily visualized. The solid vertical line is the null hypothesis results.

1. When the measure of association is an odds ratio, or a relative risk, or an incidence rate ratio, or a hazard ratio, the null hypothesis measure of association is _____________ .

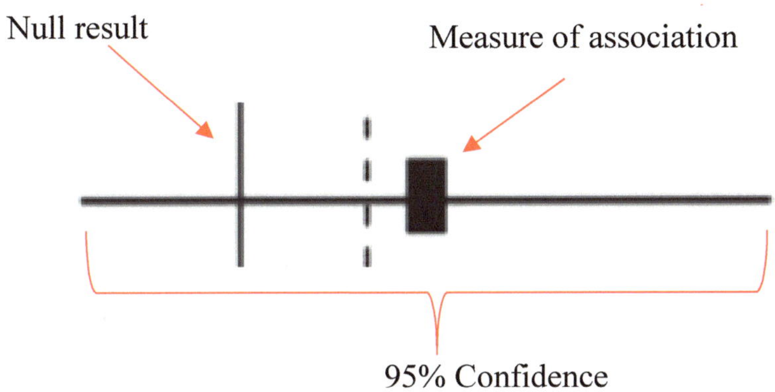

Look back up to figure B9.2. Notice that of the four individual studies, only one showed a statistically significant result (the JUPITER study). The other three studies did not show statistically significant results, because their 95% confidence intervals cross 1. And if you look up at figure B9.1, you will see that of the 13 studies included, only two show significant results.

2. Of the 13 studies included, only the ____________________ trial and the ____________________ trial showed statistically significant results. Because their confidence intervals do not cross _________ .

And now I will zoom in to the very bottom of the plot:

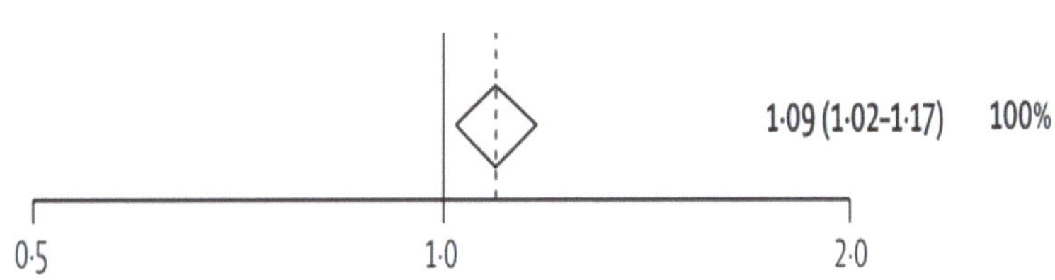

The is the "pooled" results, and the measure of association is now represented by a diamond. Notice that the pooled result is statistically significant, as it does not include 1. (The diamond shape itself does not cross 1). In the pooled result, we don't draw the horizontal lines for the 95% CI, we just use the shape itself, so the left and right endpoints of the diamond are the confidence interval boundaries).

And *viola:* even though only 2 out of the 13 trials showed significant results, when we pool them, we now have a statistically significant result!! Can you imagine why that would be the case? It is because the trials that show significant results, and the trials that *almost* show significant results are *stronger* studies than many of the trials that do not show significant results. And that is the key to meta-analyses: the individual trials are **weighted** before the results are pooled, so that the stronger trials are awarded more value more than the weaker trials. And what determines "strength?" You guessed it: the number of participants! (mostly; more below). You will notice in figure B9.1 that some of the little black blocks are bigger than others. The size of the block represents the relative weight of the trial. And so, the HPS[4] trial, the biggest block, is the strongest, and the WOSCOPS[5] trial, the smallest block, is the weakest. (You can see all the individual weights listed in the column at the far right). And you will also notice that the strongest trials have the narrowest 95% confidence intervals, and the weakest trials have the widest intervals. This is consistent with what we know about trials: the more participants, the higher the precision of our results. And the pooled result (the diamond) shows (by far) the narrowest confidence interval, again because the pooled results include many many more participants than the individual trials.

Section B9.2: Weighted mean effect size

The following is the step-by-step method of calculating the weighted mean (the pooled result) of the effect size.

Step 1: The relative weight of each trial is determined by the quality of the trial, which is often best determined by the standard error of the sample. Recall from Section B3.4 that the standard error of the difference of two means is: $SE_{(\bar{x}_1-\bar{x}_2)} = \sqrt{\frac{s_1^2}{n_1}+\frac{s_2^2}{n_2}},$

and the standard error of the odds ratio is:

$$\widehat{SE}(\ln(RR)) = \sqrt{\frac{1}{a}+\frac{1}{a+b}+\frac{1}{c}+\frac{1}{c+d}}$$

The weight of the effect is the inverse of the SE:

$$W_i = 1/SE^2$$

I should point out that this is valid only for a "fixed effect" model, rather than a "random effects" model (explained more below).

So, let's say we have three studies. Study 1 has an SE of 0.04, study 2 has an SE of 0.12, and study 3 has an SE of 0.16.

The individual weights would then be: $W_1 = \frac{1}{0.04} = 25$; $W_2 = \frac{1}{0.12} = 8.33$; $W_3 = 6.25$. You can see that study 1 is weighted a lot more than the other 2 studies because its variance was so much smaller.

To get the weighted mean, we continue:

Step 2: Multiply the weight of each study by its effect size to give the *weighted* effect. So, assume effect size of study 1 is 10, study 2 is 16 and study 3 is 14. (The effect size here would be mean differences). Study1: 25 x 10 = 250. Study 2: 8.33 x 16 = 133.3. Study 3: 6.25 x 14 = **87.5**.

Step 3: Add these all up to get the total weighted effects: 250 + 133.3 + 87.5 = **470.8**.

Step 4: Divide by the total weights. 470.8/39.6 = **11.9**

11.9 is our "mean weighted effect size." Notice that it is close to the effect size of study 1, because study 1 was by far the strongest study!

But most meta-analyses are not "fixed effect" models, they are "random effects" models, and in random effects models we add another factor in when we calculate relative weight. I will talk more about fixed vs random effects in the next section, but basically in random effects models, there is variation in effects *between* the studies, in addition to within the studies. So for random effects models, our individual weight is now:

$$W_i = \frac{1}{SE^2 + \tau^2}$$

In which τ^2 ("tau-squared") is our measure of variance between the studies. We then proceed in the manner described above.

Section B9.3: Random vs Fixed Effects models

This is somewhat of a controversial topic in the area of meta-analysis, but I will start by stating that it unequivocally should *not* be controversial. And that is because virtually every meta-analysis performed in medical research should be a random effects model. (If not *every* meta-analysis). It is extremely rare that it is appropriate to run a fixed effect model. So the only reason I am even going to mention fixed effect models is because you will still often see meta-analyses *incorrectly* run as fixed effect models, and the results are not at all trustworthy.

What is fixed effect? It means that the effect is basically the same in all studies. What do I mean by that? I would like to demonstrate with a fictitious study on the effect of an exercise program to lower blood pressure, and let's say I include 5 studies in my meta-analysis. In the trials, half the people underwent an exercise program designed to lower blood pressure, and the other half did not. Before the trial and at the end of 6 weeks, their systolic blood pressures were measured. The amount of improvement in the two groups was compared. In the very unlikely event that all five of my studies were conducted in the exact same population, under the exact same set of circumstances, I could justifiably run a fixed effect model, because I would expect the effect size would be the *same* in each of the five studies. The results of my meta-analysis might look like this:

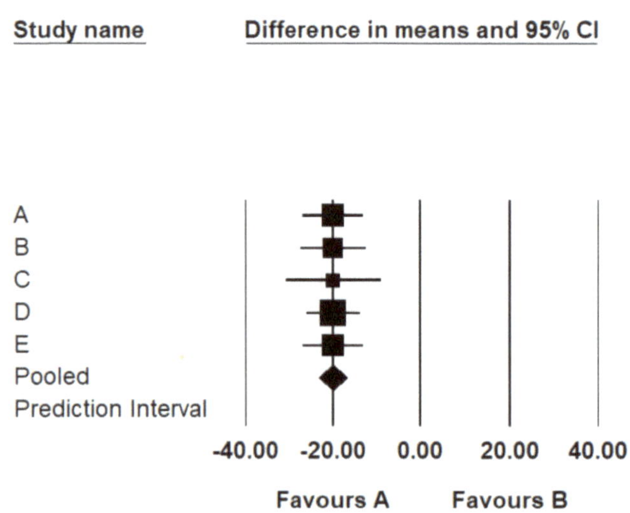

Figure B9.3

The effect size of each study is a difference in blood pressure improvement of 20 mmHg (the treatment group's blood pressure improved by 20 points more than the control group's blood pressure improved). Notice that not all the studies are completely identical: some have more participants than others and difference variances, that is why some of the boxes are smaller than others (the larger the box, the better the study and the more weight assigned to it), and the 95% confidence interval horizontal lines are a bit different: the stronger studies have a narrower confidence interval. Nonetheless, the effect size – the difference of 20 mmHg – is the same for all studies. And so the "pooled" effect size is also 20, and the pooled 95% CI (the borders of the diamond) are narrower than any of the studies, because the pooled result now has many more participants.

The only way, of course, that we could get such results is if all five of the studies were obtained from exactly the same population. For example, all the studies were done at Gold's Gym, and the participants were all men between the ages of 50 and 55 who had been gym members for 10 years, and all weighed exactly the same, etc. Now of course, even in a studies that are all from the same population like this example, we would not expect the effect sizes from each individual study to be *exactly* the same. Rather, we expect some variation due to *sampling.* That is, due to chance. Remember that no one sample is perfect, and remember that we do not care about the results of one particular study; we only care about the entire "target" population (see section E5.4). (Here, the "target" population that we care about is the entire "universe" of all males between 50 and 55 who are members of Gold's Gym!). But at any rate, remember that each individual study is only one sample of this "universe," and we would not expect the results of each individual sample to be *exactly* the same as the true effect of the universe. There would instead be some variation, just due to random error of the sample, and our results would more likely look this this:

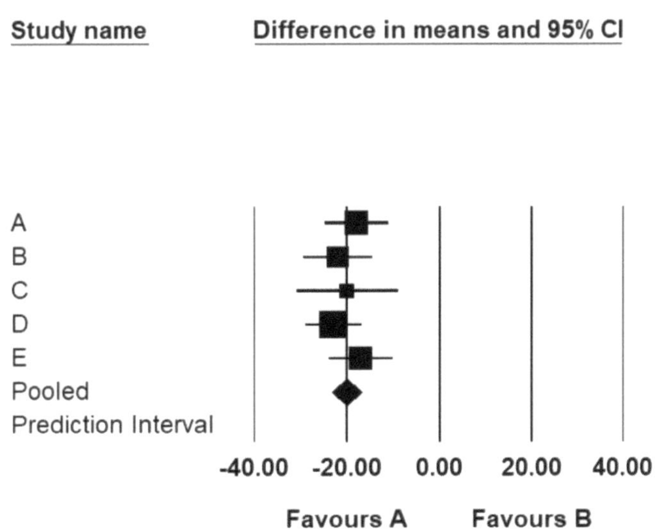

Figure B9.4

Now you see some "wobbling" around the mean effect. This is just due to chance, and is sometimes referred to as "noise." But the effect size is still *essentially* the same in each study, and so we use the "fixed effect" model.

3. In order to use a "fixed effect" model, all the studies have to be identical; the subjects, methods, process, etc, must be exactly the ____________________ in all the studies. This is extremely ___________ when conducting a meta-analysis in the real world, and so way more often we cannot use the ______________ _________________ model.

Now let us move into the real world. If we really wanted to know the effect of exercise on blood pressure, our research would extend way beyond men between 50 and 55 who are Gold's Gym members, and we would search for studies done on many different populations. And we would likely find that the effect sizes in the studies really vary: some show a small effect, some show a large effect, some show no effect, and some even show an effect that favors that placebo group. This is the real world. The variance in the effects is because the study populations are different: some of the studies were conducted on Gold's Gym members, some were conducted on elderly clients in rehabilitation facilities, some were conducted on patients of primary care doctors in a health clinic etc. The people are very different and would respond differently to any treatment. In addition, the studies would not be identical in the way they are run: the treatment protocols may differ, the data may be collected differently etc. This is the real world of meta-analysis studies. You can see there would be much less precision in our results, but the advantage is that we now can generalize our results to the target population that we really care about: the entire universe of *all adults* with high blood pressure.

And what would a "real" meta-analysis look like? Perhaps something like this:

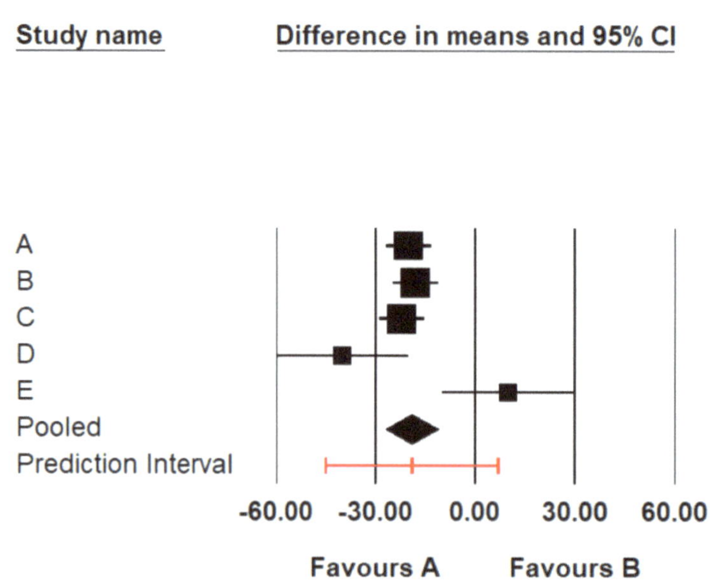

This is a "random effects model," and comes with the red line shown, which is the "prediction interval," which I will discuss below. But notice that the effects now vary quite a bit because of study D and study E. We can no longer say that the effect size is the same (or *essentially* the same) in every study. There is variation of effect size *between the studies* (called "heterogeneity") and so we must use the "random effects model" when we run our meta-analysis. In a random effects model, we care about *two* things: the mean weighted effect size *and* how much heterogeneity exists between the studies.

4. In the real world of meta-analyses, we almost always must run a _______________ ________________ model.

Again, I keep bringing this up because you will find in the literature many examples of researchers incorrectly using the fixed effect model. And I will now show you why this matters. I will run this meta-analysis again, and both the fixed and random effects results are now shown, and now with all the statistics:

Model	Study name	Statistics for each study						
		Difference in means	Standard error	Variance	Lower limit	Upper limit	Z-Value	p-Value
	A	-20.000	3.536	12.500	-26.930	-13.070	-5.657	0.000
	B	-18.000	3.536	12.500	-24.930	-11.070	-5.091	0.000
	C	-22.000	3.536	12.500	-28.930	-15.070	-6.223	0.000
	D	-40.000	10.124	102.500	-59.843	-20.157	-3.951	0.000
	E	10.000	10.124	102.500	-9.843	29.843	0.988	0.323
Fixed	Pooled	-19.624	1.963	3.853	-23.471	-15.777	-9.997	0.000
Random	Pooled	-18.925	4.052	16.420	-26.867	-10.983	-4.670	0.000

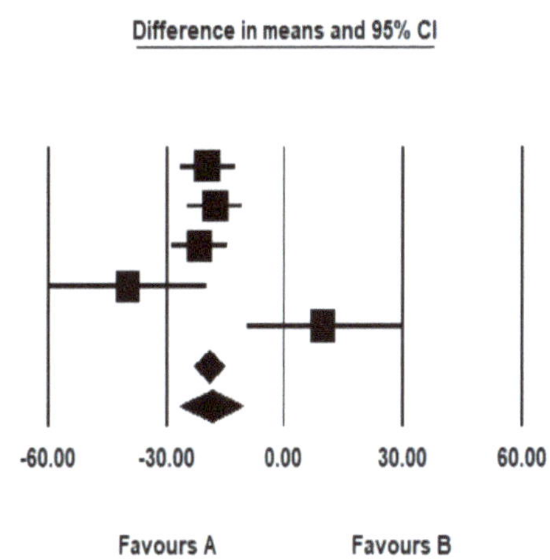

Note that although the pooled effects are similar (-19.6 vs -18.9), the 95% confidence intervals are quite different: in the fixed effect model it is much narrower. And this is the main difference between fixed and random: the fixed effect model is a lot more precise in its results, and so *much easier to show statistical significance* than a random effect model. And that is why researchers will often "fudge" the results by incorrectly using a fixed effect model!

5. Be very suspicious if you see a _______________ effect model in a meta-analysis!

Prediction interval

So let's return to the appropriate model here: the random effects model. Here it is again, with all the attached statistics:

Study name	Difference in means	Standard error	Variance	Lower limit	Upper limit	Z-Value	p-Value
A	-20.000	3.536	12.500	-26.930	-13.070	-5.657	0.000
B	-18.000	3.536	12.500	-24.930	-11.070	-5.091	0.000
C	-22.000	3.536	12.500	-28.930	-15.070	-6.223	0.000
D	-40.000	10.124	102.500	-59.843	-20.157	-3.951	0.000
E	10.000	10.124	102.500	-9.843	29.843	0.988	0.323
Pooled	-18.925	4.052	16.420	-26.867	-10.983	-4.670	0.000
Prediction Interval	-18.925			-44.911	7.061		

(Statistics for each study)

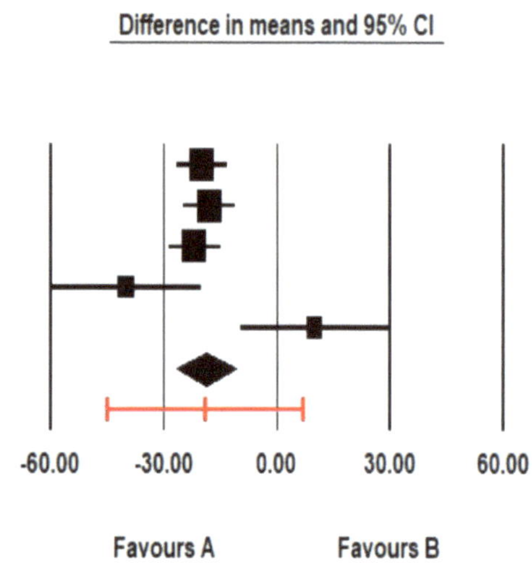

I will focus now on the bottom two rows, "pooled" and "prediction interval." The pooled result is just as before, the weighted mean of all the studies, with its 95% confidence interval. The interpretation is: we can be reasonably certain that the mean of the studies lies somewhere between an effect size of -26.9 and -11.0. And so the researchers would conclude that exercise shows a statistically significant benefit by lowering blood pressure an average of -18.9 points more in the exercise group. But our meta-analysis tells us that there is a wide range of effects since one of the studies actually showed results favoring the control group (study E has a difference in blood pressure of +10 mmHg). And so in random effects models, our primary focus should be on this "dispersion" of results. And that is what the prediction interval tells us. It is also a 95% confidence interval, but it is interpreted as: "in the whole universe of trials similar to the ones we included, we can be reasonably certain that the effect size could vary from **-44.9 to 7.06.** And in the real world, *this* is the statistic that we really need to know.

To show the importance of this, I would like to return your attention to the real meta-analysis that I started the chapter with (figure B9.1).

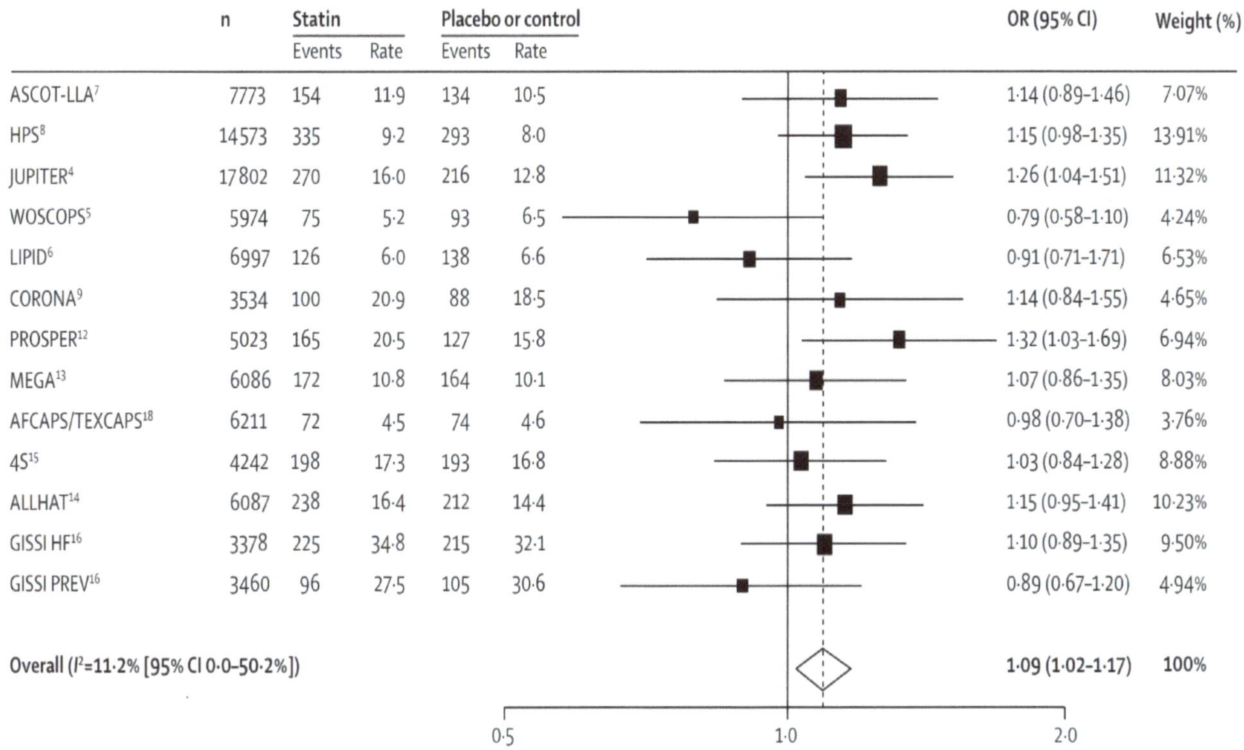

The authors concluded that there is indeed an association between statin use and the onset of diabetes because the pooled result of their meta-analysis was an OR of 1.09, and it was statistically significant because the 95% CI was from 1.02 to 1.17.

6. Since the 95% confidence interval of the odds ratio did not include _________, the authors can claim that their results were statistically significant.

And the authors did the right thing by running a random effects model, instead of a fixed effect model. But what they did not include was a measure of dispersion of results (which is often referred to as "heterogeneity."). I would like to show you what that would look like, so I re-ran the meta-analysis using R statistical software, and asked it to include the prediction interval.

Here are the results:

Study	Experimental Events	Experimental Total	Control Events	Control Total	RR	95%-CI
ASCOT-LLA	154	3910	134	3863	1.14	[0.90; 1.43]
HPS	335	7291	293	7283	1.14	[0.98; 1.33]
JUPITER	270	8901	216	8901	1.25	[1.05; 1.49]
WOSCOPS	75	2999	93	2975	0.80	[0.59; 1.08]
LIPID	126	3496	138	3501	0.91	[0.72; 1.16]
CORONA	100	1771	88	1763	1.13	[0.86; 1.49]
PROSPER	165	2510	127	2513	1.30	[1.04; 1.63]
MEGA	172	3013	164	3073	1.07	[0.87; 1.32]
AFSCAPS	72	3094	74	3117	0.98	[0.71; 1.35]
4S	198	2116	193	2126	1.03	[0.85; 1.25]
ALLHAT-LLA	238	3017	212	3070	1.14	[0.96; 1.37]
GISSI-HF	225	1660	215	1718	1.08	[0.91; 1.29]
GISSI-PR	96	1743	105	1717	0.90	[0.69; 1.18]
Common effect model		**45521**		**45620**	**1.09**	**[1.03; 1.16]**
Random effects model					**1.09**	**[1.02; 1.16]**
Prediction interval						**[0.95; 1.25]**

Heterogeneity: $I^2 = 16.9\%$, $\tau^2 = 0.0029$, $p = 0.2736$

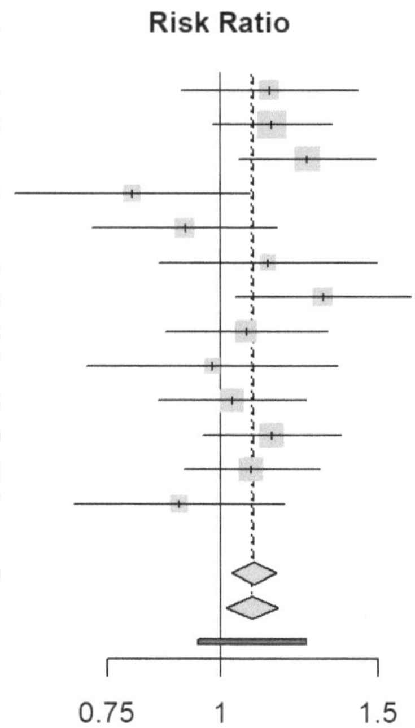

Note that the red horizontal line at the bottom, the prediction interval, spans from an odds ratio of **0.95 to 1.25.** So, in 95% of comparable studies in the "universe," the results span from an OR of 0.95 (meaning statin treatment is actually *protective* against diabetes), to an OR of 1.25 (meaning statin treatment is associated with diabetes). The authors should have made this their primary outcome, because this is a random effects model, and there is heterogeneity in the trials…they are all different and have different effect sizes! And if they did make this their primary outcome, they would *not* have declared statistical significance!

It is vital that you understand the difference between the pooled result and the prediction interval. The pooled result is the weighted mean of all the studies, and the 95% confidence interval simply tells us how confident we are in that pooled mean. The prediction interval tells us how the effect sizes vary across all the studies, because of the inherent differences in all the studies.

Section B9.4: Statistics used in meta-analyses

To begin this discussion, I will quote from the meta-analysis above:

> As in the main analysis, risk of incident diabetes with statin therapy remained higher with statin therapy than control in analyses restricted to the placebo-control trials (OR 1·10, 95% CI 1·01–1·20, I^2=21%; n=75 507).

Do you see that I^2 in there? That is the most important statistic that we see in meta-analyses, and also the most misunderstood, so it is important to discuss it, and how it's derived. It is often used as a measure of *heterogeneity* of the trials. A high I^2 (like 50% or more) is generally considered to mean that there is "a lot" of heterogeneity, and a low I^2 is generally considered to mean that there is not a lot of heterogeneity.

And there are a couple of other statistics in addition to I^2 and τ^2 which I discussed above. Here is another meta-analysis seeking to determine if a Mediterranean diet can help prevent diabetes:

> Koloverou et al. The effect of Mediterranean diet on the development of type 2 diabetes mellitus: A meta-analysis of 10 prospective studies and 136,846 participants. *Metabolism.* Volume 63, Issue 7, July 2014, Pages 903-911

Here is a quote from their results section:

> "Since heterogeneity existed among prospective studies (Cochran's Q = 21.53, df = 10, pQ = 0.01 and I^2 = 58%)…"

So we have another statistic, the Q value, to discuss as well.

Variance

So here we go. Let's go back to my initial fictious meta-analysis, the one about lowering blood pressure on an exercise program. Here are figures B8.3 and B8.4:

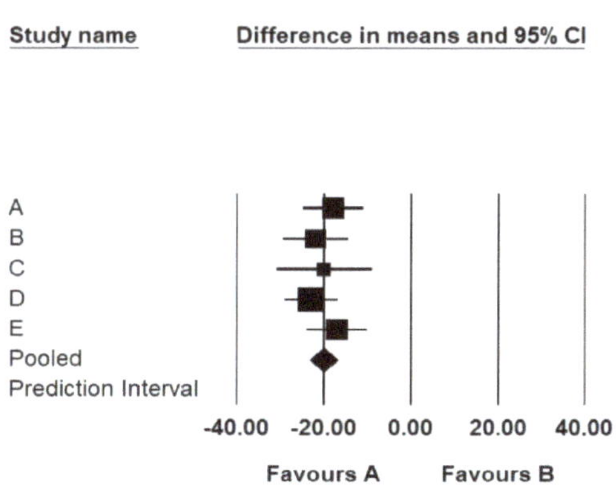

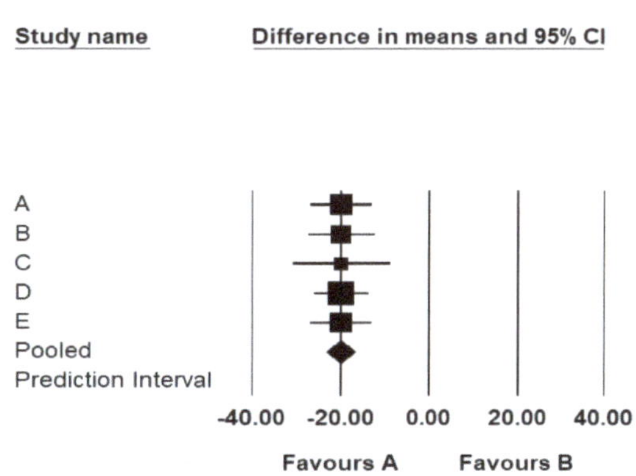

The figure on the left is the *observed* effects for a fixed effect model – that is, all the 5 studies were perfectly homogeneous in participants, methods, etc. Notice that it is not exactly the same as the graph on the right, which is the *true* effects. That is, if we were able to eliminate all the "noise" that comes from random chance, we would get the results on the right. So the reason that the left is different from the right is because we have a variance that is due to random sampling. We call this variance due to "error."

$$V_{observed} = V_{true} + V_{error}$$

In the example above, the true variance is 0 (because it's a fixed effect model), and so the observed variance is simply the variance due to error. It makes intuitive sense that the observed variance is always greater than the true variance. How much greater? Well, that depends on the quality of the studies in the meta-analysis. If the studies are all very large with small variances, the observed variance will be very close to the true variance.

Now let's imagine the more realistic scenario in which the studies in the meta-analysis are heterogeneous. So now we have a bunch of *different* true effects. And that is because the studies are all different. For example, one study was conducted on very physically fit men at Gold's Gym, one study may have been conducted on nursing home immobile patients (and a very different exercise program was of course prescribed!), one may have been conducted on overweight cigarette smokers in a nutrition clinic, etc. We would certainly expect that the effect size might well be quite different for all these studies, because they are so different. So now, we have a V_{true} that is not 0. It is some value. And so in this situation, the $V_{observed}$ is more than just the variance due to error. It is also made up of the true effect variance.

7. in meta-analyses, the observed variance is the variance of the true effects plus the variance due to ________________ .

Q statistic

The Q statistic is the sum of the squares of the differences of the effect sizes and the mean effect size. And just like variance, the total Q is the Q of the error plus the Q of the effects.

$$Q_{observed} = Q_{error} + Q_{true}$$

And the cool thing about Q is that it follows (pretty closely) the chi-square distribution. Remember the chi-square distribution (section B3.5)? The very cool thing about the chi-square distribution is that the mean of the distribution (the "expected" value) is the same as the "degrees of freedom" of the distribution.

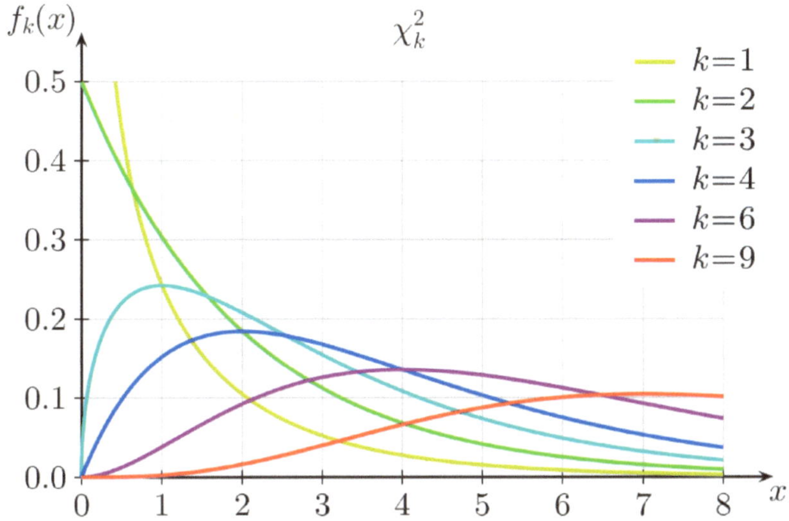

For example, the turquoise-colored distribution of k=3 has a mean value of 3; the blue distribution of k=4 has a mean of 4; the violet distribution of k=6 has a mean of 6 etc. Thus, if the variations are only due to error, then the expected Q value should be equal to the degrees of freedom! (which is the # of studies in our meta-analysis minus 1). So, in our meta-analysis that included 5 studies, we would expect Q to be 4. If it is more than 4, then we expect that indeed some effect size variation is present.

So the Q statistic is the weighted sum of all the differences of the individual effect sizes from the mean effect size, and is expected to equal (or be less than) the degrees of freedom (number of studies minus one). If the Q statistic is greater than the degrees of freedom, we expect that indeed there is some variation in the effect sizes between studies (i.e. there is heterogeneity of the studies). How much bigger? Well, of course we have a p-value for that! The p-value will tell us if the Q statistic we calculate is the same, statistically speaking, as the degrees of freedom, or if it is so different that it is unlikely due to chance alone. If the p-value is less than 0.1, we say that we can reject the null hypothesis, and there is indeed a difference…and…that means that there is heterogeneity between the studies! (But it doesn't tell us how much…the higher the Q value, we can say the more likely there is heterogeneity).

8. If the Q is much larger than the degrees of freedom, we suspect that there is some ______________________ of the studies.

The I^2 statistic

We can talk about a ratio of $\frac{Q_{true}}{Q_{observed}}$ and this is I^2. So the higher the I^2, the greater is the *proportion* of heterogeneity of the studies. But, just like Q, it does not tell us *how much* variation there is, it just tells us what the proportion is.

Remember we can't calculate Q_{true} directly, because by definition we do not know the true effects, we only know the observed effects. But we do know that Q_{true} is $Q_{observed} - Q_{error}$ and we know that $Q_{error} = k - 1$ (the degrees of freedom).

So we calculate I^2 indirectly by:

$$I^2 = \frac{Q_{observed} - (k-1)}{Q_{observed}}$$

9. The I^2 statistic tells us how much of the observed variation is due to ________________ between the studies.

The prediction interval

The best measure of how much heterogeneity exists between studies is the prediction interval. Recall that the prediction interval is denoted by the red line:

Study name	Statistics for each study						
	Difference in means	Standard error	Variance	Lower limit	Upper limit	Z-Value	p-Value
A	-20.000	3.536	12.500	-26.930	-13.070	-5.657	0.000
B	-18.000	3.536	12.500	-24.930	-11.070	-5.091	0.000
C	-22.000	3.536	12.500	-28.930	-15.070	-6.223	0.000
D	-40.000	10.124	102.500	-59.843	-20.157	-3.951	0.000
E	10.000	10.124	102.500	-9.843	29.843	0.988	0.323
Pooled	-18.925	4.052	16.420	-26.867	-10.983	-4.670	0.000
Prediction Interval	-18.925			-44.911	7.061		

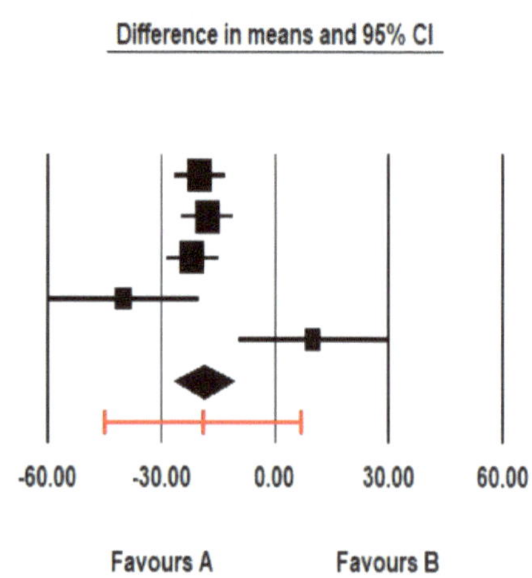

How is this calculated?

First we calculate our Q_{true}. Again, we can't calculate this directly, but we can indirectly since $Q_{true} = Q_{observed} - (k - 1)$.

Then, we can use Q_{true} to calculate our $Variance_{true}$, and then we use our V_{true} to calculate the standard deviation of the true effects. (Because recall that SD is just the square root of the variance). And then once we have the SD, our 95% prediction interval is 2 x the SD above and below the mean. (By the way, V_{true} and τ^2 are synonymous: they are the variance of the true effects.

Mistakes to watch out for

The first and most serious mistake that you will see in the world of meta-analyses is choosing a fixed effect model instead of a random effects model. And the justification that you will often see something along the lines of "the I^2 was less than 25%, meaning a very low amount of heterogeneity, and so a fixed effect model was used." Please remember that I^2 is a *proportion.* It is the proportion of the observed variation in effects that is due to heterogeneity. But it does not tell us *how much* heterogeneity is present. And remember that a fixed effect model should very rarely, if ever, be used in a meta-analysis. And in the rare case in which a fixed effect model may be justified? Well, that decision can only be made *before* the data are analyzed. The decision is not based on the results of the meta-analysis. Rather, it is based on what information we hope to gain, what conclusions we hope to draw from our meta-analysis, what is the target population of interest, what are specifics of each study included, etc.

The second mistake is that most meta-analyses will only discuss the mean effect, and not discuss heterogeneity. Heterogeneity is very important; perhaps more important than the mean effect as it tells us the *range* of effects across the studies. The range is very important for clinicians to know. They need to know that for some populations, the intervention may be helpful, but for other populations it may not be, and in some populations it may even be harmful. This information would not be available by just focusing on the mean effect. Again, please be sure that you understand the difference between the 95% confidence interval of the mean effect, which is a measure of the precision of the mean (and depends on the quality of the studies included in the analysis), and the prediction interval, which shows us the spread of the heterogeneity of the effect sizes. These two things give us entirely different information!

The third mistake you will often see is that the authors will presume that a low I^2 and a low Q value mean that there is no significant heterogeneity in the meta-analysis, or conversely, that a high I^2 or high Q means that there is a large amount of heterogeneity. This is not true. Remember that I^2 is a proportion, not a value. So a high I^2 tells us nothing about the amount of dispersion of effect sizes between studies. Only the prediction interval tells us that. And the Q value as well…if the Q value is much higher than the degrees of freedom, it tells you that heterogeneity is present, but *it doesn't tell you how much.* Only the prediction interval tells us that.

References:

[1] Ridker, PM · Danielson, E · Fonseca, FA · et al. Rosuvastatin to prevent vascular events in men and women with elevated C-reactive protein.*N Engl J Med.* 2008; 359:2195-2207

[2] Sever, PS · Dahlof, B · Poulter, NR · et al. Prevention of coronary and stroke events with atorvastatin in hypertensive patients who have average or lower-than-average cholesterol concentrations, in the Anglo-Scandinavian Cardiac Outcomes Trial–Lipid Lowering Arm (ASCOT-LLA): a multicentre randomised controlled trial. *Lancet.* 2003; 361:1149-1158

[3] Sattar, et al. Statins and risk of incident diabetes: a collaborative meta-analysis of randomised statin trials. *Lancet* Volume 375, Issue 9716p735-742February 27, 2010

[4] Collins, R · Armitage, J · Parish, S · et al., for the Heart Protection Study Collaborative Group. MRC/BHF Heart Protection Study of cholesterol-lowering with simvastatin in 5963 people with diabetes: a randomised placebo-controlled trial. *Lancet.* 2003; 361:2005-2016

[5] Shepherd et al.Prevention of Coronary Heart Disease with Pravastatin in Men with Hypercholesterolemia. *N Engl J Med* 1995;333:1301-1308.

Epidemiology/Biostats: The Problem with Statistical Significance

Well, nothing is perfect in life (in case you haven't noticed). In this chapter, which is labeled "EB" because it included both epidemiology and biostats topics, I will present the difficulties that arise with our well trusted p-values and confidence intervals in modern medical literature, due to the rather commonplace inclusion of subgroup analyses and secondary outcome analyses.

Section EB.1: Subgroup Analysis

The current ubiquity of subgroup analyses in the literature is mostly due to legislation that passed in 2012 requiring the FDA to report on how subgroups were addressed in labeling etc, prompting an action plan by the FDA in 2014 titled: "Plan to Enhance the Collection and Availability of Demographic Subgroup Data." Here is an example that is rather typical of these analyses:

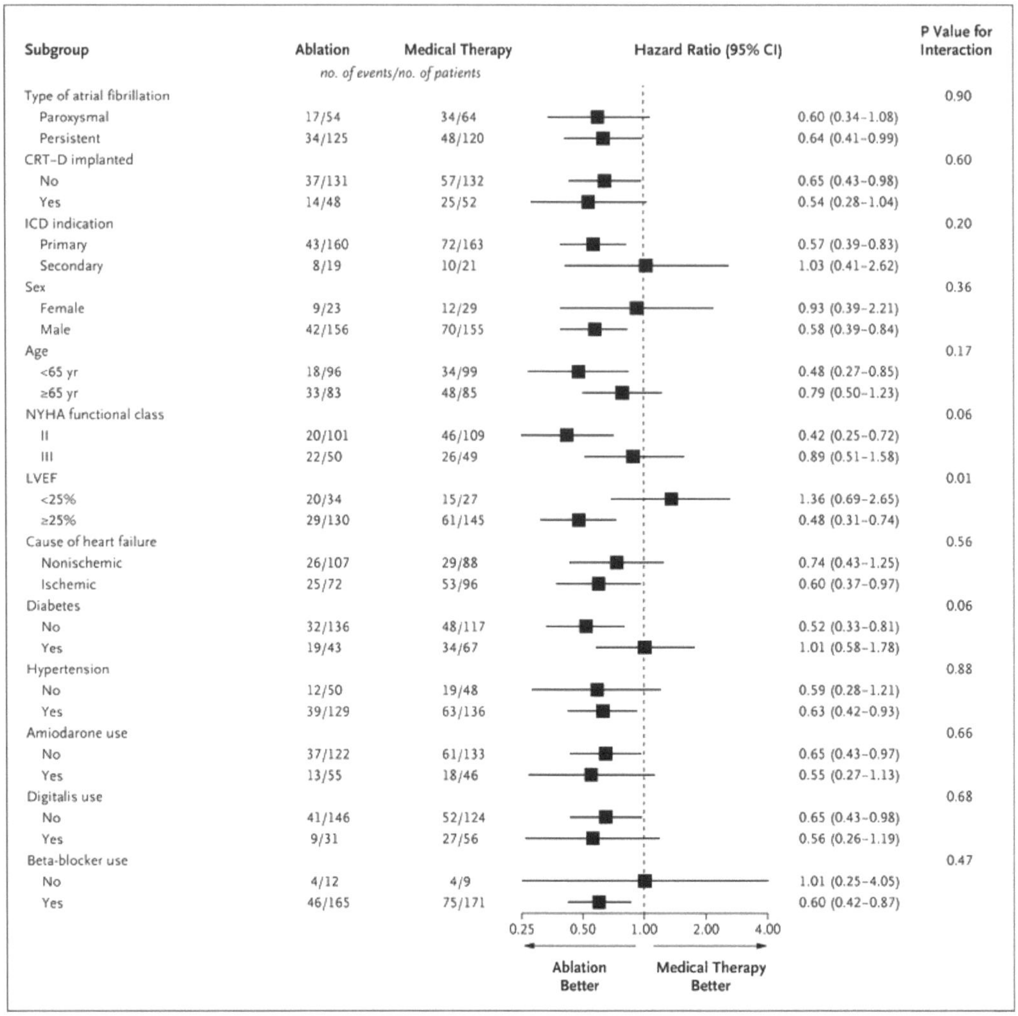

This is from *N Engl J Med 2018; 378:417-427*, and is a study comparing Catheter Ablation with Medical treatment for patients with atrial fibrillation with heart failure.

The authors first reported their end-point results as statistically-significantly favoring ablation. And then they presented the above subgroup analysis. This is a "forest plot," by the way, which I discussed in detail in the previous chapter. Authors also use this plot to present subgroup analysis. Start at the very bottom. You see the vertical hashed line at 1.00. And as we go to the left, the Hazard Ratio becomes less than one, so the treatment in question (ablation) is favored. As we go to the right, the Hazard Ratio becomes greater than one, and so the treatment is less favorable (the medical treatment is better). Now go back up to the very top. The first subgroup is type of atrial fibrillation, paroxysmal vs persistent. For paroxysmal, you see that the Hazard Ratio is 0.60, which is represented by the black square. The horizontal black line on either side of the black square is the 95% confidence interval, which spans from 0.34 to 1.08.

1. A "forest plot" is sometimes called a "_________________________________" which is really funny. A forest plot is just a pictorial representation of the Hazard Ratio (or whatever our statistical test happens to be…it could also be Odds Ratio, or Relative Risk, or whatever), accompanied by the 95% confidence interval.

Now, scroll down to "Causes of Heart Disease," divided into 2 factors: non-ischemic or ischemic. Non-ischemic has an HR of .74, with a 95% confidence interval of 0.43 to 1.25. You see that this Hazard Ratio crosses 1, so we can conclude that there is *no difference* in the treatment among people with non-ischemic heart disease. For ischemic heart disease, we see a Hazard Ratio of 0.60, with a 95% confidence interval of 0.37 to 0.97. Since, this does not cross 1, we can conclude that it is a statistically significant Hazard Ratio. The investigators might then conclude that the treatment (ablation) only works for those with ischemic heart disease. Now scroll up a bit to "sex." Look at the HR for women. It is just about 1. Clearly no difference. But there is definitely a statistically significant difference in men. So the investigators might conclude that: "Well, it appears that our treatment (ablation) is superior to medical treatment, but we only recommend it for men, and not for women; and we can only recommend it for ischemic heart disease, and not for non-ischemic heart disease." If they conclude this, they are wrong, and I know that is counter-intuitive, but that is why I am writing this chapter!

Subgroup analyses are both very informative and very problematic and I will tell you that the problems of subgroup analyses are vast and complicated, and the subject of intense debate over that past twenty years in the biostats world. Therefore, I will do my best to summarize the problems, and advise you on the practicalities, and how best to interpret these analyses. And the above is an example of the most common problem inherent in subgroup analyses: *The overall results are statistically significant, but some subgroups show no benefit from the treatment*. It is simply wrong to interpret the above subgroup analysis by stating that the treatment works, but it appears to only work for males, or for those <65 years, or several others! First thing to remember: By doing subgroup analysis, you are allowed to say that there is (or is not) a statistically significant effect in men, and that there is (or is not) a statistically significant effect in women. *But you are not allowed to say that there is a statistically significant **difference** in the treatment effect between men and women.* Does that make sense? I will give that a few minutes to sink in. So, you can say that there may or may not be a statistically significant treatment effect in men, and you can say that there may or may not be a treatment effect in women. But you cannot say that there is any difference between the two groups! So if you can't say that there is a statistically significant difference *between the two groups*, then you really cannot say anything at all about that subgroup analysis! Isn't that weird? Yes, it is weird. But it's true. Sorry. Deal with it. Remember what F. Scott Fitzgerald said in *The Crack-up*:

"The test of a first-rate intelligence is the ability to hold two opposed ideas in the mind at the same time, and still retain the ability to function."

The only useful thing to say when comparing two or more parts of a subgroup is whether or not there is a statistically significant difference *between the two groups.*

2. When doing a subgroup analysis of, say, sex, the only useful thing to talk about is whether or not there is a statistically significant difference in treatment effect between ___________ and ____________. That is really all we can talk about.

So, take men and women. Look back up at the table. Do you see the very last column titled "P-value for interaction?" Ah…that is the key thing. That is the only thing (essentially) that matters when doing a subgroup analysis. You may remember this statistic from the section on interaction (effect measure modification), section B7.4. It is the p-value for the interaction term in the multivariable regression. If the p-value is less than 0.05, then indeed the factor is acting differently on each of the subroups, and if it's greater than 0.05, then there is essentially no difference between the subroups.

3. When reading subgroup analyses, be sure to look for the "p-value for __________________." That is really the only important thing.

So, is there, or is there not, a statistically significant difference between the treatment effect among men and women? The p-value for interaction is .36. No difference at all between men and women in how they respond to treatment. And this makes perfect sense, because there is no physiologic or other plausible reason to *expect* that there might be a difference between men and women. It would indeed be a mistake to deny efficacy among a certain subgroup if there were no biologically cogent explanation as to why the treatment would only be ineffective in that subgroup. Subgroup analysis often shows variations in effects, especially if many subgroups are included, and in general, this variation does not mean a heck of a lot.

As explained by Alosh, et al:

"When a large number of subgroup analyses are conducted, and particularly when the treatment effect is not large, the probability is high that some subgroups will have treatment effect estimates in the opposite direction (favoring the control). Care should be taken to avoid misinterpreting subgroup analyses that were not included as part of a prespecified and multiplicity-adjusted statistical plan."

(Alosh, et al. Statistics in Biopharmaceutical Research. Vol 7, Sept 2015, pp 286-303.)

So as I look through this table, there is only one subgroup in which there is a statistically significant interaction. Look at LVEF (left ventricular ejection fraction). You see that for LVEF <25%, we have a Hazard Ratio of 1.36, which is greater than 1, indicating that among these patients, the treatment in question, ablation, is actually harmful. (Although we also note that the 95% confidence interval crosses 1, indicating that it is not a statistically significant finding). And now again look to the far right, where you see the P-value for interaction for LVEF is 0.01. Since that is less than 0.05, we conclude a statistically significant interaction effect of ejection fraction. There seems to be something about a low ejection fraction that truly affects the results physiologically, and this could well be plausible because ablation is a somewhat aggressive electrophysiologic procedure. It is quite possible that those who have a low ejection fraction to begin with simply have a poorer outcome with the aggressive therapy. Of course, the number of patients who had a LVEF <25% was small. Nonetheless, the statistically significant p-value for interaction of 0.01 at least warrants a comment from the authors, and there surprisingly was none.

Let's take a look at another example:

Table 2. Prespecified Primary and Secondary Outcomes and Post Hoc Additional Outcomes, According to Treatment Group, in the Intention-to-Treat Analysis.

Outcome	Chlorhexidine–Alcohol (N=572)	Iodine–Alcohol (N=575)	Relative Risk (95% CI)	P Value*
Primary outcome				
Surgical-site infection — no. (%)	23 (4.0)	42 (7.3)	0.55 (0.34–0.90)	0.02
Superficial incisional	17 (3.0)	28 (4.9)	0.61 (0.34–1.10)	0.10
Deep incisional	6 (1.0)	14 (2.4)	0.43 (0.17–1.11)	0.07
Secondary outcomes				
Median length of hospital stay (IQR) — days	4 (3–4)	4 (3–4)	—	0.24
Physician office visit — no. (%)	45 (7.9)	72 (12.5)	0.63 (0.44–0.90)	0.009
Hospital readmission — no. (%)	19 (3.3)	25 (4.3)	0.76 (0.43–1.37)	0.37
Endometritis — no. (%)	8 (1.4)	11 (1.9)	0.73 (0.30–1.80)	0.49
Adverse skin reaction — no. (%)				
Erythema at operative site	13 (2.3)	11 (1.9)	1.19 (0.54–2.63)	0.67
Skin irritation	0	3 (0.5)	—	0.08
Allergic skin reaction	2 (0.3)	1 (0.2)	2.02 (0.18–22.11)	0.56
Skin irritation or allergic skin reaction	2 (0.3)	4 (0.7)	0.51 (0.09–2.73)	0.42
Additional outcomes				
Other wound complication — no. (%)				
Skin separation	66 (11.5)	66 (11.5)	1.01 (0.73–1.39)	0.97
Seroma	24 (4.2)	28 (4.9)	0.87 (0.51–1.47)	0.58
Hematoma	7 (1.2)	5 (0.9)	1.41 (0.45–4.41)	0.56
Cellulitis	5 (0.9)	10 (1.7)	0.50 (0.17–1.46)	0.20
Fire or chemical skin burn — no.	0	0	—	—

* P values are based on chi-square tests or Fisher's exact test for categorical variables and on the Mann–Whitney U test for continuous variables.

This is from a trial comparing two different skin antiseptics for Caesarian section: chlorhexidine/alcohol and iodine/alcohol. (*N Engl J Med 2016; 374:647-55*).

The overall results of the trial revealed a statistically significant advantage of the chlorhexidine group. Now look at the subgroup analysis:

Subgroup	Chlorhexidine–Alcohol	Iodine–Alcohol	Relative Risk (95% CI)	P Value for Interaction
	no. of events/total no.			
Type of cesarean delivery				0.22
Scheduled	8/334	21/335	0.38 (0.17–0.85)	
Unscheduled	15/238	21/240	0.72 (0.38–1.36)	
Obese				0.70
Yes	18/402	30/387	0.58 (0.33–1.02)	
No	5/170	12/188	0.46 (0.17–1.28)	
Skin-closure type				0.12
Staples	9/108	9/107	0.99 (0.41–2.40)	
Suture	14/464	33/467	0.43 (0.23–0.79)	
Chronic medical condition				0.59
Yes	5/107	11/101	0.43 (0.15–1.19)	
No	18/465	31/474	0.59 (0.34–1.04)	
Diabetes				0.84
Yes	2/55	5/65	0.47 (0.10–2.34)	
No	21/517	37/510	0.56 (0.33–0.94)	

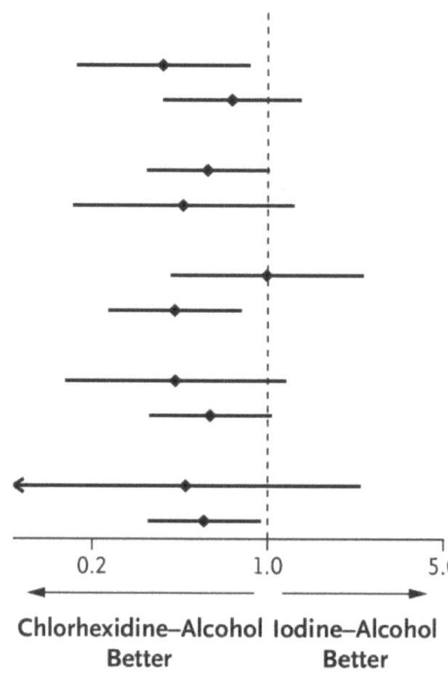

One could easily conclude looking at this analysis that the chlorhexidine group only showed an advantage in *scheduled* c-sections. (RR of 0.38). Is it then valid for surgeons to change their practice and only be sure to use chlorhexidine in scheduled c-sections, but for unscheduled c-sections they could use either one? No, of course not. Once again, it is the p-value for interaction (the last column) that is the only thing that "counts." The p-value for interaction is 0.22, meaning there is no difference at all between the "scheduled" and unscheduled" groups. And the same is true for staples vs sutures. The experimenters might conclude that chlorhexidine is better only for sutured closures, but not for stapled closures. And they might be right, but that is not proven by this data, since the p-value for interaction is 0.12.

Indeed, the investigators correctly report:

"In the subgroup analyses, four prespecified and one post hoc, the risks of surgical-site infection were lower in the chlorhexidine–alcohol group than in the iodine–alcohol group in all subgroups. The reductions in risk were not materially affected by whether cesarean delivery was scheduled versus unscheduled, by the presence or absence of obesity, by the type of skin closure, by the presence or absence of chronic medical conditions, or by status with respect to diabetes."

That being said, while they are technically correct in their conclusions, I paused a bit when I saw the staples vs sutures subgroup analysis. It is conceivable that there is effect modification here. There could well be a physiologic difference in chlorhexidine vs iodine depending on whether sutures or staples are used. And the p-value is *not that far* from .05. I think the researchers should design another study or studies specifically designed to measure a difference in chlorhexidine and iodine among sutures and staples to really examine this possible difference. Nonetheless, for the point of this chapter, the researchers were correct in stating that there was no significant difference across the subgroups.

Another thing to watch out for in the literature when dealing with subgroup analyses is when the results of the overall trial are *negative* (no statistically significant difference between the two groups), but the subgroup analysis reveals a significantly positive result in one of the subgroups. When this happens, the researchers should know that very little stock, if any, can be put in that subgroup result. Although this occurs less frequently in modern literature, it is always something to watch out for, and to be cautious about interpreting results.

Here is an example. This is from a study that compared birth weights of babies born to mothers randomized to either caffeinated coffee or decaffeinated coffee.

(*Bech, et al. Effect of reducing caffeine intake on birth weight and length of gestation: randomised controlled trial. BMJ 2007;334:409)*

The results of the study were very clear: caffeine consumption made *no difference* in birthweight, gestational age, head circumference, etc. But then they included this subgroup analysis below, and it is useful to examine this in detail.

Variable	Birth weight			Length of gestation		
	No of women*	Mean difference† (95% CI)	P value‡	No of women*	Mean difference§ (95% CI)	P value‡
Coffee consumption (cups/day) at baseline:						
<3	131	−31 (−202 to 240)	0.40	131	−2.50 (−7.4 to 2.3)	0.58
4-7	480	7 (−78 to 92)		482	−0.27 (−2.6 to 2.0)	
>7	497	57 (−28 to 142)		498	−2.06 (−4.5 to 0.3)	
Missing data	4			4		
Consumption (cups/day) of other caffeinated coffee¶:						
0	283	−9 (−125 to 107)	0.24	283	0.38 (−2.0 to 2.8)	0.35
<1	266	−39 (−150 to 72)		267	−1.45 (−0.8 to 3.7)	
1-3	271	115 (3 to 226)		271	−1.65 (−4.3 to 1.0)	
4-7	76	−120 (−354 to 113)		76	−0.41 (−5.1 to 4.3)	
≥8	21	92 (−475 to 659)		21	−4.39 (−18.1 to 9.4)	
Missing data	195	152 (9 to 295)		197	−2.40 (−8.5 to 3.7)	
Smoking (cigarettes/day) at baseline:						
Non-smoker	692	−48 (−118 to 23)	<0.001	694	−0.44 (−2.5 to 1.6)	0.25
1-10	272	36 (−78 to 149)		272	−1.80 (−4.9 to 1.3)	
>10	148	263 (97 to 430)		149	−4.19 (−8.4 to 0.01)	

Differences are for decaffeinated minus caffeinated groups.
*Number with information on all covariates and outcome measure.
†Adjusted for parity, smoking, prepregnancy body mass index, and length of gestation.
‡Test for interaction.
§Adjusted for parity, smoking, and prepregnancy body mass index.
¶Consumption at time of third interview (median 35 gestational weeks).

What is going on here? Let's just look at the left half, "birth weight." The first subgroup they decided to analyze was the amount of coffee consumed. Was there a connection (an "interaction") between the amount consumed and the difference in birth weights in the caffeinated vs decaffeinated group? This subgroup does make some logical sense, so we should probably pay it *some* attention. But lo and behold: even those who drank >7 cups a day showed no difference in caffeine vs decaffeinated. The mean birthweight difference was only 57 grams (the decaffeinated average minus the caffeinated average), and the 95% confidence interval crosses zero, so no statistically significant difference. That is certainly reassuring to the heavy coffee drinkers! But then look at the bottom section, "smoking." Those who drank >10 cups a day did have a significant difference. Babies born to the caffeinated mothers in this heavy-smoker subgroup weighed 263 gm less than babies born to decaffeinated mothers in the heavy-smoker subgroup. And the 95% confidence interval does not cross zero indicating a statistically significant result. OK, so what does this mean? *It seems to mean that we have a positive subgroup in a study that otherwise has negative results.* We must be very careful with these results, as with all subgroup analyses. Remember that the more subgroups we analyze, the greater the chance that one or more of them will show (falsely) positive results. This is due to what is known as "multiplicity," which is the inflated probability of getting a false positive result when none actually exists, as we analyze more and more subgroups. How much more?

Here is the probability of observing at least one subgroup having a significant (p <0.025) treatment effect given that the overall result was not statistically significant and the true treatment effect is 0 in all subgroups:

	Number of classification factors		
Levels per factor	1	2	3
2	0.03	0.06	0.09
3	0.06	0.11	0.15
4	0.08	0.15	0.20
6	0.13	0.23	0.30
8	0.17	0.30	0.39

Assumptions: equal numbers of subjects in each subgroup level, true treatment effect is 0 across all subgroups, classification factors are independent, normal distribution with known variance, and sample size determined so that the trial is powered for 80% with one-sided significance level of 0.025 and some treatment effect $\delta > 0$.

(Alosh et al. Statistical Considerations on Subgroup Analysis in Clinical Trials. *Statistics in Biopharmaceutical Research.* 2015; 7:4, 286-303)

This table demonstrates how frequently "false-positive" results can occur across a subgroup. It increases rather dramatically as the number of subgroups (and "levels" per subgroup) increases. In our study, for example, there are 3 subgroups with on average somewhere between 3 and 4 levels each…so in our study there is somewhere between a 15 and 20% chance that a false positive result will occur in one of the subgroups. So it is not terribly surprising that we have a positive result (among those smoking >10 cigarettes/day). So the next step, when a difference is noted, is to calculate the p-value for interaction which the researches appropriately did here. You see it in the far right "p-value". We know that this is a p-value for interaction, and not a p-value for a specific subgroup level because there is only one p-value listed for the entire subgroup. (They wrote it a little weirdly and made it a little confusing because they put these p-values horizontal from the first sub-level of the subgroup…for example, the p-value of <0.001 should have been written adjacent to "smoking" rather than adjacent to "non-smoker." By doing this they made it seem like that p-value just pertains to the "non-smoker."). But if you look at the legend below, you will see that it is indeed a "p-value for interaction". And so the p-value for interaction for cigarette smoking is significant at <0.001. This means that there indeed does seem to be some sort of biologic interaction, or effect modification of tobacco on caffeine. So, *now* what do we do, or think??

Well, the most important question to ask is: Is this something the experimenters thought about *before* they conducted the experiment? Or was this just the result of a "fishing expedition?" You can imagine that after all the time, effort, money, etc. involved in conducting a medical experiment it is rather disappointing to come up with negative results. The researchers are hungry to find "something," and thus dredge the subgroups to come with something significant that they can report on. So if the researchers truly were considering subgroup differences *before* they conduct the experiment (a priori) due to a possible physiologic effect that they were aware of, well that carries much more weight than if they just happened to stumble upon something *after* the experiment ("post hoc"). A post-hoc positive finding in a subgroup is pretty much worthless, in general. A good analogy would be shooting your arrow into a huge bale of hay that you cannot miss, and then walking up to the bale of hay and drawing a small target around your arrow and hollering, "Bullseye!"

4. When researchers report on subgroup analyses, be sure that they were considering the subgroups __ _________________.

So what I'm telling you is *even if the p-value for interaction is significant,* you have the right to think very critically about these analyses. I mentioned "multiplicity" above, which results in false-positive subgroup analyses. There has been much written on this problem, and many possible methods of "correcting" for the multiplicity problem. Some of these are as follows: the Bonferroni method, the Holm procedure, the Simes method, the Hochberg procedure, the Dunnett test, the Dunnett Stepwise test. And all the methods are somewhat valid and somewhat helpful, but all also have their weaknesses, so there is no general consensus on which method to use. Indeed, some methods may be better than others depending on the type of study, how many sublevels there are, etc..

And the problem goes in both directions: since the numbers are low in the subgroups, they are underpowered. And remember from chapter B4 that when a study is underpowered, you will have false *negative* results, that is, even if there is a correlation or an interaction, or an effect of one subgroup, the number of people in the subgroup is too small to detect it. I mean, it's a big old mess. Because of multiplicity issues, you have falsely positive results, and because of underpowering, you might have falsely negative results!

Section EB.2: Secondary Analysis

The multiplicity issue also rears its somewhat ugly head when dealing with "secondary outcomes." Remember, the more things you evaluate, the greater the chance of getting a falsely positive result. Secondary outcomes, then, run into the same problem as do subgroup analyses, the only difference being that there is no "interaction effect." The *primary* outcome of a study is what researchers are most interested in. It is their hypothesis that they set out to prove. But many time, especially if the primary outcome is not statistically significant, researchers will comment on a bunch of other possible outcomes, known as "secondary outcomes." Look at this example: This is from a study that compared prophylactic antibiotic treatment vs placebo for miscarriage surgery.

(Lissauer, et al. A Randomized Trial of Prophylactic Antibiotics for Miscarriage Surgery. *N Engl J Med 2019; 380:1012-1021)*

Table 2. Primary, Secondary, and Other Outcomes.*

Outcome	Antibiotic Prophylaxis	Placebo	Risk Ratio or Difference in Means (95% CI)†
Primary outcome: pelvic infection defined by pragmatic broad criteria — no./total no. (%)‡	68/1676 (4.1)	90/1684 (5.3)	0.77 (0.56 to 1.04)§
≥2 Clinical features and antibiotics used to treat infection	24/1676 (1.4)	41/1684 (2.4)	
≥2 Clinical features and no antibiotics used to treat infection	2/1676 (0.1)	3/1684 (0.2)	
1 Clinical feature and need for antibiotics per clinician judgment	42/1676 (2.5)	46/1684 (2.7)	
Secondary outcomes			
Pelvic infection defined by strict criteria — no./total no. (%)¶	26/1700 (1.5)	44/1704 (2.6)	0.60 (0.37 to 0.96)
Additional antibiotic use — no./total no. (%)	131/1676 (7.8)	164/1684 (9.7)	0.81 (0.65 to 1.01)
Additional analgesia — no./total no. (%)	106/1676 (6.3)	147/1684 (8.7)	0.72 (0.57 to 0.92)
Unplanned ward admission — no./total no. (%)	15/1676 (0.9)	21/1684 (1.2)	0.72 (0.37 to 1.39)
Unplanned consultation — no./total no. (%)	25/1700 (1.5)	42/1704 (2.5)	0.60 (0.37 to 0.97)
Abdominal or pelvic pain			
Presence of abdominal or pelvic pain — no./total no. (%)‖	210/1700 (12.4)	260/1704 (15.3)	0.80 (0.68 to 0.95)
Duration of abdominal or pelvic pain — days	2.9±3.0	2.6±2.8	0.3 (−0.2 to 0.8)
Vaginal bleeding			
Presence of vaginal bleeding — no./total no. (%)‖	448/1700 (26.4)	451/1704 (26.5)	1.00 (0.93 to 1.07)
Duration of vaginal bleeding — days	1.8±2.5	1.6±1.8	0.2 (−0.1 to 0.5)
Delay to usual activities			
Occurrence of delay to usual activities — no./total no. (%)‖	7/1671 (0.4)	10/1678 (0.6)	0.70 (0.27 to 1.84)
Duration of delay to usual activities — days	14.3±13.8	8.3±4.3	5.7 (−6.3 to 17.8)

* Plus–minus values are means ±SD.
† Risk ratios are presented for binary outcomes; values of less than 1 favor antibiotic prophylaxis. Differences in means are presented for duration outcomes; values of less than 0 favor antibiotic prophylaxis. All estimates were adjusted for minimization variables when possible. Because the widths of the confidence intervals were not adjusted for multiple comparisons, they should not be used to infer definitive treatment differences.
‡ For the primary outcome analysis, pelvic infection was defined by the presence of two or more of four clinical features (purulent vaginal discharge, pyrexia, uterine tenderness, and leukocytosis) or by the presence of one of these features and the clinically identified need to administer antibiotics.
§ P=0.09. P values were not calculated for secondary outcomes.
¶ For the secondary outcome analysis, pelvic infection was defined by the presence of two or more of four clinical features: purulent vaginal discharge, pyrexia, uterine tenderness, and leukocytosis. Shown are the patients included in the intention-to-treat analysis.
‖ These outcomes were not prespecified.

As you can see, the primary outcome (the occurrence of pelvic infection) gave a Risk Ratio of 0.77 (but the 95% confidence interval crossed 1 indicated a non-significant result). The authors state, correctly that:

"*We found that the use of prophylactic antibiotics before miscarriage surgery did not result in a significantly lower risk of pelvic infection than the use of placebo…*"

But now look at secondary outcomes in the table. As we scan down, we see one of them looks significant: "pelvic infections defined by strict criteria" we have a 95% confidence interval that does not cross 1. Hmmm…maybe we have a statistically significant result? Well, let's look at how many outcomes there are…there are 12 outcomes. Unfortunately, because of the multiplicity issue, there is a good chance that one or more of these will be falsely positive. And that is why the authors wrote in the legend, "Because the widths of the confidence intervals were not adjusted for multiple comparisons, they should not be used to infer definitive treatment differences." They are correct to state this; one only wishes that they did apply an appropriate correction to account for multiplicity, but they did not. At least they admitted it! And then again, in their discussion:

"*In a secondary analysis that used strict criteria to define pelvic infection, based on the CDC definition,*[23] *we found that patients who received prophylactic antibiotics had a lower rate of pelvic infection than those who received placebo, but we did not adjust for multiple comparisons of secondary outcomes.*"

Why didn't they? I don't know. And here is another: you will see a lot of this nowadays:

Table 3. Clinical Outcomes.

Outcome	Volatile Anesthetics Group (N=2709)		Total Intravenous Anesthesia Group (N=2691)		Relative Risk (95% CI)*
	Value	No. with Missing Data	Value	No. with Missing Data	
Primary outcome					
Death from any cause at 1 year — no. (%)	75 (2.8)	24	79 (3.0)	23	0.94 (0.69 to 1.29)†
Secondary outcomes					
Death from any cause at 30 days — no. (%)	38 (1.4)	0	34 (1.3)	2	1.11 (0.70 to 1.76)
Death from cardiac causes — no. (%)					
At 30 days	20 (0.7)	0	24 (0.9)	2	0.83 (0.46 to 1.49)
At 1 year	33 (1.2)	25	43 (1.6)	23	0.76 (0.49 to 1.20)
Composite of nonfatal myocardial infarction or death at 30 days — no. (%)	134 (5.0)	27	127 (4.7)	11	1.05 (0.83 to 1.34)
At least one hospital readmission during follow-up — no. (%)‡					
Within 30 days after discharge from the hospital	56 (2.1)	92	61 (2.4)	99	0.91 (0.64 to 1.30)
Between 30 days and 1 year after discharge from the hospital	222 (8.7)	154	202 (8.0)	154	1.09 (0.91 to 1.31)
Within 1 year after discharge from the hospital	257 (10.1)	153	249 (9.8)	154	1.02 (0.87 to 1.21)
Median duration of stay in intensive care unit (IQR) — nights	1.0 (1.0 to 2.0)	15	1.0 (1.0 to 2.0)	4	−0.04 (−0.18 to 0.11)§
Median duration of stay in hospital (IQR) — nights	8.0 (7.0 to 12.0)	22	8.0 (7.0 to 12.0)	14	−0.12 (−0.52 to 0.29)§

* Data are presented as relative risks for dichotomous outcomes and as absolute risk differences for continuous outcomes. The 95% confidence intervals presented in this table have not been adjusted for multiplicity; therefore, inferences drawn from these intervals may not be reproducible.
† P=0.71.
‡ Patients with missing data included patients who died, patients for whom no information on readmission was available, and patients for whom no information on vital status was available.
§ These data are absolute risk differences.

Landoni et al. Volatile Anesthetics versus Total Intravenous Anesthesia for Cardiac Surgery N **Engl J Med** 2019;380:1214-1225

In the legend: "The 95% confidence intervals presented in this table have not been adjusted for multiplicity; therefore, inferences drawn from these differences may not be reproducible." (In this study, it did not really matter anyway since none of the secondary outcomes showed a statistically significant result, but you get the point!)

Summary

Our test for statistical significance, the p-value, is very much a hot potato in the world of statistics when it is used to analyze the result of multiple layers, whether it be during subgroup analyses or secondary outcome analyses. Many experts believe the bar should be lowered, i.e. the p-values should be set lower than 0.05 due to multiplicity; others say it should be raised to account for lower numbers in the subgroups and under-powering. (Probably both are correct!!). At any rate, be sure to remember that especially when a post-hoc subgroup analysis or a secondary outcome is shown to be statistically significant, all that means is that the researchers need to follow up with another study concentrating on that particular subgroup, or that particular secondary outcome. They must attempt to confirm that result with a dedicated study. It is indeed the case that most of the time when these confirmatory studies are run the results do *not* pan out. Other than that, (if they are not planning to do confirmatory studies), then they are just noting these outcomes for interest's sake. This is especially the case when the original result shows no significance, and is unfortunately part of the bias that is so prevalent in medical literature: researchers are funded by industry, and are desperate to show *some* statistically significant result!

Epidemiology 6: Testing the Tests

The very core of what we do as medical clinicians is diagnosing disease. It is what the public expects from us, and it is what we generally consider ourselves "experts" in doing. In order to diagnose a disease, medical practitioners have only two things: 1. Our clinical judgement. 2. Tests. Therefore, in this chapter I will discuss tests in some detail. Specifically, I will analyze the tools that we have to determine how good a test is. Does it help us in our ability to diagnose disease, or not? And if it does, how much?

Section E6.1: Sensitivity and Specificity

Although you are likely very familiar with the terms "sensitivity" and "specificity," if you're like me, you may have trouble keeping their exact meanings straight. My goal in this section is to clarify this for you, once and for all!

Sensitivity

The sensitivity of a test is simply defined as *the proportion of people who test positive when they actually have the disease.*

When a patient comes to see me in the clinic, I don't know if they have the disease or not, that is what I am trying to find out! So, as clinicians, the sensitivity of a test is not very helpful to us. Clinicians need to know if a positive test *rules in* disease, or perhaps more importantly if a negative test *rules out* disease. Sensitivity does not answer these questions. And that has oddly helped me remember what sensitivity is: it is important to the manufacturer of the test ("my test is 88% sensitive in detecting disease!"), but not helpful to clinicians who are trying to figure out whether or not someone has the disease.

This little trick has prevented me from falling into the false trap of sensitivity, which is something like... "Well, if sensitivity of the test is 90% that means…if they test positive they have a 90% chance of having the disease." NO! NO! Get that out of your head permanently, and the only way to get it out of your head permanently is to remember that sensitivity does NOT help us at all in diagnosing disease. So your brain says, "Sensitivity does not help me, therefore it must mean the percent of patients who test positive when they have the disease, and NOT the other way around!

1. The sensitivity of a test is the percentage of people who ____________ positive when they actually have the disease. Therefore, the sensitivity of a test is _________ useful to us in clinical practice. I repeat: sensitivity is _________ useful to us.

So, someone comes to you with a sore throat, and you wonder if it could be strep throat. You have read that the sensitivity of a point-of-care throat swab that your office has is 80%. You remember that the sensitivity of a test is not helpful to you, so you therefore remember that *if the patient has strep throat,* there is an 80% chance that the test will be positive. Not much help.

Sensitivity is also sometimes referred to as "true positives." (It's not a "false positive" because they truly *do* have the disease, so it's a *true* positive). Somehow, though, this never helped me in remembering what sensitivity is. And the actual mathematical definition is $\frac{true\ positive}{all\ disease\ cases}$ which equals: $\frac{true\ positives}{true\ positives + false\ negatives.}$ Somehow, these never helped me either! At any rate, if the sensitivity of a test is high, that is a good thing, because it means that there are only very few "false negatives." Again, although it does not help us when the patient is in our office, it helps us after the test result comes back. So we run the test and it results negative for strep. The sensitivity of the test is 80% means that 20% of patients will be "falsely negative." So there is a 20% chance that our patient will be falsely negative, meaning that they actually do have strep, but the test failed to show it. Our test really didn't help us very much in determining if he or she actually has strep throat.

2. If the sensitivity of a test is low, say like 60%, then there are a lot of _________ negatives. That is, many patients who actually have the disease will test _________________.

(I will grant you that if the sensitivity of a test is like super high, like say 98%, it might be somewhat helpful to us, but more on this to come!)

Specificity

The specificity of a test is also not very helpful to us. It is simply defined as *the proportion of people who test negative when they actually do* ***not*** *have the disease.*

And since we *don't know if someone has the disease or not,* the specificity of a test is also not useful to us. Like sensitivity, the higher the specificity, the better. If a test has, say a 98% specificity, it means that if a patient does not have the disease, there is only a 2% chance that he or she will test positive. And so specificity is also sometimes called "true negatives." They do not have the disease, so they are truly negative. And the mathematical thing for specificity is: $\frac{true\ negatives}{total\ without\ disease} = \frac{true\ negatives}{true\ negatives+fase\ positives}$. And the higher the specificity, the smaller the amount of "false positives," i.e. those who do not have the disease but falsely test positive.

3. The specificity of a test is the percentage of people who test _______________ when they in fact do ________ have the disease. The higher the specificity, the smaller is the chance that someone will test positive when they _______ _________ have the disease.

Back to our strep throat example. The patient tested positive for strep. We read that our rapid point-of-care test has a specificity of 93%. We feel pretty good, then, that the patient really has strep throat, because the false positive rate is only 7%, meaning that there is a 7% chance that the patient actually does *not* have strep throat, even though she tested positive.

Section B6.2: Predictive values

The positive and negative predictive values are far more useful to us in a clinical setting than sensitivity and specificity. They are the flip-arounds of sensitivity and specificity. The formal definition of **positive predictive value** is:

The percentage of people who truly have the disease when they test positive.

And, perhaps even more importantly, the formal definition of **negative predictive value** is:

The percentage of people who truly do NOT have the disease when they test negative.

Ahh…yes! This is what we clinicians need! If a test has a high positive predictive value and our patient tests positive, then we know (with very good odds) that he or she does have the disease; and if a test has a high negative predictive value, and the patient tests negative, we can say (with very good odds) that we have "ruled out" the disease! So you can see why positive and negative predictive values are much more useful to us in a clinical setting than are sensitivity and specificity.

4. Positive and negative predictive values are useful to us in a clinical setting. They tell us the chance that a patient truly has the disease when testing _________________, or truly does not have the disease when testing _____________________.

Unfortunately, we usually do not know the positive and negative predictive value of a test. (Wouldn't you know!) These parameters are not something that the test makers can report. When they first test their test to get it approved by the FDA, they take a bunch of people with the disease, and a bunch of people without the disease (as defined by a positive or negative test on a known very accurate test). For example, a lab company wants to make a new point-of-care strep throat test designed for offices, because the results are available in 5 minutes. They would test, say 100 people who test positive for strep throat by the "gold-standard," which is formal throat culture, and apply their new rapid test to those people. If 82 of the people tested positive, they would say that the **sensitivity** of their test is 82%, and it has a "false-negative" rate of 18%. Then they would take 100 patients who have no symptoms (and whose formal throat culture is negative), and apply their new tests to these patients. If 98 of them tested and negative, and 2 test positive, they would say that the **specificity** of their new test is 98%, and the "false-positive" rate is 2%. But that is all they can say. They can say nothing of predictive values, because predictive values take into account the *prevalence* of disease in a particular population.

We will need to go through an example. Painful but necessary, sorry.

Assume that the lab makers report to us that the sensitivity of their test is 80% and the specificity of their test is 90%. Those are pretty good numbers. So if we have 1000 patients with sore throats and we know that the prevalence in our community of strep throat among all people with sore throats is 20%. And we set up a table as follows:

	Have Strep	**No Strep**
Test positive		
Test negative		
total		

Let us fill in the boxes. First, the totals. 1000 people have sore throats, and 20% of those will have strep:

	Have Strep	**No Strep**
Test positive		
Test negative		
total	200	800

So now let's look at those who have the disease. How many will be expected to test positive? Well, we know that the sensitivity of our test is 80%. And remember that sensitivity means the chance that if you have the disease you will test positive. So 80% of the 200 will test positive. That is 160. And 40 will test negative (will be "falsely-negative). So let's fill those two boxes in:

	Have Strep	No Strep
Test positive	160	
Test negative	40	
total	200	800

Now, 800 people do not have the disease. How many of these people will test positive? Well, the specificity is 90%. So 90% of 800 (720) will test negative, and 80 will test positive (will be "falsely-positive.")

	Have Strep	No Strep
Test positive	160	80
Test negative	40	720
total	200	800

So how do we get the predictive values? We read *across.* Remember that positive predictive value is the percentage of those who test positive who actually have the disease. Since 160 have the disease and 80 do not, we have: $\frac{160}{160+80}$ = **67%** Wow!! The positive predictive value of our rapid strep is test is only 67%. Because there is a 10% false-positive rate, and because the prevalence of the disease is low, if you test positive, you only have a 67% chance of having the disease!

And how about negative predictive value? That is, how good is the test at "ruling out" disease?

Read across the Test negative line: Of those who test negative, 720 actually do not have the disease, while 40 actually do have the disease. $\frac{720}{40+720}$ = **95%**. So the negative predictive value is good, and the test then is very good at ruling *out* disease, but not so good at ruling *in* disease. And that is the general case with predictive values. If the prevalence is low, a test is better at ruling out disease than ruling in disease.

And let us do the exercise one more time assuming an even lower prevalence, like say 5%. (And a 5% prevalence might occur for a more serious disease, so I have changed "Have Strep" to "Have disease." If the prevalence was 5%, the numbers would read:

	Have Disease	No Disease
Test positive	40	95
Test negative	10	855
total	50	950

Now we see that the positive predictive value is $\frac{40}{40+95}$ = **30%**, and the negative predictive value is $\frac{855}{855+10}$ = **99%**

If you test positive, the chance of having the disease is only 30%!

Section B6.3: Likelihood Ratios

In the world of "testing tests," Likelihood ratios are indeed miraculous. They will solve all the problems described in the previous chapter and will change the way you practice medicine. Really. I am very excited to tell you about it.

Recall that sensitivity of a test is the percentage of "true positives." And if we extend that thought, we can also say that 1– sensitivity = "false negatives". (Does that make sense? If the sensitivity is 80%, then the "false positive" rate is 20%). And the same with specificity. Since specificity is "true negatives," we can say that 1– specificity = "false positives." So keep these new definitions in mind:

The Positive likelihood ratio is just what it says: the ratio of true positives over false positives. Or, in the language of sensitivity and specificity:

PLR (positive likelihood ratio) = $\frac{\textit{sensitivity}}{1-\textit{specificity}}$

The Negative likelihood ratio is just what it says (but upside-down): the ratio of false negatives over true negatives. (The reason it's upside-down will become clear shortly!)

NLR (negative likelihood ratio) = $\frac{1-\textit{sensitivity}}{\textit{specificity}}$

5. A way to help you remember the formulae for PLR and NLR is that sensitivity is in the numerator for both. For PLR, it's just ____________________ in the numerator; for NLR it is ______ ______________________ sensitivity in the numerator.

The higher the PLR, the better the test. A test of 1 is meaningless; you really want this to be 10 or higher. The *lower* the NLR, the better the test. An NLR of 1 is meaningless; you really want this to be 0.1 or less.

6. The bigger the __________, the better the test. The smaller the ___________, the better the test.

To see the amazing capabilities of the likelihood ratios, I will next introduce the following, which is called a "Bayes' nomogram," and other times referred to as a "Fagan nomogram." Here it is:

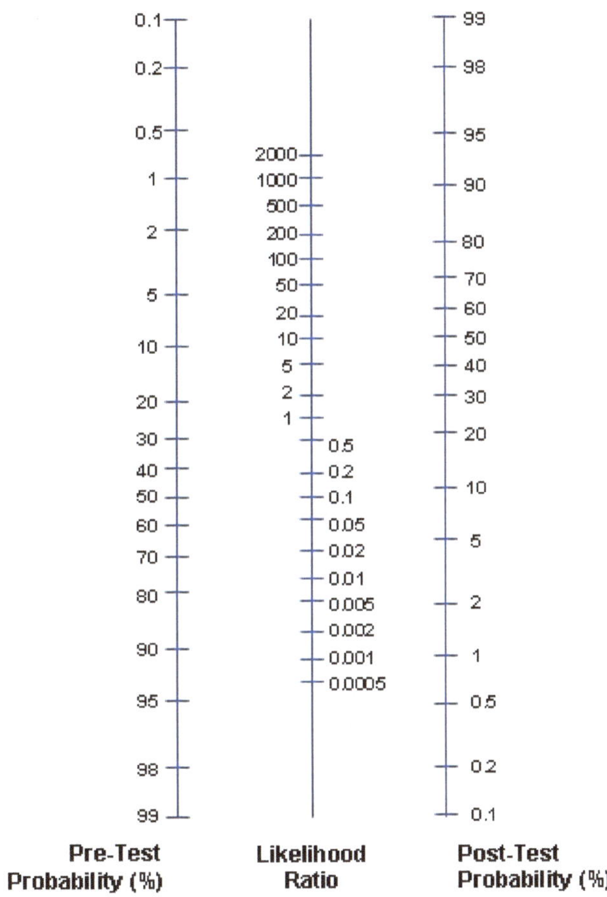

:

It is fascinating that this thing has been around forever in medicine, yet few clinicians have any experience playing around with it. It is a way to calculate the post-test probability of having a disease using the pre-test probability and the likelihood ratio of the test.

The left column is the pre-test probability, the middle column is the likelihood ratio (either positive or negative), and the right column is the post-test probability. So, what is pre-test probability? It is what you, the clinician, has decided the probability of the disease is after you have seen and examined the patient, but before you have done any tests. To estimate the pre-test probability, you take into account the history and physical and combine that with your knowledge of the disease in question, its prevalence in your community at the time, etc. The post-test probability is what the probability of disease is *after* you have done the test.

Let's take an example.

I am now going to switch diseases and use the most notorious stress-inducing diagnosis in the emergency medicine world, pulmonary embolism. The test now considered the "gold-standard" for diagnosing this condition is a specialized CAT scan know as a "CTA" or "CT-angio." In this test, a radio-opaque dye is injected into the body at the just the right rate/time that the blood vessels of the pulmonary system show up fairly well, and a radiologist is usually able to make the diagnosis by reviewing the images. Like all tests in medicine, though, it is far from perfect. While it has a specificity of 96% (very few false positives), it has a sensitivity of only 83%. (Despite its "gold-standard" status)

Let's calculate the likelihood ratios:

PLR (positive likelihood ratio) $= \frac{\boldsymbol{sensitivity}}{\boldsymbol{1-specificity}} = \frac{.83}{1-.96} = \mathbf{21}$

NLR (negative likelihood ratio) $= \frac{\boldsymbol{1-sensitivity}}{\boldsymbol{specificity}} = \frac{1-.83}{.96} = \mathbf{.18}$

So now a patient comes in and you are the clinician and you think a little bit about pulmonary embolism because the patient has a little bit of chest pain. (ED clinicians *always* think of pulmonary embolism, because it is a difficult diagnosis to make, because it can present in many ways, and because it is potentially life-threatening). After extensive history and physical, knowing the prevalence of pulmonary embolism in the community among patients who present to the emergency department, and using your twenty years' experience, you think there is a very low likelihood that the patient has this condition. You estimate that the patient has, say, a 1% chance of having a pulmonary embolism. You still wonder if you should "rule it out," because a "missed" pulmonary embolism can be disastrous, so you contemplate doing a CTA. But before you order the CTA, you look at your Bayes' nomogram. Your pre-test probability is 1%. You put our pencil on 1% on the left column, and then draw a line right through the PLR of 21, and see where it comes out on the right column. Here is the result:

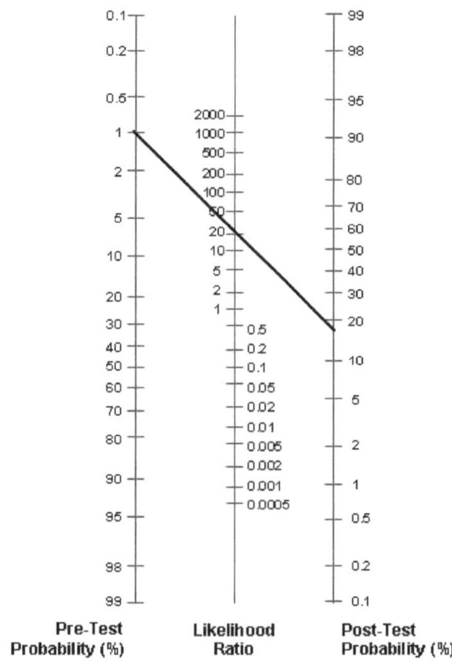

The post-test probability is only 18%! So, you wisely decide *not* to do the CTA, because even with a positive test, there is still *less than a 20% chance that the patient has a pulmonary embolism!* And that is the beauty of likelihood ratios. Even though the CTA has pretty good numbers for a test—sensitivity 83%, specificity 96%— its results are meaningless, and an expensive, potentially harmful test is wasted on this patient.

Let's switch gears to another test commonly done in Urgent Care centers and Primary Care offices. There is a rapid test for detecting influenza antigen via nasal swab; the one I am most familiar with (Sofia rapid flu made by Quidel) has a specificity of about 98%, which is good as there are very few false positives. But the sensitivity varies from 50% to 80%, depending on which study you read (be careful to only read the studies that are *not* funded by Quidel!). I will take the average, and declare that the sensitivity is 65%. That means there are a lot of false-negatives—those who actually have the disease but test negative. So let us see how this test rates. Plugging these numbers in, we get a PLR of: 32.5. The NLR is: 0.36. Right away we see that the PLR is good, but the NLR is not so good.

First case: A patient comes to you right in January, the heart of flu season, with classic influenza symptoms. I mean…fever, cough, congestion, sore throat, intense body-aches, etc. After you do your history and physical, you *just know* that this patient has the flu. Unfortunately, your medical assistant had decided to run the Sofia test before you saw the patient, and the test comes back negative. Let's look at our Bayes' nomogram, and assume there was a 90% pre-test probability.

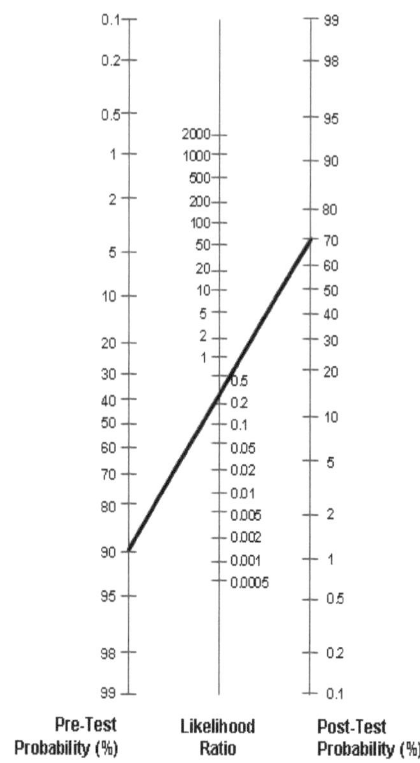

You see I started at 90% and drew a line across the NLR, and ended up with a post-test probability of 70%! So, you can see that the negative test has not helped us at all. We will still say that the patient has influenza.

The next case is one in which you are not so sure. The patient comes to you in January, but her symptoms are not quite as dramatic: she is coughing, has a low-grade fever, a moderate sore throat, but doesn't feel that terrible. She tells you she is thinking of going to work today. Well, you know you are in the heart of flu season, and you know influenza symptoms can vary from person to person, so after your history and physical, you just aren't sure if the patient has the flu or not. You estimate the pre-test probability to be around, say, 30%. Now let's see what happens when we run our test. First, a positive test: (remember we draw the line through our PLR of 32.5:

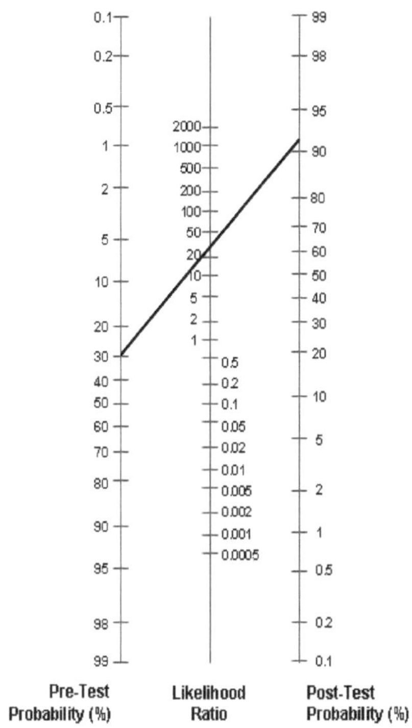

Ah! Now the test has helped us! We have a post-test probability of 92%! And what about a negative test?

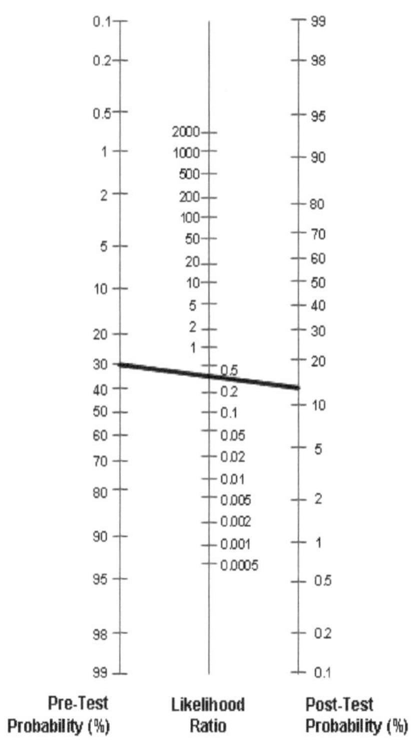

OK, so post-test probability is about 12%, so you can reasonably tell the patient it is likely that she does not have the flu.

And finally, a patient comes to you in May as flu season has pretty much wound down, with a sore throat and nasal congestion. Despite his relatively mild symptoms, he is worried he might have the flu. After your history and physical, you determine that the pre-test probability of influenza is say, 5%. The patient requests a flu swab, so you agree. Well, a negative result is easy, I won't bother showing it. What about a positive result?

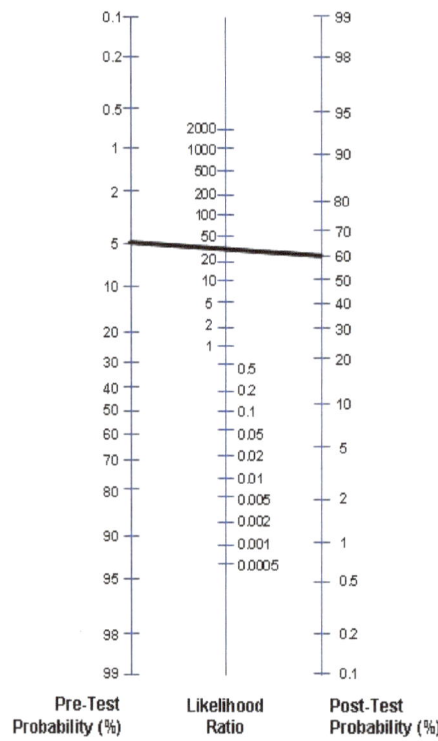

Well, now your post-test probability is 60%, and so you were likely wrong (hey, it happens!), and can tell your nervous patient that it is likely he has the flu.

And so you see, with a test like this that has a good PLR, but an OK but not so great NLR (because of a low sensitivity), the test is definitely helpful to you when you are not sure of the diagnosis (pre-test prob of 30% above); it is somewhat helpful to you when you think it is very unlikely (pre-test prob of 5% above), in that a positive test truly changed your mind; and it is not at all helpful when you were sure of the disease (pre-test prob of 90% above), as neither a positive nor a negative test changed your mind on the diagnosis.

7. No test in medicine is perfect. In general, if our pre-test probability is extremely high, we should think about __________ doing the test at all, because it is unlikely that either a positive or a negative test will change our minds.

And that is the beauty and elegance of likelihood ratios. Recall that in the last chapter I mentioned the inherent weakness of using predictive values, because they do not take into account at all your pre-test probability. "Wait; I was sure that patient had the disease!!" With likelihood ratios, you do not have to worry about that. Your pre-test probability combines everything: history, physical, "gestalt," prevalence of the disease etc. And the great thing is that all you need to know is the sensitivity and specificity of a test, and you can calculate your likelihood ratios. And, of course, there are Bayes' nomogram calculators easily found on the internet, if you don't like having a piece of paper and drawing lines! And you can find likelihood ratios for many different tests, and also for physical exam findings, and history findings on-line at sites like www.thennt.com

Summary of Epidemiology 6

The main point of this chapter is relative lack of value in sensitivity and specificity, and the relative wealth of value in predictive values. But if there is one thing in this book that I hope will change your practice, it is using likelihood ratios and Bayes' nomogram to help in your clinical decision making. Have fun!!

Answers to Questions

Biostats I: Populations and Samples

1. spread out
2. thinner (narrower)
3. 95
4. sample; population
5. standard deviation; number of participants; population
6. lower; less
7. normally
8. means
9. 2.54; 5.38
10. decreases; narrow

Epidemiology 1: Types of Studies I

1. related
2. exposure; outcome
3. rare
4. time; money
5. outcome
6. shot; causality
7. ecological fallacy

Epidemiology 2: Types of Studies II

1. evenly
2. participants
3. retrospective cohort

Biostats 2: Comparing Continuous Outcomes

1. statistically significant
2. zero; non-significant
3. standard errors
4. 5; reject; statistically
5. One
6. Different; reject
7. Reject

Epidemiology 3: Measures of Association

1. risk; risk
2. exposure; outcome
3. greater; less
4. outcome; exposure
5. risk difference
6. exposure; entire
7. time
8. greater; low; high
9. does

Biostats 3: Comparing Categorical Outcomes

1. mean
2. trials
3. proportion
4. log; antilog
5. independent
6. continuous; categorical
7. 10; exact

Biostats 4: Power; Type I and II errors

1. small
2. are the same
3. student's t
4. decreases
5. β; II; reject
6. rejected; not

Biostats 5: Non-inferiority Trials

1. is
2. less
3. M (or δ or NI)
4. lLess; non-inferiority
5. placebo; null hypothesis
6. no difference
7. meta-analysis
8. superior; inferiority
9. variability
10. easier
11. intention-to-treat analyzed

Epidemiology 4: Bias

1. association
2. odds ratio
3. a/c; b/d
4. relative risk
5. risk; risk
6. either
7. toward; away; toward
8. selection bias
9. statistically significant

Epidemiology 5: Confounding and Effect measure modification

1. not; unevenly
2. matching; one to one
3. cohort
4. inactivity; cancer; cigarette smoking
5. 10; confounder
6. closer to
7. confounders
8. interaction; effect measure modification
9. case-control
10. confounder; effect measure modification; interaction
11. less

Biostats 6: Regression

1. related; 1; 0; -1; +1
2. cannot
3. x; y; independent; dependent
4. slope
5. population; confidence
6. R^2; correlation coefficient; variation
7. odds ratio
8. dependent; independent

Biostats 7: Multivariable regression

1. y-intercept; slope
2. variables; coefficients; computer
3. variable; variables
4. predictors (or independent variables); outcome
5. adjusted
6. confounder
7. x_2; x_2; x_1
8. linear
9. confounder
10. interaction

Biostats 8: Survival Analysis

1. y; x
2. 50; surviving
3. censored
4. better; worse; event
5. log-rank
6. better
7. time; risk; risk
8. incidence rate
9. linear
10. dependent
11. independent
12. hazard; ratio
13. eliminate

Biostats 9: Meta-analysis

1. one
2. JUPITER; PROSPER
3. same; unusual; fixed effect
4. random effects
5. fixed
6. one
7. error
8. heterogeneity

Epidemiology/Biostats1: The Problem with Statistical significance

1. blobbogram
2. men; women
3. interaction
4. a priori

Epidemiology 6: Testing the Tests

1. test; not; not
2. false; negative
3. negative; not; do not
4. positive; negative
5. sensitivity; 1 minus
6. PLR; NLR
7. Not

INDEX

www.ingramcontent.com/pod-product-compliance
Lightning Source LLC
LaVergne TN
LVHW070933210926
848482LV00003B/232
* 9 7 9 8 3 4 9 2 7 1 4 8 9 *